DEPRESSION AND DEMENTIA: PROGRESS IN BRAIN RESEARCH, CLINICAL APPLICATIONS AND FUTURE TRENDS

DEPRESSION AND DEMENTIA: PROGRESS IN BRAIN RESEARCH, CLINICAL APPLICATIONS AND FUTURE TRENDS

S. N. Sarbadhikari
Editor

Nova Biomedical Books
New York

Library of Congress Cataloging-in-Publication Data
Available upon Request

ISBN: 1-59454-114-0

Published by Nova Science Publishers, Inc. ✢ New York

CONTENTS

PREFACE

There are two things which I am confident I can do very well: one is an introduction ... stating what it is to contain and how it should be executed in the most perfect manner; the other is a conclusion, showing from various causes why the execution has not been equal to what the author promised to himself and the public.

Samuel Johnson

Editing a book now has become both easy and difficult. The Internet makes Communication very easy in the global village. On the other hand, this has led to an ever increasing activity for exchanging new ideas, and in the process, time is running short. Initially I had got positive response from some other authors who had kindly agreed to contribute to this book and enrich its value. However, their other academic commitments could not make it possible. I am greatly thankful to all the contributors who have kindly taken some time out from their very busy schedule to write here. Meeting the deadline set by the Publisher and also managing all our academic and personal commitments require extraordinary jugglery from all.

Needless to say, the vast area of brain research and applications that the book aimed to address is beyond the scope of a single monograph. On the other hand editing a multi-volume edition would have demanded even greater efficiency in time management. Therefore, this is a trade off between the possible information that could have been gathered and the time allotted for it. The book is intended to target researchers, as well as clinicians, to give a quick overview of the present state of art in depression and dementia. Young students and researchers will be able to benefit from this volume, which also contains an extensive bibliography that can direct them to specialized references for satisfying their further queries.

I shall be happy to receive feedback from the readers (through snail mail or email).

I should not fail to put it on record the invaluable time spared by Dr. Anindya, my wife and Ms. Sohini, my daughter to complete this work.

I must thank the Publishers, especially Dr. Frank Columbus, for their constant empathy and support.

Suptendra Nath Sarbadhikari
Ettimadai
August 9, 2004

SUMMARY

Most of the mechanisms of brain action, in health, as well as diseases like depression and dementia, are nonlinear. The psychomotor theory can shed some light on the brain-mind-body interaction in health and disease. Specific neurotransmitters through their different receptor subtypes ultimately act along some final common pathway, in a lateralized fashion to produce depression and dementia. The currently available neurochemical and genetic evidences and their correlation with life events from population based studies, may be useful in screening susceptibility to dementia and depression. Further, criteria may be set up for susceptibility to these diseases and they might help designing early interventions in prevention of depression and dementia. The breakdown of the BBB (Blood brain barrier) through Heat Shock Protein (HSP) is also responsible for many neurodegenerative diseases. Aggressive and individualized management of patients suffering from depression and dementia may be the most promising gift of medical science and technology to humanity. Nonlinear dynamic analysis (NDA) of EEG (electroencephalography) may aid in the differential diagnosis of dementias. However, the methodologies have to be standardized further to make it clinically acceptable universally. ERPs (event related potentials in EEG) can be of great help in diagnosis and also assessing prognosis of dementias. Finally, fusion or hybrid techniques, especially those incorporating fMRI or functional magnetic resonance imaging (along with qEEG or quantitative EEG) can be of immense help in diagnosing, managing and predicting the prognosis of depression and dementia.

This book elaborately discusses the above issues and tries to bring a useful update in the area of depression and dementia.

BIOGRAPHICAL SKETCH OF THE EDITOR

SUPTENDRA NATH SARBADHIKARI

After graduating in Medicine and Surgery from Calcutta University in 1989, he has done his residency in General Internal Medicine and in Psychiatry. He has been awarded a PhD, in Biomedical Engineering, on neural network aided analysis of electrophysiological signals in stress and exercise, from the Institute of Technology, Banaras Hindu University, Varanasi, in 1995. He has delivered invited talks in many national and international conferences. He has written four guest editorials for the *Journal of the Indian Medical Association*. He is a life member of the Indian Medical Association, Indian Association of Medical Informatics and also of the Biomedical Engineering Society of India. Presently he is an Associate Professor of Biomedical Engineering, Amrita Institute of Technology, Ettimadai, Coimbatore-641105 AND Amrita Institute of Medical Sciences and Research Centre, Elamakkara, Kochi-682026, India. Prior to that he was an Assistant Professor in the School of Medical Science & Technology, Indian Institute of Technology, Kharagpur. Earlier he was attached to the Department of Physiology, Sikkim Manipal Institute of Medical Sciences, as an Assistant Professor in Biophysics, and also as a Visiting Faculty at the Sikkim Manipal Institute of Technology. His research interests include electrophysiological investigations in different states of health and disease, application of e-Health, and also automated diagnostic systems for various medical conditions. He has been awarded the prestigious "Shri Shyam Lal Saksena Memorial Award 2000-2001" from the National Academy of Medical Sciences (India), for research in Biomedical Engineering. Presently he is the Associate Editor of the Indian Journal of Medical Informatics and is also writing a textbook "A Short Introduction to Biomedical Engineering". As a member of the DOEACC Committee on Bioinformatics, he has been instrumental in designing and developing the syllabus on Medical Informatics for the proposed C-level (M. Tech. equivalent) Bioinformatics Course under the Department of Information Technology, Ministry of Communications and Information Technology, Government of India. He has

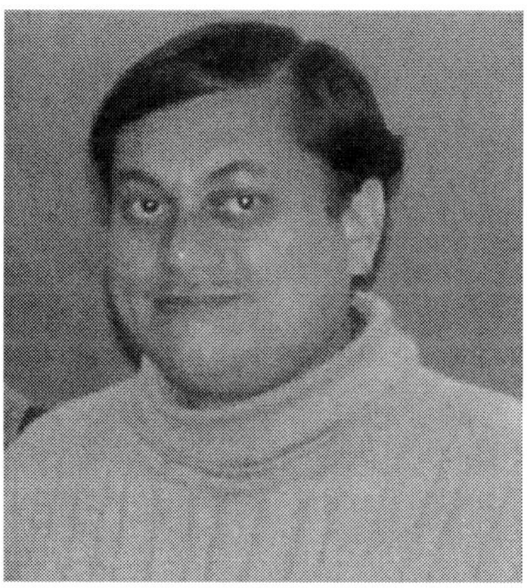

regularly conducted general and medical quiz at national level. His name is being regularly selected for inclusion in the Marquis Who's Who in the World, USA, since the 15th edition, 1998.

Homepage: (1) www.geocities.com/drsupten
(2) http://medicineonearth.com/display.php?id=1642

In: Depression and Dementia
Editor: Suptendra Nath Sarbadhikari, p. 1-20
ISBN 1-59454-114-0

Chapter 1

FRONTIERS OF RESEARCH IN NEUROSCIENCES AND PSYCHIATRY

N. Pradhan,* G. R. Arunodaya** and T. N. Sathyaprabha***

*Department of Psychopharmacology,
**Department of Neurology,
***Department of Neurophysiology,
National Institute of Mental Health \& Neurosciences,Bangalore-560029,INDIA}

ABSTRACT

Living systems are inherently nonlinear and complex in nature. However, surprisingly many biologists and medicine professionals are unaware of the power, magic and beauty of nonlinear science that underlies living processes. The recent developments in the physics of complex systems encompassing nonlinear dynamics and the theory of chaos have considerably altered our perception and analysis of many complex systems, including that of the human brain. This new scientific revolution has silently pervaded all disciplines and emerged as the frontier of research today. It is also heralded as the third most important discovery of man after relativity and quantum mechanics. This article attempts to give an overview of "Nonlinear Phenomena" and its significance for understanding human brain functioning. The importance of emerging trends of nonlinear dynamics and chaos to neurobiology is presented and discussed in the context of various states of consciousness, behavior and psychopathology. It reviews the physical and dynamical aspect of brain's electrical activity from this new perspective and indicates possible future directions. It is intended as an introduction to Nonlinear dynamical analysis of complex brain signals in neuro-psychiatric research.

Key Words: Nonlinear dynamics, Chaos, EEG, Phase-space, Attractor dimension, stochasticity, determinism, Behavioral states.

INTRODUCTION

Neurodynamics remains as a complex problem in brain science where myriads of cellular processes are interlinked in producing the marvels of human brain capable of thinking and creativity. The recent developments in nonlinear dynamics and theory of chaos have heralded new understanding of many biological processes (Golberger et al 2002). These have found applications in many fields of neurobiology. Significant meaning could be derived by nonlinear dynamical modeling of random like neuronal firing patterns with respect to novel stimuli, learning and memory. Nonlinear dynamics has been very successful in predicting the behavior of the heart, slow changing autonomic activities, other time varying biological signals and patterns of neural activity. The neurobiology of the various states of brain activity is being explored through the application of nonlinear dynamics (Galka, 2003). Modeling and prediction of dynamical behaviour of brain processes through neural net and chaotic dynamics are taking the place of standard signal detection and probability theories of learning and cognition. Even centers of nonlinear studies have come into existence because of the promises these theories hold in understanding complex systems. The dynamics that drives the brain from one state of activity to another has become the focus of current research in systemic neuroscience. These developments have been crucially linked to the availability of supercomputing platforms in research institutions. The increase in computer resources has opened up new areas of research and applications that were either unknown or inaccessible earlier. Many recently identified thrust areas in brain and behavioral sciences are totally dependent on the computational power available to a group or to a researcher. This has resulted in a novel and qualitative change in the outlook of investigating the brain and its functions. The analysis of neuronal conglomerative behaviour is greatly dependent on the availability of expensive high speed computers that explains the fewer numbers of studies in this area. However with rapid developments in VLSI technology very high speed computing and systems being available on table top to scientists, explosive publication in this area is in sight. This review presents the emerging scenario in neurobiology while rapid applications of nonlinear science are taking place in almost all fields of science. It critically appraises the recent developments in neurodynamics with respect to the various states of brain activity and application to psychiatric diagnosis and treatment evaluation. It also describes the concepts of nonlinear dynamics that are of practical importance in the analysis and interpretation of brain functions (Jansen,1991, Pradhan and Naryana Dutt, 1993).

THE EEG: BRAIN ACTIVITIES ARE NOT RANDOM PROCESSES

The complicated dynamical behaviour of the brain activity is reflected in the recording of its electrical activity as electroencephalogram (EEG). On the basis of neurophysiological, clinical and experimental investigation, EEG has been regarded as a paraphenomenon of integrated brain metabolic processes. The EEG reflects the activities in the underlying brain structure and particularly in the cerebral cortex. These signals are recorded by means of electrodes externally placed upon the intact skull. The nature of these signals varies over different parts of the scalp and is dependent upon various factors. It has been observed that the frequency content of EEG is of importance in its assessment and hence extensive studies have been made based on the frequency analysis of EEG. Thus we find frequent mention being made in EEG literature about four rhythmic activities characterized by their frequency bands that are designated as delta (0.5 to 3 Hz), theta (4 to 7 Hz), alpha (8 to 13 Hz) and beta (14 to 30 Hz). The alpha and beta are normal rhythms. The delta and theta activities are associated with altered states of consciousness or pathological conditions. While EEG changes, in some instances, are associated with specific patterns or with transients such as spikes or sharp waves, most of the changes represent alterations in the amplitude and frequency of the EEG rhythms. In view of this, EEG has become a research tool in neurophysiology, psychophysiology and psychopharmacology and its use is well established in monitoring sleep, depth of anesthesia and cessation of brain function. The status and changes in EEG are important in a wide range of normal and pathological conditions such as brain maturation, local and generalized changes from mass lesions, diffuse pathological conditions, metabolic disturbances and coma states resulting from a variety of causes. The disappearance of EEG activity in cases of cerebral silence is diagnostic of brain death.

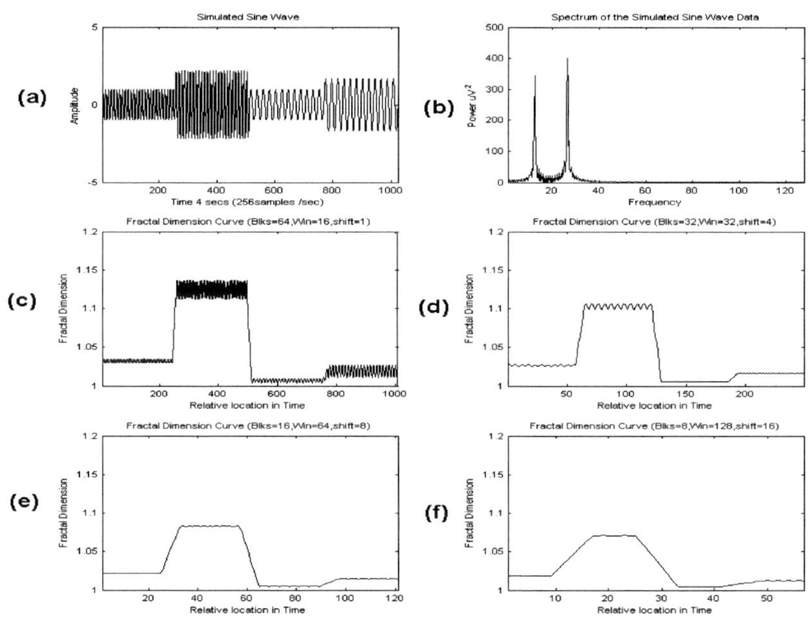

Figure 1 (a) Model data of sinewaves having two different frequencies and two different amplitude patterns, (b) The power spectrum only detecting the two frquencies but not the changing patterns in the signal, (c, d,e,f) The moving fractal dimension curve showing the points of changing patterns in the signal (at locations sample no 256, 512,768).

Since the frequency contents of EEG signals are of importance, spectral estimates by Fourier analysis are widely used to study the pattern features of EEG signals and in the analysis of EEG background activity. However, spectral methods are heavily dependent on the statistical predictability of the process. Nonperiodic signals such as transients, brief seizures etc. get superimposed on EEG and severely delimit the spectral methods of analysis. Moreover, spectral methods may fail to detect occasional spikes of low amplitude. One does not get adequate discrimination from the power spectrum; where a low amplitude, long duration alpha like activities may yield the same magnitude of power as that of a short duration alpha burst of higher amplitude. In view of these limitations, spectral methods are not suitable for detecting the time varying dynamical property of brain activity. The progresses of nonlinear dynamics in the past decade has made it possible to think of modeling the brain as a continuous, spontaneously changing, nonlinear dynamical system (Baser, 1983). Grassberger and Procacia have further developed the tools to model experimental data as the output of nonlinear dynamical system (Grassberger and Procaccia, 1983). Examples of model data made of sine waves have been shown in (Fig.1). It reflects the inability of spectral methods to detect the changing patterns which is otherwise evident.

In reviewing the patterns of brain electrical activities, it is seen that the beta and alpha dominant oscillations appear similar to random signal activities (Fig2). The nature of their historagms appear similar to gaussian distrubution. The spectral plot of random signal is flat and and is seen to be diifferent from alpha and beta activities. But it is difficult to distinguish the spectral patterns of closely overlapping alpha and beta activities. The non-random nature of brain signals are evident from the differences in autocorrelation function and phase-space plots. Even, the pattern of phase space plot are distinct for beta and alpha activities. The spectral power of background EEG signals decreases with increasing frequency. Hence, it appears that the EEG has certain scaling property and may be fractal in character.

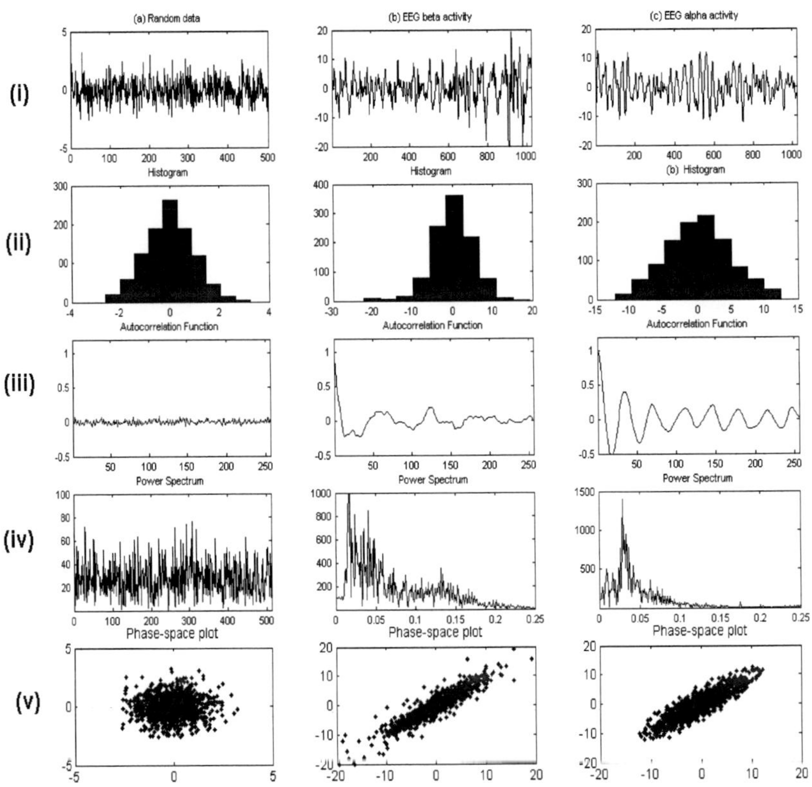

Figure2 (a) show the property of a random process like (i) the time series, (ii) the statistical distribution in histogram, (iii) autocorrelation function and (iv) powerspectrum (v) phase-space plot and similar properties of EEG (b) β and (c) α activities.

BRAIN ACTIVITY IS A NONLINEAR DETERMINISTIC PROCESS

The random-like nature of EEG has been attributed in the past to very complex dynamics of brain where stochastic description was inevitable. In contrast, nonlinear dynamics views such time series as being deterministic and of relatively low dimension, with their 'complexity' being due to their inherent nonlinearity (Snoog ans Stuart, 1988). The simplicity of the new description lies in the fractal nature of EEG which implies self-similar character with a scaling property. Structurally it is similar to simple recursion in both time and space. Nonlinear systems are capable of so-called chaotic behaviour, in which time series predictability fall off exponentially as a function of time. Despite this temporal unpredictability, the deterministic nature of chaotic time series allows a great deal of information to be recovered regarding their dynamics, for example, their phase (state) space dimensionality etc. This deterministic viewpoint for understanding brain functions has implications for visual (phase space representation of EEG) and quantitative EEG interpretation. The awareness that a relatively simple nonlinear system may account for the EEG features seen in normal and pathological brain wave recordings could force a re-evaluation of current presentation of EEG in clinical practice (Watt and Hameroff, 1988). Furthermore, the chaos conjecture has made it possible to actively search for a neurophysiologically realistic model. The extensive work done by Freeman and associates in modeling the olfactory system by chaotic dynamics and predicting the cooperative behaviour of the network has put the conjecture of nonlinear dynamics of brain function and the generation of the complex patterns of EEG on a firm ground. Replacing the phenomenological approach by model-driven approach should result in a better understanding of a chaotic time series like EEG and its transitions.

The implication of chaotic dynamics for EEG is that this seemingly disordered process can be explained by a relatively few terms. The richness of this procedure and the real theoretical power of this approach is based on mathematical theorems (e.g., Takens embedding theorem) which suggest that if any signal variable can be measured with sufficient accuracy, frequency and duration, then quantitatively meaningful statements can be constructed concerning the dynamical structure of the entire system from the behaviour of that single variable. One of the quantitative measures of a complex dynamical system is that of dimension, which refers to the ability of a space to contain a set of points (reconstructed phase space vectors). However, the implications and understanding of dimensionality to the brain electrical activity in various behavioral or experimental states have yet to be fully articulated. The theory of chaotic dynamics has developmental links to the nonlinear thermodynamics of far from equilibrium conditions described by Prigogine and the catastrophe theory of Rene Thom and topology and fractal geometry of Mandelbrot(B.Mandelbort). These theories along with high speed supercomputing platforms have opened new techniques to investigate nonlinear phenomena experimentally that were deemed to be "too complex". Two examples (1) a simple nonlinear operation with feed-back onto itself and its recursion giving rise to a strange attractor and (2) three coupled nonlinear systems producing phase-space behaviour with chaos are shown in (Fig.3).

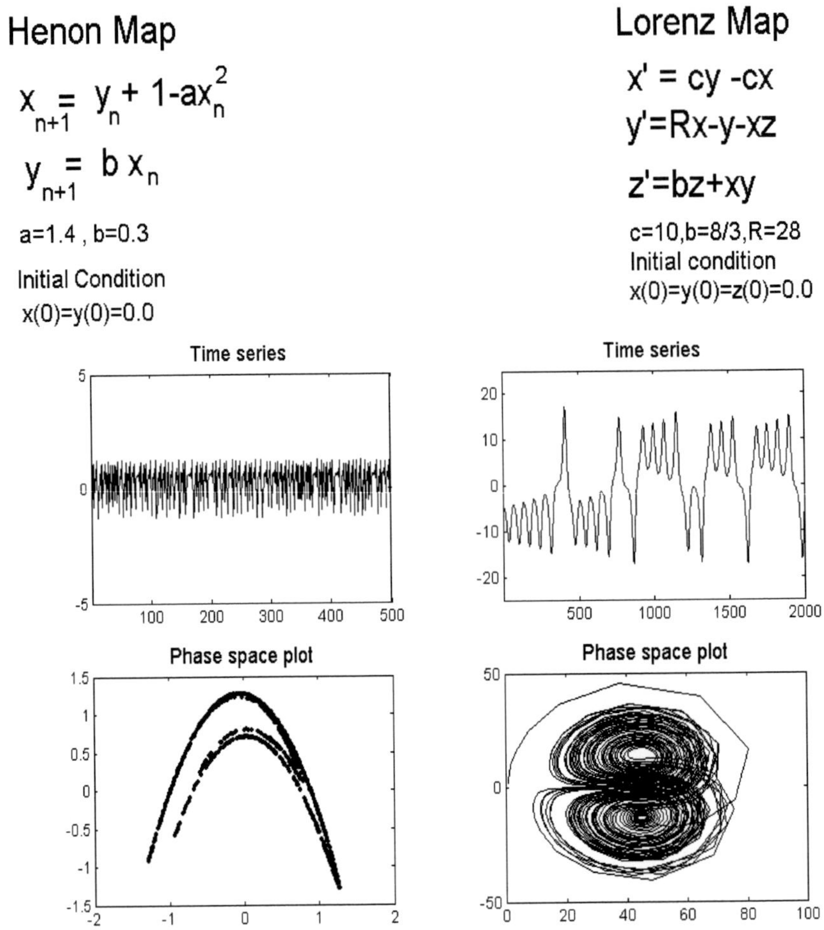

Figure 3 shows the strange attractor of (a) Henon map arising out of non-linear recursive operations and (b) Lorenz map produced by coupling of 3 differential equations.

DYNAMICAL INVARIANTS OF BRAIN ACTIVITY

The dynamical parameters of attractor dimension or Correlation Dimension (D2) and fractal dimension (D1), information dimension, Lyapunov exponents along with the trajectory behaviour through Poincare's sections, phase-space plots and recurrence plots are the starting points in understanding and interpreting the ensuing brain state (Galka,2003). The primary analysis as to the nature of underlying processes of brain activities in the various states is to determine whether the brain states are the outcome of a chaotic or stochastic process. Theoretical investigations are under progress in this field in various labs. It has found recent applications in experiments of chaninging brain states such as sleep, convulsions, electronvulsive therapy and anaesthesia. (Pradhan and Dutt, 1992).

The debate of stochasticity vs determinism in nature is one of the fundamental questions facing man for centuries. It is not only a serious mathematical problem but has profound philosophical implications. It has been realized that researches in nonlinear dynamics and chaos may help in future in understanding brain processes involved in perception, thinking, problem solving and creativity; therefore, its implication for psychiatric research is understandable. Recently the EEG from normal brain states and in various pathological and altered states have been subjected to the formalisms of nonlinear dynamics. Very preliminary reports are available. The correlation Dimension (D2) of EEG in a cognitive behavioral state (Table 1) and in various sleep stages in schizophrenia (Table 2) is given. However, the dynamical parameters mentioned above need evaluation for a proper modeling and analysis of the nature of underlying processes of brain activities in different brain states and rules governing their transitions.

Table 1. Correlation Dimension of Brain EEG activities Under different Tasks.

EEG Channel	Eye Closed	Eyes Open	Mental Arithmetic	Motor task	Photic Stimulation	Auditory Clicks
F3	4.7272 ±0.4161	4.5583 ±0.5280	4.5332 ±0.9660	3.9626 ±1.0638	4.9379 ±0.8222	4.7599 ±0.7479
C3	4.5882 ±0.3982	4.9576 ±0.5054	4.3776 ±0.8747	4.1197 ±1.1507	5.0717 ±0.7922	4.9207 ±0.5503
P3	3.9619 ±0.4541	4.5731 ±0.4085	3.9304 ±0.5087	3.6051 ±0.6479	3.8568 ±0.2198	4.0782 ±0.4277
O1	3.9605 ±0.3328	3.9154 ±0.4355	4.4239 ±0.5753	3.7564 ±0.9959	5.1735 ±0.7990	3.9861 ±0.3850
F4	4.8614 ±0.3578	4.8064 ±0.5291	4.1273 ±0.7014	3.9311 ±1.0599	5.0370 ±0.8678	4.2961 ±0.5704
P4	4.1670 ±0.4130	4.2723 ±0.3463	4.2267 ±0.6862	3.6798 ±0.7791	4.5484 ±0.8570	4.5546 ±0.5122
C4	4.6638 ±0.4793	4.5127 ±0.4668	4.2116 ±0.7326	3.6019 ±0.6597	4.6223 ±0.9742	4.6931 ±0.6001
O2	3.8394 ±0.5132	3.7717 ±0.4224	4.3662 ±0.5443	3.4241 ±0.5640	4.7106 ±0.8233	4.0291 ±0.5446

All significant differences in correlation dimension (D2) was seen with task across channels (MANOVA)

Table 2. Attractor Dimension (D2) of sleep Activities in Schizophrenia

	II	**III**	**IV**	**REM**
Schizophrenia (n=6)	8.33±0.85	7.36±1.08	5.89±0.84	8.58±0.73
Control (n=7)	8.70±0.31	7.84±0.50	7.38±0.38	8.95±0.69
Significance	ns	ns	$p < 0.005$	ns

Analysis of the Stochastic or Deterministic Nature of the EEG

Generally two methods are employed to determine the properties of the time series. The standard spectral estimates and the attractor dimension are used to evaluate the deterministic or stochastic nature of the process representing the data. For a stochastic signal, the plot of log

C(r) vs log (r) may never converge. Secondly, the power-law features can determine the fractal nature of a signal. The fractal refers to geometric structures with the property of self similarity at all size of scales. The definition need not be reserved for deterministic structures but may also be applied to stochastic structures whose statistical properties exhibit scale invariant self-similarity. Furthermore the concept may be extended to time series where there are fluctuations on multiple time scales. The most commonly and widely used technique to investigate whether a signal is time scale invariant is spectral analysis. If a signal is fractal and thus time-scale invariant, the amplitude of its power spectrum will decrease with increasing frequency, falling off as $1 \over {f^a} $ where is α a positive number i.e. power spectrum scaled by an inverse powerlaw. The time histories with apparently similar spectra do not necessarily have the same dimensionality. The EEG in various states of brain activities have been found to be a broadband noise. Human EEG has a $1\over f $ like power spectrum scaling and follows the inverse power law (Prichard, 1992). The attractor dimension or correlation dimension of a time series can be estimated from the correlation integral of the phase-space vectors.

The Concept of Attractors

Different kinds of attractors are known. A closed curve, e.g. the phase-space representation of a sinusoid, is called a limit cycle. The sum of two sine waves with incommensurable frequencies results in a torus in phase space. Two arbitrarily close points of a limit cycle will continue to stay close as time increases. However, a subset of a phase space is called a strange attractor if initially arbitrary close points get macroscopically separated after sufficiently large time intervals (examples Henon and Lorenz maps, Fig.3). In this case, similar causes do not produce similar effects. This important property is called sensitive dependence on initial conditions, which means unpredictability is a basic feature of strange attractors. On the contrary, the phase-space representation of noise never converges to a lower dimensional subset. Noise always penetrates the entire phase space. Therefore a stochastic process cannot define any attractor.

Specific Properties of Attractor Dimensions D2

For a better understanding of the interpretation of the attractor dimension or correlation dimension D2, we will outline some features of D2 based on theoretical data. If an attractor is a closed curve in phase space (limit cycle), its correlation dimension is D2=1.00. A sine wave is the simplest example of a limit cycle. Moreover, the sum of two sine waves with commensurable frequencies also defines a limit cycle. On the contrary, the sum of two sine waves with incommensurable frequencies results in a torus with a dimensionality of D2=2.00.

These examples demonstrate the advantage of the nonlinear analysis versus conventional spectral analysis. Whereas the power spectrum of the sum of two sine waves (incommensurable frequencies or not) remains in two different peaks in the frequency domain, the evaluation of the correlation dimension shows the differences. The calculation of D2 from a time series consisting of a certain frequency and its harmonics gives a value of

D2=1.00. If the signal consists of two or three incommensurable frequencies, the correlation dimension is D2=2.00 or D2=3.00, respectively.

As mentioned above, the phase-space representation of a stochastic signal does not result in the convergence of the trajectory to an attractor. This means that the dimensionality of white noise is infinite. All strange attractors encountered upto now have a fractal dimension, which means that their dimensionality is noninteger. Strange attractors can be identified with the properties of deterministic chaos. The main advantage of dimensional analysis is the investigation of time series with apparently noiselike spectra. If the phase-space representation of such signals converges to an attractor, its dimensionality is a finite number. Otherwise, the investigated time series has stochastic properties and cannot be considered as a signal from a deterministic system.

Fractal Dimension, the Geometric Measure of a Curve

The concept of fractal can be extended to a signal which is a non-self-crossing curve. Fractal is a complex shape and Mandelbrot has argued that there is a natural dimension in which each fractal sits most parsimoniously (Madelbrot, 1983). This fractal dimension, D, is represented by an individual number (often a fraction) that can be used as a fundamental quantification of even the most complex shapes like coastlines, shapes of clouds, landscapes etc. Here we consider the geometry of the waveform as a space filling property of the signal in a plane (2D). A running fractal dimension can give an idea about the changing patterns of brain activity during the entire recording period (Pradhan and Narayan Dutt, 1993). It is a computation intensive task to calculate a running attractor dimension from the multidimensional phase space as the dynamics evolves with time. However, the attractor dimension (embedding of data into multidimensional phase space) may be determined for a large bulk of data segment. Alternatively, a 2D fractal procedure may help dissecting out the points of transitions in an entire record. The 2D fractal map may then be thoroughly scrutinized for any transition. In this procedure, the waveforms are seen as planar curves that proceed monotonically forward and their fractal dimension range between D=1.0 for straight line, to somewhat less than D=1.5 for certain highly spiked waves. True waveforms can never become sufficiently convoluted to fill a plane; thus waveforms will never have fractal dimensions approaching the dimensionality of a plane namely, D=2.0. This is demonstrated in Fig.1. It shows, how this simple algorithm can detect changes in time series not possible by spectral methods.

Lyapunov Exponent - a Measure of Sensitivity to Initial Conditions of the System

In a linear process starting from two nearby initial conditions the two nearby points in phase-space stay close as the system evolves. However, in nonlinear systems this is not guaranteed. Although all trajectories of a chaotic attractor converge to a subset of phase space, inside the attractor two neighboring trajectories may diverge. The Lyapunov exponents are average exponential rates of divergence (positive) or convergence (negative) of nearby trajectories in phase-space. Any attractor with at least one positive Lyapunov exponent is defined to be chaotic with the magnitude of the exponent giving the time scale on which the system dynamics becomes unpredictable. It is a measure of sensitiveness to initial conditions and almost has been synonymous as the definition of chaos. A number of neurodynamical studies involving evaluation of Lyapunov exponents of brain signals are available (Pradhan and Naryan Dutt, 1993 for review).

Chaotic Dynamics and Brain Functions

It is yet to be seen how chaos may be linked to consciousness and cognition (Jansen, 1991, Melancon,2000, Faure and Koru 2001). The fact that chaotic dynamics plays a vital role in the generation of a complex pattern like EEG has been shown by the work of Freeman and his colleagues (Freeman,1990, Freeman and Skarda, 1985, Freeman, 1986, Freeman et al 1988, Skarda and Freeman, 1987). In their studies of EEG recordings made simultaneously from 64 electrodes in the olfactory bulbs of rabbits, they have shown that behavioural information is carried by a globally distributed spatial pattern of amplitude. This carrier is shared by the entire bulb and reflects cooperative neural dynamics within the bulb responsible for perceptual recognition and memory. To analyze the dynamics of the system, Freeman developed a chaotic model using sets of coupled nonlinear ordinary differential equations (Freeman, 1987). Their solutions simulated the various EEG patterns observed experimentally and thus established to a large extent the physiological mechanisms by which these patterns emerged. From these observations and models they concluded that chaotic olfactory dynamics in the olfactory bulb support a global attractor that affords quick access to and dissemination of information.

While it is not proven mathematically whether or not this brain activity is chaotic, experimental results argue convincingly that chaos plays an indispensable role in brain functions. Spatial pattern changes occur almost instantly over the entire bulb and take place so fast that the information transmitted to the cortex can be integrated there without degradation of phase lags. This is a very important property for the management of neural information by the brain, and it provides the most compelling evidence we have to date for the genesis of chaos by the olfactory system. Chaos provides a mechanism of sensitization in the system for rapid, controlled changes under small perturbations. Chaotic dynamics also desynchronize potentially fatal periodic cortical behaviours by a low-dimensional control and suggest a mechanism whereby the basic housekeeping tasks of exercising neurons to select input. Researchers must be aware that chaotic dynamics can do what other forms of dynamic activity cannot.

A low dimensional chaotic pattern has been created by coupling the firing pattern of three neurons together (Rapp et al ,1989). The cooperative behaviour is unpredictable in its detail, "but it has tendencies for implicit ordering (limit cycle) of activity." This model predicts the experimental finding of Freeman et al., cited above (Freeman and Skarda, 1985). It shows how chaotic neural firing is transformed into an order in a collective way momentarily when an appropriate stimulus is presented. In fact, the whole system had the appearance of a limit cycle with a different limit cycle pattern for each odour. If the rabbit was introduced to a scent it had never smelt before, the bulb gave out bursts of chaotic activity. If the new odour showed up several times, the bursts gave way to a signature waveform pattern with a specific pattern for its limit cycle. Possibly the familiar smell becomes embedded in the fractal pattern of the bulb's low-level chaos, where it is available to be "recalled" through neuron feedback coupling. In these experiments the limit cycle "recognition" of familiar smells was a momentarily organized ripple.

The dynamical analysis of EEG in epilepsy shows highly periodic behaviour. The tendency to desynchronize to a low order chaos is broken down in epilepsy. The firing pattern of cells falls into a rigid order of periodicity (limit cycle) for a longer time. When cells that oscillate at one frequency are coupled with cells that oscillate at another frequency, the first frequency cuts out. This pattern repeats, creating "traveling and rotating waves" that are essentially the same as the scroll-like waves of the Belousov-Zhabointsky reaction. The lack of chaos and persistent long order is the cause of epileptic discharge (Freeman,1986, Niederhauser et al 2003). This delicate balance of order and chaos in the cooperative processes of neuronal activities can be investigated by calculating the attractor dimension and plotting the phase-space trajectory. Reports of such investigations have shown the changing pattern of low order chaos in the brain in various states like coma, deep sleep and alpha rhythm (Babloyantz, 1991). It can be seen that the complex EEG patterns have much in common with fractals and the measure of the attractor dimension has significant discerning properties (Widman et al 1999).

The mathematical tools developed for the analysis of complex dynamic systems, namely the computation of the correlation dimension, D2, can be used to reveal differences in the state of the neuronal networks as these become involved in epileptic seizure activity (Lehnertz et al 2002,Aproti et al 2003). It has been found that during an epileptic seizure the EEG signals present lower correlation dimensions, D2, than during the waking state, confirming previous studies (Babloyantz and Desstxhe, 1986, 1987). It is conjectured that the dimension of the brain's strange attractors could provide a measure of the depth of various stages of sleep (Babloyantz et al 1985,Widman,1999). But no analysis of the nature of the changes from desynchronized behaviour to synchrony and back has been made. In a similar investigation, scientists at the Center for Nonlinear Studies at Los Alamos have worked out the fractal dimensions for strange attractors associated with different levels of anesthesia (Watt and Hameroff, 1987). The group also think it may be possible to develop a computer analysis of EEG recordings to characterize different forms of seizure. In addition, it has been shown that during an epileptic seizure the different areas of the brain from which EEG signals were recorded did not show a reduction of D2 in the same way in a kindling experiment (Dvorak et al,1986). Indeed a low D2 value was observed initially only in entorhinal cortex and fascia dentata. In the course of the seizure, the EEG signal recorded from ipsilateral hippocampus showed a low D2, but contralateral hippocampus tended to a low value only late in the seizure, while the value of D2 of the signal recorded from cortex increased appreciably and became more irregular. This time sequence of changes in D2 suggests that the recruitment of different areas into the seizure takes place according to a given sequence: first the cortex and facia dentata, then the ipsilateral hippocampus later the contralateral hippocampus, while the cortical changes in the late phase to a much less regular pattern (Jing and Takigawa, 2000).

Some criticisms are encountered in interpreting the correlation dimension of EEG signals. Even when the numerical procedure has been optimized to reduce artifacts, a signal can only be distinguished from random noise if the corresponding correlation dimension is clearly lower than that of the control signal. In such a case, the signal can be considered to be generated by a chaotic system (Dvorak et al 1986). We should add that the fact that EEG signals may not be distinguishable from random noise, as during rest and locomotion, does not imply that the biophysical process underlying EEG generation is necessarily random in nature, but it may have such a high degree of complexity that only a description in terms of random noise is justified (Dvorak et al 1986, Pijn et al 1991, Esteller et al 1999). The results of these studies are compatible with the interpretation that when a given brain area displays epileptiform seizure activity the state of the underlying neuronal networks may be described by a low dimensional chaotic attractor. The way in which D2 decreased from the high values in the pre-seizure epochs to the low values during seizure indicates how the different areas become gradually recruited into the seizure indicating a global coupling process. Indeed a clear transition from a very high to a low correlation dimension was found for all the areas at the moment that they became involved in the seizure activity. It may be expected that similar spatiotemporal patterns of transitions may be found for seizures recorded intracranially in man. This needs to be further investigated. If this proves to be the case, the computation of the correlation dimension may likewise be of help for the localization of an epileptogenic focus in epileptic patients, particularly in combination with the nonlinear regression analysis and the estimation of time delays. Further investigation is necessary to validate this conclusion in a large sample of human EEG data, and to determine which parameter, correlation dimension as used here, or Lyapunov exponents as used by Iasemidis et al. are the most appropriate, both in terms of sensitivity and specificity, to detect the onset of epileptic seizure activity (Iasemidis, et al, 1990, 2001, Gamundi et al 2000). The 3D phase-portrait of EEG is characteristically different in epileptic seizure and is of greater diagnostic significance than a 2 D phase portrait of seizure activity. There is a characteristic limit cycle behaviour in the phase-space plot. The pattern appears similar to the phase-space plot of alpha activity. However, it has been amply demonstrated that the correlation dimension is lower during seizure (D2=2.05) than that of alpha activity (D2=6.1).

Application of Chaos Theory in Psychological and Psychiatric Research

Scientists have also explored complex brainwaves for the fractal signs of high-level thinking or even creativity. The change in the correlation dimension has been seen during intensive cognitive activities (Gregson et al, 1990, Nan and Jinghua,1988). The analyses of the complex dynamic activities of cortical areas have shown hypofrontality in psychiatric condition of schizophrenic disorder (Elbert et al, 1992). The dimensional complexity shows a very pronounced difference between different groups of schizophrenics in the topographical pattern: this measure generally gives larger values at the frontal than at the central sites in schizophrenic patients, whereas the reverse fronto-central gradient is exhibited by control subjects. Eight of the twelve patients were beyond the range of control values for this fronto-central difference to conclude that the finding of a higher frontal than central dimensional complexity indicates a specific characteristic in schizophrenic patients. The failure to uncover distinct patterns in alcoholic and demented patients may point to such a specificity, which, however, await further validation. If we compare this result with the repeatedly reported increased activity of slow EEG frequencies in schizophrenics, the fact that additional information is provided by the dimensional complexity measure becomes obvious. Although both results are statistically significant, the increase in the slow-frequency band has no topographical specificity and the overlap in the range of single-subject values between the patients and the control subject is considerable (Pradhan et al , 2000, Malik et al 2000). Nonlinear EEG analysis is of value in understanding both developmental and degenerative processes in brain. It may shred light on therapeutic responses and the degree of cognitive decline in dementia (Gallois et al 2003).

Hjorth has represented the EEG signal in time domain by three parameters viz., activity, mobility and complexity. Activity deals with variance of the amplitude fluctuations, mobility with measure of mean frequency and complexity with the ratio of the mobility of the first derivative of the signal to the mobility of the signal itself (Hjorth, 1970). A fronto-central difference was also depicted by the Hjorth complexity measure, suggesting more regularity in the appearance of brain waves over frontal areas in patients than in controls. Although it is possible to detect such a difference by visually examining the EEG traces, one would not easily predict that the higher regularity in the physical appearance of EEG-traces could indicate a more complex dynamic as expressed by the measure based on the attractor property. This fronto-centrally positive gradient of the fractal dimensionality of the EEG-attractor in schizophrenics indicates more intricacy of the brain dynamics (but not necessarily of the brain waves) over frontal than central areas. None of the dynamic measures correlated with the neuroleptic dosage. However, Itil also reported no effect of medication on alpha activity in patients (Itil, 1977). Although the absence of correlation of between dosage of medication and measures of EEG activity cannot be taken as a proof of the absence of drug effects, it is tempting to speculate that the presently observed patterns of complexity measures in patients cannot easily be attributed to effects of medication but adhere to the psychotic processes. However, this speculation must be substantiated by future comparisons of medicated and unmedicated patients. Surprisingly, the distinctive EEG patterns in schizophrenic patients were also not related to the measures of symptomatology, affective flattening and cognitive impairment. It may well be that these measures do not map abnormalities in the frontal and/or temporal brain dynamics in a comparable manner. Although the present results are certainly preliminary, in particular because a new methodology was applied to EEG analysis in schizophrenics, their clarity encourages further investigation of the complexity of electrocortical responses in schizophrenics.

Two views of the cerebral cortex have a long-standing tradition. In one view the structural diversity of different areas and the bulk of connections being short in range divides the cortex into various subsystems. In an alternate view, statistical similarities, like the density of synapses, dendrites, and the existence of long-range connectivity and plasticity can be considered evidence for the system operating as a whole (Braitenberg,1986). Often the solution to this problem seems to be dialectic in nature: there is some truth in both views, and like an electron, appearing one time as a wave, another time behaving like a particle, we may observe the cortex functioning as a whole system at one time, or separating into subsystems, according to different experimental conditions. This hypothesis receives support from the data reported by Lutzenberger et al. (Lutzenberger et al, 1992). Although resting conditions or imagery of pleasant scenes yielded the same dimensional complexities at every electrode site, specific sensory tasks produced distinct patterns with different attractor dimensions across the scalp. When such differences are observed, we have reason to assume that the underlying dynamics must differ, thus arising from different systems at play at a time. The presently observed fronto-central gradients in patients classified as suffering from schizophrenia suggest that the frontal and the central dynamics are dissociated even in the relaxed waking state when a coupling occurs in the control sample. Thus the physiological and pathological states of brain activity can be understood as the output of a system associated with the degrees of freedom characterized by its correlation dimension. This can lead to various mathematical modelings and prediction of the EEG in other experimental states.

The sequential dynamics of EEG is neither linear nor stationary and so what is of interest here is the relative susceptibility of attractor to driving the trajectory to various transitional states. The phase space plot and the recurrence plot can assess the instabilities and hidden periodicities in the EEG (Babloyantz, 1991). Even the simple phase portraits of different EEG activities exhibit different patterns. The degree of synchrony can be inferred from the nonlinear analysis. The 2D phase-space plots of alpha activity and beta activity of awake state can be easily visualized (Fig.4).

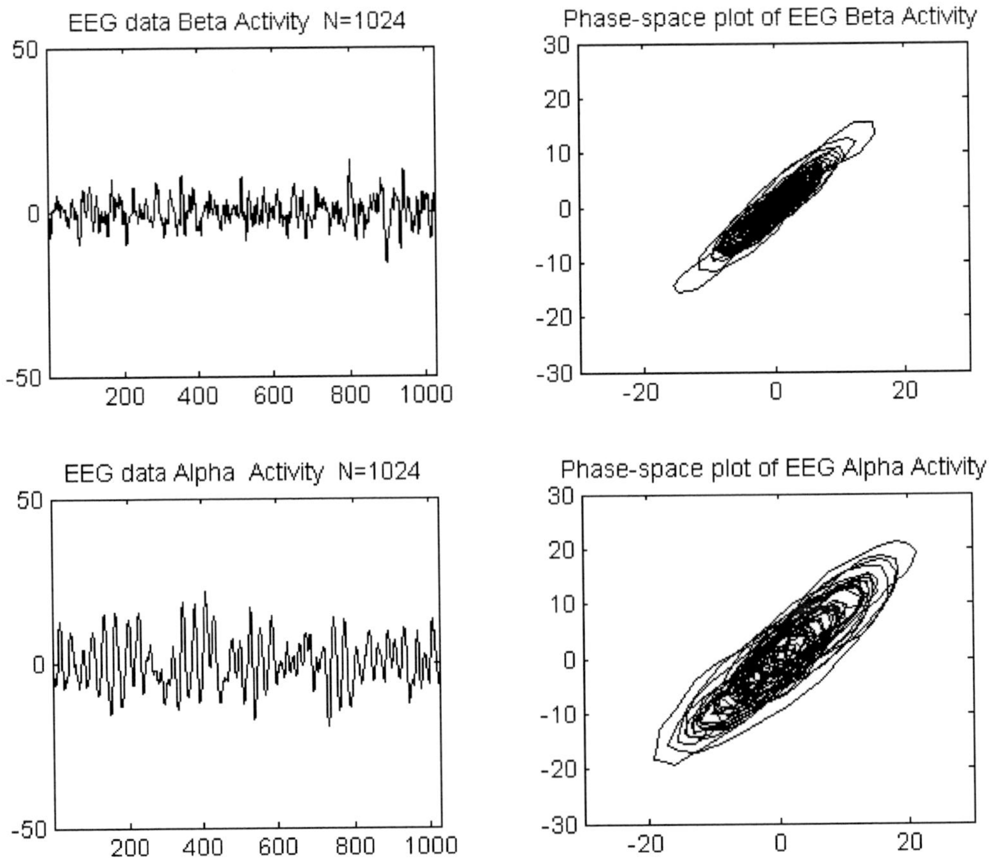

Figure 4. Shows the phase-space behaviour of β and α EEG activities.

The limit cycle pattern of alpha activity can easily be discerned in contrast to that of beta activity. The correlation dimension values of alpha activity are lower (D2=6.1) than that of beta activity that are almost of ultra high dimension, with the values ranging from 10 to 17. Another important question is whether the information one gains from the estimation of dimensionality of an attractor increases our knowledge about a system's dynamics than what we gain from power spectra. The question has been addressed by Roschke and Aldenhoff who have shown that the time series obtained from auditory cortex and hippocampus of a cat's brain during slow-wave sleep having similar spectral properties had the dimensionality of the cortex D2=5.63, and that of the hippocampus D2=4.58 (Roschke and Aldenhoff,1992). It is hoped that nonlinear dimensional and trajectory analysis may become another tool for discriminating various normal and pathological states as has been the spectral methods. The nonlinear dynamics being a model driven approach gives a more direct way of causal links between psychological processes and the neuronal substrate than does the simple representation of EEG in the frequency domain (Gregson et al,1990).

Most of the efforts have been made towards the determination of Correlation dimension of EEG tracings recorded from subjects in different neurophysiological states. Babloyantz and coworkers have studied the attractor dimension for wakefulness, sleep, epilepsy and Creutzfeld-Jacob disease [Babloyantz, 1989, Babloyantz, 1991, Babloyantz and Desstxhe,1986, Babloyantz and Desstxhe,1987, Babloyantz et ,1985). They have reported that the dimension increases with the level of mental activity. Subjects in stage IV sleep had dimension of 4 but during alert and resting state the dimension are reported to be 6. A dimension close to 10 has been reported for persons engaged in mental tasks. The Creutzfeld-Jacob disease reportedly has a dimension less than stage 4 sleep, and attractor dimension was close to 2 in petitmal seizure. Variations have been noticed in the slope determination of log C(r) vs log r, which may be the probable reason for widely varying estimations of attractor dimension (Jansen,1991). The number of data points is crucial to the estimation of attractor dimension. A guideline for selecting the number of data points and delay has been suggested (Fraser and Swinney,1986, Simm et al, 1987). Researchers have mainly focused on the absolute value of D2. It would be better to concentrate on how D2 changes in response to different states of brain activity. The concept of moving fractal dimension may be useful in this context (Pradhan and NarayanDutt,1993, Simm et al, 1987). The state of brain activity can be monitored through the moving (continuously changing) fractal dimensions of the EEG. The moving fractal dimension is effective in detecting changes in the background EEG activity. An example is given in Fig.2 which shows a segment of EEG signal with intermittent bursts of alpha activity. Its corresponding moving fractal dimension clearly shows the points whenever there is a change in the pattern of the EEG.

Future Scope

Now there has been a beginning to exploit chaotic dynamics to understand the underlying neuronal process of oscillatory behaviour of the brain. The future of this endeavour may lead to the development of predictive models to forecast the time series at the transitional states and in experimental conditions. It is now clear that EEG is produced by deterministic chaos. The basic idea has been to embed the data in a phase space that maximizes determinism and then use numerical techniques to build a nonlinear dynamical model to the map that sends the current state to the future. When random-like behaviour is encountered due to low dimensional chaos, our short term forecast can be several orders of magnitude better than those of the standard linear methods. Many adhoc nonlinear representations of coupled chaotic maps that could fit to the observed experimental data may be seen in the near future. The error estimations of parameter quantification may suggest that the use of higher order approximation techniques can give significant improvement in computing quantities such as fractal dimension or Lyaponov exponents. Furthermore, forecasting provides strong selfconsistency requirements on the identification of chaotic dynamics. The basic principle underlying these methods are similar to those of neural nets but are more straight forward.

The globally coupled nonlinear dynamical systems have remarkably rich behaviour and exhibit successive phase transitions among coherent, ordered, intermittent and turbulent phase, as the nonlinearity increases (Kaneko,1990). The dynamics of the emergence of ordered states out of chaotic background states can be modeled suitably by coupling one dimensional maps (Phillipson,1988). Coupled nonlinear oscillators with global feedback can represent diverse and complex dynamical systems such as evolutionary dynamics and economics. A globally coupled map is a dynamical system of N elements with discrete time. The dynamics consist of local mapping and interactions among all elements. It is known that a globally coupled map has two tendencies; destruction of cohesion by chaotic instability in each element and synchronization by global averaging(Watters,2000). This formalism may be of value in modeling the transitional states in EEG.

The behavioural transitions from one state to other are reflected in the change in the dimension and trajectory of the EEG signals at these instants of time (Pradhan and Sadasivan, 1996). However, the chaotic dynamics should predict those transitions at these cross sections. A predictive model may be built to forecast the time series data in different behavioural states. The predictability may be tested by taking the real recorded data with reference to the statistical properties of these data. The nonlinear forecasting has been performed for epidemics by Sugihara and May by means of simplex method from a general method described by Farmer and Sidorovich (Farmer and Sidorovich, 1987). An adaptive nearest neighbour estimate for prediction is an efficient forecasting strategy that uses the D2 value of the present data sets using the same procedure.

Neuroscience being the thrust area and neurodynamics being the most complex problem, the importance of nonlinear dynamics is self-explanatory. Chaotic dynamics is fundamentally a different approach to understand brain functions. Deterministic mathematical models of neural systems can give rise to complex chaotic dynamics in the absence of stochastic fluctuations in the variables of brain potential to the system. Chaotic dynamics are expected in nonlinear feedback systems possessing time delays and are expected in recurrent inhibition and from the periodic forcing of neural oscillators. The implications of chaotic dynamics and mathematical modeling of brain activity in transitional states may throw new ideas in our understanding of brain and behaviour.

CONCLUSIONS

Few biologists will dispute that at the simplest level, many biological systems exhibit nonlinear dynamics. Nonlinear dynamics is an emerging new approach to neurobiology and theoretically it is superior to the traditional methods of analysis by time domain or spectral methods. It has given rise to a fundamentally different approach to computerized EEG analysis and is making its way into the laboratories. The study has clinical implications for visual and quantitative EEG interpretation. The insight that a relatively simple nonlinear system may account for the EEG features seen in normal and pathological brain wave recordings could force a re-evaluation of current visual EEG interpretation practice.

Specifically, a reorientation to temporal relationships between paroxysms, rather than focusing on their morphology may be called for. Furthermore, the chaos conjecture has made it possible to actively search for a neurophysiologically realistic model of EEG generation (for example, the extensive work done by Freeman and associates on modeling the olfactory system). Replacing the phenomenological approach to EEG interpretation by a model-driven approach should result in a better understanding of EEG waveforms and rhythms. The developments in nonlinear dynamics and its application to EEG may be helpful for realistic modeling of various neuro-oscillatory phenomena. It may help in the construction of physiologically realistic mathematical models that simulate brain activities and allow prediction as to how they may be affected by experimental manipulations. Nonlinear dynamics may produce tools for feature extraction, EEG data compression and analysis. Its methodology is also of importance in analyzing other oscillatory and transitional states of brain activity seen in epilepsy, task loaded attentional states, cognitive task performance and in various states of consciousness and behaviours which have been most difficult to be discerned in background EEG activities. This newly gained insight of chaotic dynamics of brain is a significant departure from the earlier stochastic visualization. It appears that nonlinear dynamics is going to be the method of studies of complex systems and their experimental time series.

In short, this paper reviews the physical and dynamical aspects of brain's electrical activity from the new perspective of nonlinear dynamics and indicates possible future directions in realistic modeling and simulation of brain functions in various experimental conditions. The importance of the emerging trends of nonlinear science to neurobiology has been highlighted. These mainly serve to illustrate the progress being made and to indicate the need for further work. The rapid advances in nonlinear science and computer technology will make the processed EEG an increasingly viable tool in research and clinical practice.

Acknowledgment The work has been supported by a grant from Dept. of Biotechnology (BT/R\&D/09/48/92), Govt. of India.

REFERENCES

Aporti, F., Ferro-Milone, F., Cananzi, A., Minelli, T.A., Nofrate, V., and Pascoli, D. *Sampling dependence of EEG nonlinear and fractal structures in healthy subjects and Alzheimer patients*, International Nonlinear Sciences Conference, Research and Applications in the Life Sciences, INSC, Vienna, Austria (2003).

Babloyantz, A. Estimation of correlation dimension from single and multichannel recordings-a critical review.*Springer Series in Brain Dynamics*. Vol.2, 122-130, Springer Berlin, New York (1989).

Babloyantz, A. Evidence of slow brain waves: a dynamical approach. *Electroenceph. Clin. Neurophysiol.*, Vol. 78, 402-405 (1991).

Babloyantz, A and Desstxhe, A, Low dimensional chaos in an instance of epilepsy. *Proc.Natl.Acad.Sci.USA.*, Vol. 83, 3513-3517 (1986).

Babloyantz, A. and A.Desstxhe, A. Strange attractors in the human cortex. *Springer Series in Synergetics*. Vol 36, pp. 48-56, Springer, Berlin Heidelberg, New York (1987).

Babloyantz, A., M.Salazar, J.M. and Nicolis, C. Evidence of chaotic dynamics of brain activity during the sleep cycle. *Phys. Lett., Vol. 111A*, 152-156 (1985).

Baser, E. Synergetics of neuronal populations: A survey on experiments. In: E.Baser, H.Flohr, H.Haken and A.J.Mandell (Eds.)*Synergetics of the brain, Springer Series in Synergetics of the Brain*, pp. 190-200, Springer Verlag, Berlin (1983).

Braitenberg, V. Two views of the cerebral cortex. In: G.Palmand A.Aetsten (eds) *Brain Theory*, Springer, Berlin, Heidelberg, New York, pp. 81-96 (1986).

Dvorak, I., Siska, J., Wackermann, J., Hrudova, L. and Dostalek, O.C. Evidence for the interpretation of the EEG as a deterministic chaotic process with a low dimension. *Activitas Nervosa Superior,* Vol. 28, 228-231 (1986).

Elbert, T., Lutzenberger, W., Rockstroh, B., Berg, P. and Cohen, R. Physical aspects of the EEG in schizophrenics. *Biological Psychiatry*, Vol. 32, 595-606 (1992).

Esteller, R., Vachtsevanos, G., Echauz, J., Henry, T., Pennell, P., Epstein, C., Bakay, R., Bowen, C. and Litt, B. *Fractal dimension characterizes seizure onset in epileptic patients*, in Proc. IEEE International Conference on Acoustics, Speech, and Signal Processing (ICASSP'99), Vol. 4, 2343-2346, (1999).

Farmer, J.D. and J.J.Sidorovich, J.J. Predicting chaotic time series. *Phys.Rev.Lett.* Vol. 59, 845-848 (1987).

Fraser, A.M. and Swinney, H.L. Independent coordinates for strange attractors from mutual information. *Phys.Rev.A*, Vol. 3, 1134-1140 (1986).

Freeman, W.J. Simulation of chaotic EEG pattern with a dynamical model of the olfactory system. *Biol. Cybern.*, Vol. 56, 139-150 (1987).

Freeman, W.J. *On the problem of anomalous dispersion in chaoto-chaotic phase transitions in neural masses and its significance for the management of perceptual information in brains. Springer Series in Synergetics,* Vol. 45, 126-142, Springer, Berlin Heidelberg, New York (1990).

Freeman and C.A.Skarda, Spatial EEG patternss, non-linear dynamics and perception: the neosheringtonian view. *Brain. Res. Rev. Vol. 10*, 147-175 (1985).

Freeman, Pettitmal seizure spikes in olfactory bulb and cortex caused by runaway inhibition after exhaution or excitation. *Brain Res. Rev. Vol. 11*, 259-284 (1986).

Freeman, W.J. Yao, Y. and Burke, B. Central pattern generating and recognising in olfactory bulb: a correlation learning rule. *Neural Net., Vol. 1,* 277-288 (1988).

Faure, P. and Korn.H. Is there chaos in the brain? I. Concepts of nonlinear dynamics and methods of investigation. Comptes Rendus de l'Academie des Sciences Serie III - *Sciences de La Vie - Life Sciences, Vol. 324*, 773-793, (2001).

Galka, A. *Topics in Nonlinear Time Series Analysis With Implications for EEG Analysis*, World Scientific Publishing, Singaoore, 2003.

Gallois, P.H., Forzy, G., Leduc, J.J., Andres, F., Peyrodie, L., Lefebvre, E. and Hautecoeur, P. Comparison of spectral analysis and non-linear analysis of EEG in patients with cognitive decline, *Clinical Neurophysiology, Vol. 32(5),* 297-302 (2003).

Gamundi, A., Van Rijn, C.M., Pereda, E., González, J., Nicolau, M.C., Rial, R.V.I., AND Coenen, A.M.L. *Non-linear and fractal dynamics of absence-like phenomena (SWDs) in WAG/Rij rat EEGs.* Sleep-wake Research in the Netherlands, Vol. 11, 58-64. (2000).

Goldberger, A.L, Amaral, L.A, Hausdorff, J.M., Ivanov, P., Peng C.K. and Stanley, H.E. Fractal dynamics in physiology: alterations with disease and aging. *Proc Natl Acad Sci U S A, Vol. 99 Suppl 1*, 2466-72 (2002).

Grassberger, P. and I. Procacia, i. Characterisation of strange attractors. *Phys.Rev.Lett.*, Vol. 50, 346-349 (1983).

Gregson, R.A.M., Britton, L.A., Campbell, E.A. and Gates, G.R. Comparison of the nonlinear dynamics of electroencephalogram under various tasks loading conditions: a preliminary report. *Biol. Psychology, Vol. 31*, 173-191 (1990).

Hjorth, B. EEG analysis based on time domain properties. *Electroenceph. Clin. Neurophysiol., 29*, 306-310 (1970).

Iasemidis, L.D., Sakellres, J.Ch., Zaveri, H. and Williams, W.J. Phase space topography and Liapunov exponent of electrocorticograms in partial seizures. *Brain Topography, Vol. 2*, 187-201 (1990).

Iasemidis L.D, Pardalos. P., Sackellares , J.C., and Shiau, D.S. (2001) Quadratic binary programming and dynamical system approach to determine the predictability of epileptic seizures. *J Combinatorial Optimization Vol. 5*: 9-26.(2001).

Itil, T.M. Qualitative and quantitative EEG findings in schizophrenia. *Schizophrenia Bulletin, Vol. 3,* 61-75 (1977).

Jansen, B.H. Quantitaitive analysis of electroencephalogram: Is there chaos in the future? Int. *J. Biomed. Comput., 27*, 95-123 (1991).

Jing, H. and Takigawa, M. Comparison of human ictal, interictal and normal non-linear component analyses, *Clinical Neurophysiology Vol. 111* , 1282-1292 (2000).

Kaneko, K. Globally coupled chaos violates the law of large number but not the central-limit theorem. *Physic. Rev. Lett., 65*, 1391-1394 (1990).

Klonowski, W., Olejarczyk, E. and Stepien, R. Complexicity of EEG-signal in Time Domain - Possible Biomedical Application. *Experimental Chaos*, 2001

Lehnertz K, Andrzejak, R., Arnhold J, et al. Nonlinear EEG analysis in epilepsy: its possible use for interictal focus localization, seizure anticipation, and prevention. *J Clin Neurophysiol, Vol. 18:* 209-22 (2001).

Lutzenberger, W., Elbert, T., Birbaumer, N., Ray, W.J. and H.Schupp, H. The scalp distribution of the fractal dimension of the EEG and its variation with mental tasks. *Brain Topography, Vol. 5,* 27-34 (1992).

Mallik, S.K., Chandrasekharan, M.K. AND Pradhan, N. *"Nonlinear Phenomena"* INSA Volume, New Delhi (2000).

Melancon, G., Joanette, Y. and Belair, J. Chaos, brain, and cognition: Toward a nonlinear order? *Brain and Cognition, 42*:33-36, 2000.

Mandelbrot, B. *Fractal geometry of nature* , Freeman, New York (1983)

Nan, X and Jinghua, X. The fractal dimension of EEG as a physical measure of conscious human brain activation. *Bull Math Biol., Vol. 50,* 559-565 (1988).

Niederhauser, J., Esteller, R., Echauz, J., Vachtsevanos, G. and Litt, B. "Detection of seizure precursors from depth-EEG using a sign periodogram transform, " *IEEE Transactions on Biomedical Engineering, Vol. 51*, 449-458 (2003).

Phillipson, P.E. Map models for emeregence of ordered states out of chaos.*Phys. Lett. A, Vol. 133,* 383-390 (1988).

Pijn, J.P., Van Neerven, J., Noestr, A., and Lopes da Silva, F.H. Chaos or noise in the EEG signals: Dependence on state and brain site.*Electroencephalogr Clin Neurophysiol., Vol. 79*, 371-381 (1991).

Pradhan, N. and D.Narayana Dutt, D. Use of running fractal dimension for the analysis of changing patterns in electroencephalogram. *Compt. Biol. Med., Vol. 23*, 381-388 (1993).

Pradhan, N. and Narayana Dutt, D. A nonlinear perspective in understanding the neurodynamics of EEG, *Comput.Biol. Med., Vol. 23*, 425-442 (1993).

Pradhan, N. and Sadasivan, P.K. (1996). The nature of dominant lyapunov exponent and attractor dimension curves of EEG in sleep. *Comput. Biol. Med., Vol. 26,* 419-428 (1996).

Pradhan, N., Rapp, P.E. and R. Sreenivasan, (Eds.), *Nonlinear Dynamics \& Brain Functioning.* Nova Science Publishers, NY, USA (2000).

Pritchard, W.S. The brain in fractal time: $1/f$-like power spectrum scaling of the human electroencephalogram. *Int. J. Neurosc., Vol. 66,* 119-129 (1992).

Rabinovich, M.I., Varona, P. and Abarbanel, .H.D.I. Nonlinear cooperative dynamics of living neurons. *International Journal of Bifurcation and Chaos, Vol. 10*, 913-933(2000).

Rapp, P.E., Bashore, T.E., Martinerie, J.M., Albano, A.M., I.D.Zimmerman, I.D and A. Mees, A. *Dynamics of brain electrical activity. Brain Topogr., Vol. 2,* 99-118 (1989).

Roschke, R. and J.B.Aldenhoff, J.B. A nonlinear approach to brain function:*Deterministic chaos and sleep EEG. Sleep, Vol. 15,* 95-101, (1992).

Simm, C.W., Sawley, M.L., Skiff, F. and A.Pochelon, A. On the analysis of experimental signals for evidence of deterministic chaos.Helv. *Phys., Vol. 60,* 510-551, (1987).

Skarda, C.A. and Freeman, W.J. How brain makes chaos in order to make sense of the world. *Behv. Sci., Vol. 10,* 161-195, (1987).

Snoog, A.C.K. and Stuart, I.J.M. Evidence of chaotic dynamics underlying the human alpha-rhythm electroencephalogram. *Biol. Cybern., Vol. 62*, 55-62, (1988).

Watt and S.R.Hameroff, S.R. *Phase space analysis of human EEG during general anesthesia.* In: S.H.Koslow (ed), Perspectives in Biological Dynamics and Theoretical Medicine. New York: Academy of Sciences, pp. 286-288, (1987).

Watt, R.C. and Hameroff, S.R. Phase space electroencephalography: a new mode of intraoperative EEG analysis. *Int. J. Clin. Monit. Comput., Vol. 5,* 3-13, (1988).

Watters, P.A. Time-invariant EEG power laws. *International Journal of Systems Science (Special Issue on Emergent Properties of Complex Systems), Vol. 31,* 819-826, (2000)

Widman G., Bingmann D., Lehnertz, K. and Elger, C. Reduced signal complexity of intracellular recordings: a precursor for epileptiform activity? *Brain Res, Vol. 836*, 156-63, (1999)

In: Depression and Dementia
Editor: Suptendra Nath Sarbadhikari, p. 21-53
ISBN 1-59454-114-0

Chapter 2

PSYCHOMOTOR THEORY MIND-BRAIN-BODY TRIAD IN HEALTH AND DISEASE

Üner Tan
Cukurova University, Medical School, Department of Physiology,
Adana, Turkey
E-mail: unertan@cu.edu.tr
Tel: +90 322 3387348
Fax: +90 3386847

ABSTRACT

In this study the authors outline the grounds of a new theory, to explain the mind-brain-body triad in health and disease. This is the *psychomotor theory*. First, he briefly analyzes the historical development of the relationship between mind and brain, which is being discussed over more than a few thousand years. The tight junctions between psychological and motor systems were subjected to a detailed analysis using examples in health and disease. The feedback circuits between mind, brain, and body were shown to occur within the mind-brain-body triad, in normal states, and psycho-neural diseases. It was stated that psychiatric signs and symptoms are coupled with motor disturbances; neurological diseases are coupled with psychological disturbances; changes in cortical and spinal motor-system activity may influence mind-brain-body triad, and *vice versa*. Accordingly, a psychomotor theory was created to explain the psychomotor coupling in health and disease, stating that, not the mind-brain duality or unity, but the mind-brain-body triad as a functional unit is essential in health and disease, since mind does not end in the brain, but further controls movements, in a reciprocal manner; mental and motor events share the same neural substrate, cortical and spinal motor neurons; mental events emerging from the motoneuronal system is strongly coupled with the unity of the mind-brain-body triad.

Psychomotor means "....of or relating to movement or muscular activity associated with mental processes, especially affects, as in psychomotor slowing associated with depression" (The American Heritage Dictionary of the English Language, fourth edition, 2000). I will refer "Psych" for mind, and "motor" for the motoneuronal system in brain and spinal cord.

According to Hebb (1980), "*broadly speaking, the mind is that which controls behavior*" (p.3). The psychomotor system is related to mind/body (or mind/brain) problem, which has a relatively long history, and is being discussed since more than a few thousand years. The mind/body problem concerns with determining the relationship between body and its mind.

If mind and brain are the same, why do we think they may be different? If they are different, why are they different, can they interact, if so, how? The psychomotor theory is an attempt to explain the possibilities of mind/brain unity and/or the mind/brain duality in relation to motor system in humans. To understand this theory, we have to analyze the historical development of the relationship between mind *and* brain, at least briefly.

Historical Development of the Mind/Body Concept

Probably the first systematic concept of mind and body originates from *Plato* (429-347 BC), a Greek philosopher. He identified mind with soul. According to Plato, the world of forms is the real world (nonmaterial), while the visible world (material) is only its copy; truth resides in the world of forms; opinion is stuck in the visible world; intellect is immaterial because forms are immaterial. Plato speaks of the soul as imprisoned in the body, but he does not explain what binds soul to a particular body.

Aristotle (384-322 BC) did not agree with Platonic forms. He believed in body and soul by saying that the soul is the form of the body: a person's soul is no more than his nature as a human being. Although his theory seems to be materialistic for many interpreters, he argued that the intellect must be immaterial (a kind of dualism).

The first systematic study of the mind/body relationship originates from the seminal work of *Rene Descartes* (1596-1650), a French mathematician, philosopher, and physiologist, also known as *Cartesius*. He published the world's first essay on physiological psychology, *De Homine*, in Holland about 1633 on the condemnation of Galileo. Until Descartes, there was no metaphysical split between mind and body. His ideas about the mind/brain duality and the mind/brain interactionism were outlined in his book: the rational soul (mind) is distinct from body, but makes contact with it at the pineal gland; body affects mind, mind affects body or mental events can cause physical events and vice versa. This is called "interactionism" or "Cartesian dualism". This was the dualist-interactionist theory of mind. Descartes believed that pineal gland was the only contact side of the mind, since this gland was not bilaterally duplicated, being uniquely human. He arrived at a single principle: *If I deceive, "I" must exist, which is known as "cogito ergo sum", (I think, therefore I am).* A type of dualism is *Epiphenomenalism,* which also separates the mental and physical events, but argues that physical events have mental effects, but not vice versa; *mind is seen only as a by-product of brain*; mental events cannot affect physical ones.

Baruch Spinoza (1632-1677) argued that there are not really two substances, but two attributes of the same substance; reality is, therefore, a case of two perspectives on the same thing: physical matter perceived thorough senses, and mental stuff experienced by mind.

Spinoza abandoned Descartes` two-substance view in favor of double-aspect theory, which is based on the notion that the mental and physical events are different aspects of the same substance (God). The essential substance, God, is the universal essence or nature of everything that exists.

Psychophysical Parallelism, which is usually traced to *Gottfried Wilhelm Leibniz* (1646-1716), retains the mind-body dualism, but avoids any assumption of causal mind/body connection. It states that events so totally different from each other cannot affect one another.

Parallelists simply argue that every mental event is linked to a physical event so that when one occurs, so too does the other. Leipniz rejected the interactionism, since it would be impossible to conceive of material particles passing from one substance to the other. In brief, the psychophysical parallelism states that mind and body exist in a harmony that has been pre-established by God from the moment of creation.

All the above mentioned views are pointing out some distinction between mind and body. Conversely, to avoid the mind/body problem, one must deny this distinction. In the history, this denial has taken different forms. For instance, *immaterialism* best represented by *George Berkeley* (1685-1753) denies even the possibility of mindless material substance in his *A Treatise concerning the Principles of Human Knowledge* (1710). According to Berkeley, there is no mind/body duality since what we think of as body is merely a perception of mind.

Materialism dating to antiquity holds that matter is fundamental. Everything depends on matter. Materialism completely denies the existence of mental events. In a less extreme form, materialism describes mental events as dependent on bodily events, but does not deny their existence. This view was offered a century after Descartes by *Julien Offray de la Mettrie* (1709-1751). La Mettrie was born in Brittany and studied medicine at Paris. Because of public outcry over his materialism, he self-exiled to Holland, where *he published L`homme machine, that was* publicly burned and La Mettrie was forced to seek protection from Frederick the Great at Berlin, where he continued to publish on various topics, until his death in 1751. Actually, L`homme machine was a ground-breaking work, which maintained an antimetaphysical tone, and accentuated that the mental processes are identical with their physiological causes. Moreover, this book introduced the notion that conscious and voluntary phenomena are distinguished from involuntary and instinctual activities by the complexity of their mechanical substrate. *Pierre Jean Georges Cabanis* (1757-1808) argued that *"to have an accurate idea of the operations from which thought result, it is necessary to consider the brain as a special organ designed especially to produce it,* ***as the stomach and the intestines are designed to operate the digestion, and the liver to filter bile****..."*.

The 19th century heavily engaged with the mind/body problem. Progress was made in understanding *the localization of cerebral function, based on the idea that the brain serves as the organ of mind.* It was generally accepted that mental events (beliefs, mental suggestions, psychic traumas and the like) may cause radical alterations in the state of the body. At the same time, the nature of functional nervous disorders was also made progress. In 1870, An English Philosopher, *Shadworth Holloway Hodgson* (1832-1912) published a two-volume work, *The Theory of Practice,* introducing the term *epiphenomalism.* In the Theory of Practice, Hodgson has argued that the feelings have no causal efficacy; just as the stones are held in place and not by the colors, events in the nervous system from an autonomous chain independent from accompanying mental states, which are present only as "epiphenomena", incapable of reflecting back to affect the nervous system. *In support, Thomas Henry Huxley* (1825-1895) presented his most influential papers (On the hypothesis that animals are automata and its history) in front of the British Association for the Advancement of Science, in 1874. In brief, he pointed out that states of consciousness are merely the effect of molecular changes in brain....; animals are, therefore, conscious automata.

In 1874, another influential book was published by *William Benjamin Carpenter* (1813-1885), who studied medicine at Bristol, University College London, and Edinburgh, opposed to the epiphenomalism of Hodgson and Huxley. Carpenter wrote, *"Nothing can be more certain than that the primary form of mental activity, --Sensational consciousness--, is excited through physiological instrumentality".* A certain physical impression is made, for example, by the formation of a luminous image upon the Retina of the Eye....Light excites nerve-force, and the transmission of this nerve-force excites the activity of that part of the Brain which is the instrument of our Visual Consciousness. Now in what way the physical change thus excited in the Sensorium is translated (so to speak) into that psychical change which we call seeing the object whose image was formed upon our Retina, we know nothing whatever; but we are equally ignorant of the way in which Light produces Chemical changes...And all we can say is, that there is just as close a succession of sequences – as intimate a causal relation between antecedent and consequent – in the one case, as there is in the *other.* Interestingly enough, Carpenter has further suggested "the like Correlation may be shown to exist between mental states and the form of Nerve-force which calls forth Motion through the Muscular apparatus...*each kind of mental activity, --Sensational, Instinctive, Emotional, Ideational, and Volitional, -- may express itself in Bodily movement...".* Unfortunately, after 241 years from Descartes` De homine to Carpenter's Principles of "Mental Physiology", the primary objection to interactionism made little progress.

In 1871, John Tyndall wrote *"the passage from the physics of the brain to the corresponding facts of consciousness is unthinkable. Granted that a definite thought, and a definite molecular action in the brain occur simultaneously; we do not posses the intellectual organ, nor apparently any rudiment of the organ, which would enable us to pass, by a process of reasoning, from the one to the other".*

The most important brain child of *Dual-aspect monism* was *George Henry Lewes* (1817-1878), a writer, actor, biologist, philosopher, and a psychologist. His book, *Physiology of Common Life*, converted the young Pavlov to be a physiologist, and his five-volume book, *Problems of Life and Mind* (1874/1879) was a major contribution to psychology. *The "Physical Basis of Mind*" was the third volume of *Problems of Life and Mind.* According to his theory (*neutral monism or dual-aspect monism)*, there is only one kind of "stuff" and that mind and body differ only in the arrangement of that stuff or in the perspective from which it is apprehended; when seen from the subjective point of view (e.g., thinking), the psychophysical series is mental, and when seen from the objective point of view (e.g., when one observes what happens during thinking), it is physical.

Within the 19th century the mind/brain problem was especially important because physiologists and psychologists focused on the nature and cerebral localization of mind. *In fact,* we can find ideas about functional localization throughout antiquity. For example, we can find ideas about soul globally localized to the brain, in work of Pythagoras, Hippocrates, Plato, Erisistratus, and Galen, among others. The pneumatic physiologists located the mental capacities to the fluid of the cerebral ventricles, till the book *"De functionibus systematis nervosa"* was published by *Jiri Prochaska* in 1784, and the interest had shifted to the brain stem and cerebrum.

Among the 19th century achievements, the most impressive one is the localization of function to various brain regions. The most famous man of this era is *Franz Josef Gall* (1758-1828) born in Baden and studied medicine at Strasbourg and Vienna. He was impressed as a child by variations in facial and cranial appearance of his friends with unusual talents. His first lectures aroused opposition on the grounds of his presumed materialism, and in 1805, he had to leave Vienna, and after two years he arrived in Paris. Gall believed that there are correlations between character and the external craniological signs: the size and shape of the head reflect the size and shape of the underlying portions of the brain; mental abilities are innate and fixed, and the development of an innate ability is a reflection of the inherited size of its brain. In doing so, a well-developed ability can be predicted from a particularly prominent area of the cranium (functional localization of an ability in the cranium). Although Gall's correlational approach was eventually abandoned in favor of experiment, his accomplishments in the history of functional localization cannot be underestimated; he was the founder of the biologically based, functional psychology. Interestingly enough, more than 200 years later, it was found that the cognitive abilities may be predicted from the craniofacial measurements (see Dayi et al., 2002).

The first experimental demonstration of localization of function in the brain was first realized by *Marie-Jean-Pierre Flourens (1794-1867),* using the method of complete isolation of brain part to be removed: a successive slicing through the cerebral hemispheres produced diffuse damage to all of the higher mental functions. Fluorens concluded that

> "higher mental functions such as perception, volition, and intelligence are spread throughout the whole brain, operating together as a single factor, the entire cerebrum functioning in a unitary fashion (unitary soul and an indivisible mind); the brain is the organ of a unitary mind, it could not, therefore, be functionally differentiated."

The first specific demonstration of sensory-motor function originates from Alexander Bain (1818-1903), who also created a valuable survey of mind/body views (Mind and body. The Theories of Their Relation, 1873). His important contribution was the sensory-motor associationism (associationist psychology), which was analyzed in *"The Senses and the Intellect"* (1855) and *"The Emotions and the Will"* (1859). Before Bain, the movement and action with regard to the analysis of sensation was neglected. Bain brought the new physiology of movement into relation to an associationist account of mind. He defined volition as the compound of spontaneous movements and feelings; the coordination of motor impulses into purposive movements results from the association of ideas with them.

In 1855, as Bain published "The Senses and the Intellect", Herbert Spencer (1820-1903) published "The Principles of Psychology". Spencer was born in Derby (England) and largely self-taught. As he was 17 years old, he worked as a railway engineer; in 1848, he started to work as an editor and then as a free-lance writer and reviewer. Spencer discovered a cephalograph to achieve more reliable cranial measurement. Bain had introduced movement to the sensations of associationism and arrived at the first fully balanced sensory-motor associational view; Spencer grounded psychology in evolutionary biology. For Spencer, mental phenomena are adaptations, i.e., incidents of the correspondence between the organism and its environment; mental and physical life are simply species of life, mind evolves continuously from physical life, reflexes from irritations, instincts from compound reflexes, conscious life and higher mental processes from instincts:

> "If higher mental activities are the end product of a continuous process of development from simple irritation through reflexes, there is no justification for drawing a sharp distinction between mind and body; The brain is a physical system and the cortex is the most developed level of th*e brain"*.

Otherwise, the mind/brain duality continued for two centuries and supported the notion that mental processes must function according to principles entirely different from those of brain itself.

To overcome the last obstacle to extension of the *sensory*-motor view to the cortex, we needed the following period. *Paul Broca* (1824-1880) born in France studied medicine at the Hotel Dieu in Paris. He was an original member of the Societe d`Anthropologie and a founder of the Revue d`anthropology and the Department of Anthropology at the University of Paris.

In 1861, Broca set in the audience as Ernest Aubertin presented a paper citing several striking cases to argue a craniological case for cerebral localization of spoken language. Aubertin was a student of Jean Baptiste Bouillaud. As early as 1825, Bouillaud provided clinical evidence to support Gall's view that the articulate language is localized in the anterior lobes of the brain. This hypothesis was kept alive for almost 40 years. Aubertin claimed that he will give up his belief in cerebral localization if even a single case of speech loss could be shown without a frontal lesion. Broca had decided to take up Albertan's challenge. His speechless patient ("*Tan")* had died from gangrene on Boca's surgical ward. Broca published this case, presenting a detailed account of his post-mortem examination of Tan's brain. He found a superficial lesion in the left frontal lobe. This finding was confirmed a few weeks later by another case with a similar lesion. This was the first report about the localization of the articulate language in the anterior portion of the brain. However, to be sure, the cerebral cortex should be explored experimentally in normal subjects. The technique was introduced by *Gustav Theodor Fritsch (1838-1927) and Eduard Hitzig (1838-1907).*

Firtsch and Hitzig, in 1870, published a classic paper, providing evidence of cortical localization of function. Namely, using galvanic stimulation of the dog brain, they *provided first evide*nce that areas of the cerebral cortex are involved in movements of the contralateral extremities. These results established *electrophysiology* for the experimental exploration of cortical localization of function, which demonstrated the participation of brain in motor functions. At approximately the same time in England, *John Hughlings Jackson (1835-1911)started b*rain from a different direction. He was a physician at the National Hospital for the Paralyzed and Epileptics, Queen Square. *His ideas can be summarized up as follows*:

> "All complex mental phenomena are made up of these simple elements – from the simplest reflex to the most sublime thoughts; all functions and faculties can be explained in these terms….It is asserted by some that the cerebrum is the organ of mind, and that it is not a motor organ. Some think the cerebrum is to be linked to an instrumentalist, and the motor centres to the instrument – one part is for ideas, and the other for movements. It may, then, be asked, How can discharge of part of a mental organ produce motor symptoms only?...But of what `substance` can the organ of mind be composed, unless of processes representing movements and impressions…? Are we to believe that the hemisphere is built on a plan fundamentally different from that of the motor tract?...Surely the conclusion is irresistible, that mental symptoms… must all be due to lack, or to disorderly development, of sensori-motor processes."

With Jackson, the theoretical analysis of cerebral localization reached its full development in 19th century. These results were fully confirmed by his friend and colleague, *David Ferrier (1843-1928), who usin*g controlled ablations and faradic stimulation of the brain, succeeded in mapping sensory and motor areas across a wide range of species. This was the dominant paradigm for explanation in both physiology and psychology.

The concept of subconsciousness emerged in the 19th century. This was an epoch of trance and trauma (functional nervous disorders). The most prominent scientist of this area *was Franz Anton Mesmer (1734-1815)*, born in a German town, and studied medicine at the University of Vienna with a dissertation on the influence of the planets on human disease.

Mesmer had a patient, Madame Oesterlin (27 years), who suffered from recurring physical ailments. On the 28th of July 1774, he asked his patient to swallow a solution containing iron and affixed magnets to her stomach and legs. Her symptoms began to disappear, and she completely recovered with continued treatment. Unfortunately, the results were not confirmed by others and Mesmer had to leave for Paris, where he further developed his "magnetic cure". However, he also had to leave Paris after several spectacular therapeutic failures, and died near the place of his birth.

In the history of Western philosophy, one of the most influential philosophers is *Immanuel Kant (1724-1804),*who was born, lived, and died at Koenigsberg, East Prussia. During his life he did not travel more than forty miles from his birth place. His most original contribution is his "Copernican Revolution": the representation that makes the object possible rather than the object that makes the representation possible; the human mind is an active originator of experience rather than just a passive recipient of perception; perceptual input must be processed (recognized), otherwise it would be a noise or nothing. Kant argued that mind plays an active role in constituting the features of experience, limiting the mind's access to the empirical realm of space and time; "thoughts without content are empty, intuitions without concepts are blind." In the philosophical classic, *Critique of Pure Reason,* he asserts that our perceptual apparatus is able of ordering sense-impressions into intelligible unities, lead us to conclude through "pure reason" that the intelligible unities, such as God, freedom, and immortability, do exists. Kant did not describe himself as "dualist", in contrast to Plato who believed that there is a world beyond the material world, soul or mind, he insisted that none of reality exists; reality and all that is in it, including human beings are part of this outer world, all part of a dream world. Kant argued that the universe did not consist of matter but of for*ces. Kant pro*posed that the objective reality is the essential structure of the knowing mind. Only objects of experience can be known, whereas things lying beyond experience are unknowab*le. The unk*nowable "things-in-themselves" can be neither confirmed nor denied, nor can be scientifically demonstrated. Accordingly, he showed in the Critique of Pure Reason that the great metaphysical problems, such as God, freedom, and immortability, cannot be solved by scientific thought.

During this time period, another philosopher of mind, *Johann Friedrich Herbart (1776-1841)* concerned with the new scientific psychology, making a critical distinction between ideas above and below the threshold of consciousness. He was a transitional figure between Kant and Fechner; he was not able to link his philosophy of mind to the physiology of the brain. Evangelista Purkyne (1787-1869) and Ernst Heinrich Weber (1795-1878) made fundamental contributions to the experimental phenomenology of sensation, and Johannes Mueller (1801-1858) elaborated the doctrine of specific nerve energies, suggesting the nervous system as intermediary between mind and the world. Weber described the *just noticeable difference*, which refers to the smallest perceptible difference between two sensations. He played an important role in the emerging science of psychology. Weber provided evidence for the relationship between variations in physical and mental events.

According to Mueller, the mind is directly aware of the states of the nervous system. That is, *the nervous system plays a role as an intermediary between the world and the mind* and thus imposes its own nature on mental processes. After that, the quantitative measurement of the mind/body relationship emerged in Fetcher's psychophysics.

The experimental psychology formally started with *Gustav Theodor Fechner (1801-1887).* Before that, there was only psychological physiology and philosophical psychology. Fechner was born in Prussia. At 16, he began to study medicine at the University of Leibzig; after MD he began to study physics and mathematics. He suffered a nervous collapse, in 1840, as his article on subjective afterimages appeared. He had a painful injury to his eyes while gazing at the sun during his research. This resulted in temporary blindness and prostration. He resigned his position and his interests changed to metaphysics. In 1848, he returned to the University as a professor of philosophy; he write a book, Nanna, Ueber das Seelenleben der Pflanzen, which contained his first philosophical treatment of the mind/body relation *(monistic-dual aspect,* pan-psychical mind/body view). Fechner wanted to demonstrate the unity of mind and body empirically by relating increase in bodily energy to an increase in mental intensity.

Between 1851 and 1860, he worked on the measuring sensation indirectly a just noticeable difference between two sensations. Working out this subject, he concluded his book, *Elemente der Psychophysik.* His aim was to establish an exact science of the functional relationship between physical and mental phenomena, and formulated his famous principle that the intensity of sensation increases as the log of the stimulus ($S = k \log R$). In doing so, he believed that he had arrived at a fundamental philosophical truth: mind and matter are simply different ways of conceiving of one and the same reality. Mental events were shown not only be measured, but also brought into relation to physical phenomena; psychophysics became of the methods of the newly emerging scientific psychology. *Wilhelm Wundt (1832-1920),* physiologist, also rejected a metaphysical foundation of psychology. Wundt argued that the limitations of the direct study of consciousness can be transcended using genetic, comparative, statistical, historical, and particularly experimental methods. Only in this way, it would be possible to understand the conscious phenomena as "complex products of the unconscious mind".

Hermann Ludwig Ferdinand von Helmholtz (1821-1894) born in Postdam (Germany), graduated in medicine at 21 years age, interested in physiological basis of animal heat. He calculated the conduction velocity of a nervous impulse, by stimulating nerves at various distances from a muscle and measuring the time it took for muscle contraction, and introduced the technique for measuring the reaction time into physiology. Between 1865 and 1868, another great physiologist, *Franciscus Cornelis Donders (*1818-1889) developed and assimilated the reaction-time, the time taken up by mental operations, measurement to psychology. Donders separated the time taken to respond to a stimulus under conditions of choice and non-choice. In doing so, Donders calculated the time interval taken by the decision process. His discoveries with respect to mental reaction times exerted a major impact on his contemporaries and reaction time is installed, along with psychophysics, as a method of choice in the early experimental psychology.

The most influential neurophysiologist and philosopher of the 19th century is *Sir Charles Sherrington (1857-1952),* who completed his medicine study at the Royal College of Surgeons. First he worked on the effects of excisions of parts of the cortex of the dog brains. In 1885, he went to Spain to study an outbreak of cholera; in 1886 he visited Venice to investigate this disease, then he took the material to Virchow in Berlin for further examination. As he was in Spain, he was influenced by the Spanish Neurologist Ramon y Cajal, and took up the study of the spinal cord, and began to study the spinal reflexes. After passing of the man of genius on March 4, 1952, Sherrington left us more than 350 works on the foundations of our knowledge of the functioning of the brain and spinal cord. His work *Integrative Action of the Nervous System (1906)* is still a source of inspiration to physiologists all over the world. Sherrington did not retire from the Chair of Physiology at Oxford until 1935 at the age of seventy-eight. After making experiments with cats, dogs, and monkeys, he became a philosopher and interested with the mind/body relationship. He had a dualist position in the mind/body controversy. Five days before his death, he said to Sir John Eccles, one of his prominent pupils: "For me know, the only reality is the human soul."

According to the results of the experiments performed on decerebrate cats, dogs, and monkeys, he suggested that reflexes must be regarded as integrated activities of the total organism (total integration), not as the results of isolated reflex arcs. In accord, he demonstrated the "reciprocal innervation of muscles" (Sherrington's law): when one muscle (e.g. extensor) is stimulated, the opposite muscle (e.g. flexor) is simultaneously inhibited.

In the 1880's Cajal demonstrated that neuronal extensions (axon endings) do not physically touch one another – they are separated by a gap called *"synapse"*. Sherrington proposed (1906) that neurons communicate via synapses. He measured the total distance that an impulse travels from sensory receptor to spinal cord to muscle and calculated the speed of the nerve impulse, and found that the speed of conduction through a reflex arc is slower that along a single axon; therefore there must be some delay at the synapses. The other important findings are as follows. Schiff-Sherrington reflex: rigid extension of the forelimbs after damage to the spinal cord; Liddle-Sherrington reflex (myotatic reflex): contraction of the muscles in response to its being stretched; the law of reciprocal innervation (Sherrington's law II).

According to Sherrington,

> "....mind is attached to a voluntary motor act performed with skill. "What the mind is concerned with is not the act but the aim. It is more aware of the finger-part than the rest because the fingers` part stands nearest to the aim...Clearly we must not suppose 'life' and `mind` are one and the same. The finite life is a phenomenon accessible to sense; the finite mind is not." What is most important for the subject of the present work is that "mind, recognizable mind, seems to have arisen in connection with the motor act. Where motor integration progressed and where motor behavior progressively evolved, mind progressively evolved."

One of Sherrington's most notable students was the Canadian neurosurgeon *Wilder Penfield (1891-1976).* His main goal was to establish a neurological institute with surgeons, laboratory researchers, physiologists, and scientists in neurology. After a decade, he succeeded in establishing the Montreal Neurological Institute in 1934. In the 1950s, Penfield was trying to treat epileptic patients, removing or destroying the brain tissue responsible for seizures. His technique was often successful. He made a dramatic discovery at the same time: stimulating only the temporal lobe elicited meaningful, integrated responses such as memory, including sound, movements, and color. These memories were distinct from usual memories which were unremembered under ordinary circumstances. If he stimulated the same area again, the same memory appeared again. He believed that he found a physical basis of memory (engram). He also interested in "mind"; until his death in 1976 questioned the scientific basis of mind –whether there is a scientific basis for the existence of the human soul--:

> "Throughout my own scientific career, I, like the other scientists, have struggled to prove that the brain accounts for the mind. But now, perhaps, the time has come when we may profitably consider the evidence as it stands, and ask question: Do brain mechanisms account for the mind?. Can the mind be explained by what is now known about the brain? If not, which is the more reasonable of the two possible hypotheses, that man's being is based on one element, or on two?"

First, Penfield offered an entirely mechanistic interpretation of the brain functions. But subsequently, he was convinced that this mechanistic and monistic view cannot explain the facts: "something else finds its dwelling place between the sensory complex and the motor mechanisms."

As Penfield worked during his training with Sir Charles Sherrington and for a short period under Santiago Ramon-y-Cajal in Spain he believed that mind will be entirely explained in terms of physics, chemistry, and electricity. But later, he thought that this mechanistic and monistic view did not adequately account for the facts. He had a surprising and remarkable experience as a form of double consciousness in one of his subjects during temporal lobe stimulation. The patient was aware of his immediate surroundings (operating room, the surgeon, and his assistants), and at the same time he re-enacted scene from the past with vivid sounds etc. Another patient from South Africa was also aware of his environment in the operating room, but he was, at the same time, laughing with his cousins on a farm in South Africa. According to Penfield, the mind of the patient was independent as was the mind of the surgeon listening and understanding him: "thus, my argument favors independence of mind-action." Penfield concluded that the stimulus was responsible for a kind of TV program the subject watched objectively, while the subject's mind was directing to record the events in the room around him. Just as we can objectively watch a TV program in the company of others whose presence we are fully conscious of, so here were two different types of consciousness. Similar observations repeated again and again for hundreds of patients. He emphasized that it is the mind that must first program the computer brain which has no ability to make totally new decisions for which it is programmed. Stimulation of the same point in the temporal cortex induced the same scenes. This was repeatable; in one subject this occurred sixty-two successive times. However, in another subject, the stimulation of the same area caused four apparently unrelated responses. First he heard "footsteps", secondly "a company of people in the room", thirdly "like being in a gymnasium", and finally "a lady talking to a child at the seashore". The experiences were not as a kind of hallucination but as a real life. In the end Penfield concluded that "it is easier to rationalize man's being on the basis of two elements than on the basis of one."

In 1961 Penfield demonstrated the reality of active mind or free will. He stimulated an area in the cerebral cortex with a single electrode using an electric shock at 60 Hz frequency and 2 volt intensity. When the neurosurgeon applied this stimulation to the motor area, the opposite hand moved, as expected. Surgeon asked the patient, why he moved his hand. The response was: "I did not do it, you made me do it. "It may be said that the patient thinks of himself as having an existence separate from his body". Penfield goes on: "Once When I warned a patient of my intention to stimulate the motor area of the cortex, and challenged him to keep his hand from moving when the electrode was applied, he seized it with the other hand and struggled to hold it still. Thus one hand, under the control of the right hemisphere driven by an electrode, and the other hand, which he controlled through the left hemisphere, was caused to struggle against each other. Behind the brain action of one hemisphere was the patient's mind. Behind the action of the other hemisphere was the electrode."

Sherrington's mind/body dualism was followed not only by Penfield in Canada, but also by another pupil, a worthy successor, Sir John Eccles (1903-1997). Eccles is recognized for his remarkable and outstanding impact on the neurosciences for more than six decades. Moreover, his essays on the mind/brain interaction generated considerable interest and debate. He studied science and mathematics at Melbourne High School, before entering the University, shared the State geometry prize and gained a Senior Scholarship to the University. He was deeply interested in mathematics, but chose medicine to study. He was interested in Darwin's Origin of Species in the first-year zoology course, and in philosophy dealing with the mind-body problem. Because the unsatisfactory explanation of the interaction between brain and mind, he decided to be a neuroscientist. In Oxford, he spent two years studying for the Final *Honors* School in Physiology and Biochemistry; he read the neurophysiological, biochemical, philosophical, and theological books. He worked with R. Granit on the crossed extensor reflexes using an optical isometric myograph. In 1935, Sherrington retired and was replaced by J. Mellanby. Eccles was disappointed and was also concerned about the increasing political uncertainty in Europe. He resigned his Oxford appointments and went to Sydney with this family in 1937. Eccles resigned in 1943, however, because of a debate between him and hospital board, and accepted the Chair of Physiology in Otago (New Zealand), where he recorded ventral root responses to dorsal root stimulation, dorsal root potentials upon dorsal-root stimulations, which were described by Barron and Matthews in 1938. The results were consistent with an electrical hypothesis of synaptic and neuromuscular transmission, as published in Nature (1945).

Eccles encountered K.R. Popper in New Zealand. He was deeply impressed by Popper's philosophy: "the scientific hypotheses should be clearly formulated and testable by experiment; the strength of a hypothesis depends upon the failure of rigorous investigation to falsify it rather than on evidence which apparently supports *it"*. He had a long lasting debate with Dale about the origins of the synaptic transmission. Eccles insisted of electrical transmission in contrast to Dale who insisted of chemical transmission. Eccles stated his hypothesis of electrical excitatory transmission at central and ganglionic synapses, and the neuromuscular junction, proposing a number of physiological and pharmacological experiments. Accordingly, he tested this hypothesis in 1946 with C. McC. Brooks by recording the monosynaptic excitation from the spinal motoneurones. The results were interpreted as consistent with his electrical hypothesis, and were published in Nature.

In 1949, Eccles restated his electrical hypothesis using synaptic excitation and inhibition in the spinal cord. However, his studies with Kuffler and others have convinced him in 1948 that transmission at the neuromuscular junction was a chemical process mediated by Ach. In 1951, he considered his hypothesis to have been falsified, and accepted that spinal excitation and inhibition were both chemical in nature. After this year, he accepted an invitation to Canberra. He was involved in the mind/brain problem at the same time. His dualistic view, a neurophysiological hypothesis of will, was first published in Nature, had created intense discussion. His lectures were published in 1953: The Neurophysiological Basis of Mind: The

Principles of Neurophysiology. After 1952 onwards for nearly 13 years, Eccles was most productive in Canberra: 74 investigators from 20 different countries worked with him, during this time. He later wrote:

"Without doubt it was the high point of my research career, my 14 golden years, scientifically speaking ..." He had six large research laboratories, with co-workers interested in neuropharmacology and neurochemistry. In 1958, he recorded the dorsal root potentials intracellularly from intraspinal afferent fibers, and prolonged EPSPs from dorsal horn interneurones involved in DRPs. The period of 1961-1965 was full of papers (29 full papers, 13 review articles and one book) dealing with presynaptic inhibition. In the ventrobasal complex of the thalamus he made two interesting observations: a recurrent inhibition and large post-inhibitory `rebound` depolarizing responses with superimposed bursts of action potentials (rhythmic thalamic activity). Eccles' last period of experimental neuroscience concerned with the cerebellum, began in Canberra in 1963 and continued in USA until his retirement in 1975. The results were published in a series of articles in Nature and in a book, "*The Cerebellum as a Neuronal Machine*".

An important factor in Eccles' decision to leave Australia was his feeling of intellectual isolation, especially concerning his philosophical interest in mind-body interaction. His last experimental paper was about the hippocampal inhibition. In 1975, Eccles voluntarily retired and moved to Contra in Swiss, where he dedicated himself to work on the mind/brain problem. "How the Self Controls its Brain" was published in 1994. Throughout his mental life, he has been a dualist, searching for mechanisms by which mind and brain interact. However, only 18% of his 568 publications dealt with this subject. In "The Self and Its Brain", he summarized his views:

> "It is a very strong dualism and raises the most severe scientific problems in relationship between the world of matter-energy, and the world of states of consciousness that is referred to as the self-conscious mind. Briefly, the hypothesis states that the self-conscious mind is an independent entity that actively engages in the reading out from a multitude of active centers in the modules of the liaison areas of the dominant cerebral hemisphere."

He also suggested that the mind-brain liaison function in both directions, from the brain to the mind in perception and from mind to brain in willed action;

> "the self-conscious mind interacts with the brain on aggregations of cortical pyramidal cell dendrites. "

Eccles actively participated in the experiments from 1927 to 1975. He had a strong motivation and stamina for an outstanding scientific career. He also owed much of his success to his productive research teams. He was a prolific writer with 568 items, including 19 books. His experiments usually began early in the morning each week, often lasting 16-20 hours, occasionally extending into the following day. He always had the best equipment in his laboratories including the first-class electronic and mechanical workshop personnel and facilities. As Eccles decided to move to Chicago in 1966, his wife preferred to stay in Australia, and their marriage was dissolved in 1968. In the same year Eccles married Helena, a neurophysiologist who collaborated with him from 1966 until he completed experimentation in 1975, after which they moved to Switzerland, where Eccles continued to work on the mind-brain problem. Until well beyond his 90th year, he had a long series of books, articles, reviews, comments, book reviews, and obituaries, which all were hand-written. He was always assisted in these activities by his wife Helena. He had bad health, however, from 1994, and he died in 1997 in the Hospital La Carita in Locarno.

The dualist-interactionist view of the mind-brain problem underwent to a considerable change by *Roger W. Sperry (1913-1994)*, who offered the most contemporary hypothesis on this subject. He was born in Hartford (USA), stayed in Oberlin for an MA in Psychology (1937), and received his PhD (1941), in Zoology under Paul A. Weiss at the University of Chicago. He argued that the basic structure of the mammalian central nervous system is hard wired, and unmodifiable by training. He was uncomfortable with the idea that electrical fields or waves were critical for neocortical processing. He demonstrated in monkeys that motor coordination remained unaffected after multiple transactions of sensorimotor cortex. He is famous with the *"split-brain"* experiments. In commisurotomized animals, restriction of sensory input on one cerebral hemisphere was shown to limit the learning activities to that hemisphere; the other brain half was capable of learning but remained naïve to those tasks until trained; the learning curves for each hemisphere were the same; it was as if two separate brains were housed within a single cranium. Sperry carried out much work during 1950s and 1960s on the split-brain preparation. Then, Sperry studied the effects of commissurotomy on perception. The left brain was found to be involved in analytical, sequential, and linguistic processes, and the right brain in holistic, parallel, and spatial abilities. Moreover, the combined effect of bi-hemispheric activity was more than the simple additive effects of the two separate hemispheres. Sperry then began to explore the emergence of consciousness from the unified brain:

> "I have never been satisfied with the materialistic or behavioristic thesis that a complete explanation of brain function is possible in purely objective terms with no reference whatever to subjective experience, i.e., that in scientific analysis we can confidently and advantageously disregard the subjective properties of the brain process....The mental forces are inseparably tied to the cerebral structure and its functional organization...In contrast to mind-brain identity theory, in the present theory the conventional differences between mind and brain are accepted and emphasized...The brain process consists of a multilevel hierarchic compound of entities and events from subatomic up through cerebral circuit and cognitive levels, is composed mostly of nonconscious elements that are common both to conscious and nonconscious brain processes....The brain process and the conscious processes are inseparable but different. The difference between mind and brain is the kind which exists between an emergent property and its infrastructure...Subjective experience in this interpretation is conceived to be an emergent dynamic property of cerebral excitation, inseparable from the material brain process, but different from and more than, the collected sum of the physicochemical components...The conscious experience is a property of, and cannot exists apart from the cerebral substrate."

According to Sperry, emergence occurs when, for instance, subparticles, atoms and molecules, create a new entity with new properties formerly nonexistent in the universe. Sperry did not see this as dualism, which describes the mind as a separate entity outside the brain. Consciousness emerges from the creativity of cerebral networks as an independent entity, which (mind or consciousness) continually feeds back to the brain, causing new dynamic processes in the brain, feedback (downward causation) with newly emergent states, and so forth.

Before leaving the developments in mind's history, I have to mention Democritus (460-370 BC), a contemporary of Socrates, whose ideas represent the first formal attempt to create materialism: everything – even the soul – is composed of atoms (indivisible matter). He argued the impossibility of dividing things ad infinitum. According to this materialist view, the origins and character of human consciousness (soul) were atoms: the human soul consists of atoms of fire, made up of these special atoms of a certain variety, which are lively and easily entering the body in our breathing. The small atoms of soul are distributed throughout the body, so that atoms of soul and body alternate: "the soul has two parts; the one, which is rational (logicos) is located in the heart, while the unreasoning part is dispersed throughout the body". So, Democritus can be described not only as a materialist but also a monistic atomist. However, we see the traces of dualism in his mechanistic theory, since he did not neglect the conscious experience.

Materialism (physicalism) refers to the idea that we are completely physical beings; there is no mind separate from brain; the concepts of a soul or mind are only mythical; every event including mental phenomena may be explained by matter and motion. Materialism is the simplest explanation of reality: no psychic or spiritual truths exist independent from the physical world. Philosophical materialism claims that there is only one substance in the universe: physical, empirical or material; everything is matter and energy; consciousness is an emergent property of the physical brain. The existence of a supernatural God is denied, but God is identified with the material universe, as in Pantheism. Materialism originated in ancient Greek philosophy, in China, and India, during the 6th century (BC). Analytical materialism deals with the so-called mind-brain problem: whether or not human consciousness can be explained by scientific laws. In the 1960s and 1970s, it was argued that the brain and mind are the same material things. Reductionist materialism claims that the mind is identical to the brain in all respects; mental states are identical to brain states; mental processes are reducible to physical facts. Functionalism states that mental events are functional states of the brain; environmental stimuli are linked with mental states (interconnected functions), and behavioral responses (output). Behaviorism, eliminative materialism, claims that there is no mind; our vague talk about feelings, thoughts, desires, etc should be eliminated from our vocabulary and replaced with scientific terms referring only to brain states. Property dualism says that there are no mental substances, but there are nonphysical properties of physical matter. Epiphenomenalism is similar to property dualism, and states that mental states are mere nonphysical by-products or effects of neural firings in the brain. These latter philosophies all agree that human consciousness is irreducible to natural processes.

Mind-Brain-Body Triad in Health

From the beginnings of ancient history there is *dance* as an expression of God. Through movement and sound, this created a connection to spirit. Spiritual dancing is a cross-cultural phenomenon. The purpose was to enter the consciousness (mind), or become the spirit of the sun, moon, and/or various animals. Dance was used to promote spiritual and physical health, and vitality. An ancient dance type, trance dance, was a healing vehicle through which people could communicate with their spirit. Today, there are dance/movement therapies, which are the psychotherapeutic processes improving the emotional states, cognition, and the social and physical integration of the individual.

Dance is the esthetic expression of mind in bodily movement. Dance originates in a discrete bodily-kinesthetic "intelligence" (Gardner, 1993); skilled movements is a form of thinking (Bartlett, 1958; Fisher & Bidell, 1998); movement is predominant in all forms of human intellectual activity (Laban, 1975; Laban & Lawrence, 1974). Rhythmic movements in dance inject itself into all cognitive actions including our mind and self-conscious brain. Indeed,

> "self-generated movement is the foundation of thought and willed action, the underlying mechanism by which the physical and psychological coordinates of the self come into being" (Wilson, 1998, p. 291).

The mind/body approach is represented in the scientific literature by yoga, martial arts, and mind/body fitness instruction. Yoga creates a mind/body connection by using awareness of the breath and concentration of the mind. In the mind/body approach, exercises are taken from yoga, tai chi, aikido, and from dance movement therapy, to enhance awareness of breathing, increase ability to breathe, experience the interplay among the physical, mental, and emotional, and spiritual aspects of well-being, feeling powerful, and feeling graceful (Eckstein & Keeling, 1991). Considering breath and mental activity, it was interestingly found that the nonverbal IQ (Cattell's Culture Fair Intelligence Test) increased with tidal volume of the lungs in human subjects (Tan et al., 2003). It was also reported that aerobic dance is beneficial in the therapy of anxiety (Kern & Baker, 1997). In accord, exercise has been reported to have tranquilizing and antidepressant effects on participants (Berger, 1984).

In addition to voluntary active movement as occurred in dance, the gentle rhythmical movements performed with hands on a subject can induce positive and long-term change*s* (*s*ee Blackburn, 2003): The clients, though passive, would become aware of very pleasurable sensations in their bodies, who learnt then to replicate these movements for themselves. This method was proven to be effective not only in healthy subjects, but also in patients with cerebral palsy, post-polio-related paralysis, muscular dystrophy, and Parkinson's disease. This method of manual therapy and movement re-education was called *Psychophysical integration: . "the body must be accompanied by profound shifts in the mind".* In accord, Blackburn (2003) states:

> "There is an underlying assumption that everything that takes place in the body is reflected in the mind and vice versa. We can describe the mind as a continuum of awareness that is distributed throughout the body to the cellular level, physically linked through neural transmitters. Although we often regard the body and mind separate entities, they are one soma or functional unit....The sensations in the body, imparted by the movement, become the medium for reaching or changing the mind of the client (psychophysical integration)".

Dance was recognized as a therapeutic agent first after 1930s (dance therapy or dance/movement therapy). It was used in the treatment of anxiety disorders (Leste & Rust, 1990), Parkinson's disease (Westbrook & McKibben, 1989), addictions (Murray-Lane, 1995; Rose, 1995), multiple personality disorder (Baum, 1995), and learning difficulties

(MacDonald, 1992). Cohen and Walco (1999) reported that even in cancer cases the dance movement/therapy may have beneficial effects on the cognitive, emotional, and social activities.

The above reported studies suggest that "movement" may occupy a central position in cognitive actions. There is an information-processing system relating to movement and cognitive actions, such as planning, reasoning, and emotion (see Leiner et al., 1989). The cerebellum known to be involved only in voluntary and involuntary motor control also plays a major role in thought itself (Leiner et al., 1986); the resulting information-processing system may be essential for the manipulation of kinesthetic mind. In accord, it was posited that thinking is an advanced form of skilled behavior that evolved from earlier forms of flexible adaptation to the environment (see Barlett, 1958). Interestingly enough, it was reported that mental practice alone may improve physical skills (Hinshaw, 1992; Ogles et al., 1994).

Disorders in the fronto-thalamo-cerebellar circuit may cause "cognitive dysmetria" or problems in information processing which may play a role in the origins of schizophrenia and other mental illnesses (see Andreasen et al., 1998). The spinal cord, as a part of the central nervous system should also involved in this network. Namely, in schizophrenia patients, the spinal motor asymmetry disappeared after chlorpromazine treatment (Tan & Gurgen, 1986). The "cerebellar cognitive affective syndrome" is associated with disturbances in language (e.g., agrammatism), personality (e.g., blunted affect), spatial cognition (e.g., deficits in visuospatial memory), and executive functions (e.g., difficulties in planning); cerebellar lesions are linked to disturbed affect, and problems in cognitive processing, especially in posterior lobe lesions (see Seitz, 2000).

> The parallel evolution of the frontal lobe regions (speech?) and hands in hominids suggests motor activity as the basis of human intelligence (see Seitz, 2000).

There are more examples indicating the psychomotor coupling in the human body. For instance, there are cognitive (e.g., dementia and depression) as well as motor deficits in defects of basal ganglia, substantia nigra, locus coeruleus, and raphe nuclei of the brain stem. These symptoms are characteristic for Parkinson's disease exhibiting an increase in inhibitory signals leading to a decrease in cortical excitation and movement (see DeLong, 1990), and for Huntington's disease exhibiting a reduction in inhibitory action leading to an increase in cortical excitation and movement (Middleton & Strick, 1994). Cerebellum is now known to play an important role, along with basal ganglia, in planning, regulation, and attention (Akshoomoff & Courchesne, 1994); the developmental deficits in cerebellum may lead to poor social and cognitive development even in the absence of an hippocampal damage.

The posterior parietal cortex, another motor region, is responsible for creating a frame of reference (*i.e.*, spatial, visual, vestibular) for movement (Willingham, 1998). Ito (1993) suggests that

> "there is no inherent distinction between thought and movement at the level of the brain; both can be controlled by identical neural systems." "Therefore concepts and ideas can be manipulated just as are body parts in motion" (Seitz, 2000).

The same representations are shared among our body maps, spatial maps, the representation of number on a number lime (Dehaene, 1997). In "arithmetic epilepsy", there are rhythmic discharges of the body. The parietal lobes and the intraparietal sulci are involved in finger movements during finger counting and finger calculation, a cross-cultural stage in the learning of numbers by children (Butterwork, 1999). In Gerstmann syndrome, deficits in the left inferior parietal region , is characterized by difficulties in writing, distinguishing left from right, and acalculia: writing, finger movements, and mind share the same neural substrate, a motor-accentuated system. Seitz (2000) concluded that

> "..human consciousness may arise not just from some novel feature of human brains, but way of the body's awareness of itself through its exteroceptive and proprioceptive senses. Indeed, the body structures thought as much as cognition shapes bodily experiences."

It was found using neuroimaging techniques that there are networks of widely separated discrete areas involved in viewing faces, reading words or orienting to sensory even*ts*. *How*ever, the results did not seem to be able to explain the links between cognition, emotion, and behavior in relation to brain mechanisms (see Uttal, 2001). In fact, the real question is whether the function of these cerebral areas can be used in the analysis of mental function.

Contemporary researchers have recently proposed that there are two distinct cognitive systems (Dual-process theory; see Evans, 2003): System 1 describes a form of universal cognition shared between humans and animals (instinctive behaviors controlling specific behaviors); System 2 evolved much more recently than System 1 (volitional) is thought to be uniquely human, and permits abstract thinking not present in System 1. Briefly, the dual-process theories of thinking and reasoning propose the presence of two minds in one brain.

The spinal motor system is also involved in cognitive actions. Paillard (1955) found that the number of motoneurones increased during mental arithmetical calculations: the T-reflex amplitude enhanced, but there was no change in the H-reflex (Hoffmann reflex, a counterpart of the monosynaptic stretch reflex) amplitude. Considering handedness, Davis (1937) reported that arithmetical calculations produced EMG gradients in the right forearm extensor muscles in right-handers. As well known, the paired Hoffmann reflex produced by double shock stimulation of the tibial nerve provides a measure of motoneuronal excitability under a variety of experimental and clinical conditions. It is also a useful tool in examining the neurophysiologic basis of alterations in reflex response in different states of awareness.

Using this technique, Wallace et al. (1984) found that the facilitation period of the paired H-reflex recovery curve may be a useful indicator for the academic achievement. Accordingly, Tan (1991) reported that there is an inverse correlation between the latency of the Hoffman reflex recorded from the thenar muscles of the right and left hands and nonverbal IQ: high IQ was associated with fast motoneurones, and vice versa. Concerning the more peripheral nervous system, Tan (1996) found that the sensory and motor median-nerve conduction velocity was positively linearly correlated with IQ (Cattell's Culture Fair Intelligence Test) in men, and negatively linearly in women. Tan concluded that "..the conduction speed of the input-output channels of brain as an information processing unit may differentially contribute to intelligence, depending upon sex." An eminent 19th century physiologist, Edouard Pfluger (1853) argued that

> "an animal with a transected spinal cord has two separate consciousnesses."

With regard to the `mind-body` relation, Dayi et al. (2002) reported that Cattell IQ (nonverbal) linearly increased with the right- minus left-face width in left-handers, and negatively correlated in right-handed men and women; verbal ability inversely related to right- minus left-face width in right- and left-handed men, but directly correlated in right-handed women; the mental rotation ability positively and linearly correlated with the right-minus left-face width in left-handers and right-handed women. The authors concluded that

> " the structural functional coupling revealed in the present work may have its origins in parallel development of the craniofacial skeleton and brain under the influence of homeobox genes."

Moreover, IQ is closely related to spinal-motor activity, assessed by Hoffmann reflex in humans (Tan, 1989a); IQ also related to hand skill in right- and left-handed subjects (Tan, 1989b,c; Tan 1990).

MIND-BRAIN-BODY TRIAD IN DISEASE

Parkinson's Disease (PD)

PD is a disorder of motor system exhibiting a triad of akinesia, rigidity, and tremor. It is, however, accompanied by non-motor manifestations, such as neuropsychiatric, perceptual, and cognitive deficits. James Parkinson described melancholia in his original report concerning the disorder referred to his Name. Depression is one of the major non-motor symptoms occurring in 4% to 75% of patients with PD (Allain et al., 2000; Ranoux, 2000). The surveys, however, suffer from a number of methodological flaws (see McDonald et al., 2003). Parkinson's disease is characterized by a series of motor system disturbances, such as tremor, rigidity, slowness of movement, and abnormalities of posture. In addition, there are nonmotor symptoms like mood changes, and cognitive deterioration. In many countries including US, approximately half of PD patients had depressive symptoms (see McDonald et al., 2003). "The diagnosis of depression in PD is particularly difficult because,…., the symptoms of PD overlap with the symptoms of depression" (McDonald et al., 2003). Parkinson patients often have psychological disturbances, which include psychomotor slowing, concentration difficulty, depressed mood, and diminished sexual activity. Their facial appearance typically resembles to that in melancholics; apathy, concentration, and memory problems associated with dementia can frequently be described as comorbid depression. Various depression scales were used to assess depression in PD, but there is no scale specific to comorbid depression in PD; the accurate diagnosis of depression in PD is complicated by various factors; the DSM diagnostic criteria for major depression do not adequately describe the PD patients with subsyndromal depression (see McDonald et al., 2003). The prevalence of depression in PD remains controversial.

Motor Neuron Disease (MND)

A motoneuronal disease with mental disorders is *the amyotrophic lateral sclerosis* (ALS), which is simply called as *Motor Neuron Disease,* which actually comprises a series of motor neuron disorders, such as progressive bulbar palsy, amyotrophic lateral sclerosis, spinal muscular atrophies, Kugelberg-Welander syndrome, Duchenne's paralysis, Werdnig-Hoffmann disease, Juvenile spinal muscular atrophy, and infantile spinal muscular atrophy. MNDs may affect the upper (from brain to medulla or spinal cord) and lower motor neurons (from spinal cord to skeletal muscles). As a result of MND/ALS, the skeletal muscles weaken and lose their ability to move; many muscle groups may be affected, including those which control swallowing and breathing as well as muscles in the arms, legs, back, and neck. Generally, the terms MND and ALS are used interchangeably. As early as in 1932, a combination of MND with mental symptoms was reported, and psychic disturbances accompanying ALS were reported in 19th century (see Bak & Hodges, 2001). The most common psychiatric symptoms observed in MND are emotional changes including depression, manic-depressive illness, and emotional irritability, at times culminating in violent and uncontrollable outbursts of rage. Emotional symptoms are often observed with other changes in personality and behavior, ranging from suspiciousness to outright delusions and hallucinations, including psychotic symptoms such as paranoid and catatonic schizophrenia (see Bak & Hodges, 2001). Since the MND frequently occurred with cognitive impairment, it was considered as a multiple system disorder. Barson et al. (2000) found 8% of patients 22% of patients with MND were diagnosed with dementia. Most studies on mental functions in MND concentrated on the dramatic decline seen in MND/dementia complex. The other cognitive functions not related to dementia are also being studied nowadays in MND patients. Interestingly, Abrahams et al. (1997) suggested a link between the presence of the pseudobulbar palsy and the severity of cognitive deficits; the motor component of dementia in MND mostly involves the bulbar and proximal upper limbs, and dementia shows similarities with the frontal variant of frontal-lobe dementia, which also shows motor abnormalities. The cognitive symptoms in MND/dementia almost always precede the motor symptoms; the opposite is quite rare. The reason of this process is unknown. Cooper et al. (1995) found ubiquitin-positive tau-negative intraneuronal inclusions in hippocampus and spinal cord, one of the features of MND/dementia complex.

Ito et al. (2001) reported a motor neuron disease with presenile dementia as well as bilateral degeneration of the pyramidal tract on cranial MRI. Portet et al. (2001) found that 48% of their patients with MND/ALS were cognitively impaired, exhibiting memory impairment, alteration in judgment and reasoning, etc. The authors concluded that there is a continuum between MND/ALS and fronto-temporal lobe dementia. The continuum hypothesis was also supported by Wilson et al. (2001), who reported diffuse intraneuronal Ub inclusions in cortical, hippocampal, and subcortical regions in MND-patients with cognitive impairment.

> Interestingly, the spinal cords of the patients with parkinsonism/dementia complex with or without ALS, or Alzheimer disease contained neurofibrillary tangles, as also found in cortical gray matter of patients exhibiting Alzheimer disease and ALS/dementia complex (Schmidt et al., 2001). Furthermore, the fronto-temporal dementia exhibiting ubiquitinated inclusions in hippocampus and fronto-temporal cortex may involve lateral

corticospinal tracts and spinal motor neurons typical of MND. This is consistent with the hypothesis that the pathological changes of pure MND and MND with dementia form a spectrum, and show that pathological involvement of the motor system may occur in MND-dementia without clinical evidence of MND (Holton et al., 2002).

MND with dementia can also include degeneration of the striatonigral and pallidoluysian systems, in addition to neuronal loss in the upper and lower motoneuronal system and fronto-temporal cortex (Sudo et al., 2002). However, not all the MND cases exhibit dementia.

To understand the relation of MND to cognitive disturbances, more specific and more sensitive neuropsychological test batteries must be used to detect and study the entire disruption of cognitive processes in dementia related to MNDs (Moretti et al., 2001).
In fact, there are accumulations of argyrophilic tau immunoreactive inclusions in neurons of spinal cord, brain stem, and neocortex in tau Tg mice, similar to human taupathies; since the inclusions were most abundant in the spinal motor neurons, the taupathy in these mice resembles ALS/PDC (amyotrophic lateral sclerosis/parkinsonism dementia) wherein tangles are abundant in spinal cord (see Trojanowski et al., 2002).

Both Alzheimer's and Parkinson's diseases could share the same neural substrates, i.e., morphologically homogenous groups of subcortical neurons extending from the midbrain to the top of the spinal cord, including the locus coeruleus and raphe nuclei, as well as the basal forebrain and substantia nigra. Because of the existence of a diffuse projection from brain stem origins to the remote areas of the brain and spinal cord, Woolf (1996) introduced the term "global neurons". This system might be extended to motor neuron disease, which can, like Parkinson's disease, co-exits with Alzheimer-like features (Massman et al., 1996); motor neurons comprise part of the "global cell population". Indeed, the common pathological association for the Alzheimer's and Parkinson's disease is also demonstrated for the motor neurons (Bataille et al., 1998). Accordingly, Greenfield and Vaux (2002) proposed that these three major neurodegenerative disorders can be associated by a common mechanism.

Restless Legs Syndrome (RLS) and Periodic Limb Movement Disorder (PLMD)

RLS (nocturnal myoclonus) is a disorder characterized by disagreeable leg sensations, usually prior to sleep onset, that cause an irresistible urge to move the legs. The cause is not know*n. It is* often accompanied by "creepy-crawly" sensations in the lower legs that make the person uncomfortable unless the legs are moved. Patients with RLS exhibit major depression and those with PLMD exhibit generalized anxiety disorder, according to the results of EEG mappings (Saletu et al., 2002).

Psychiatric Disorders

In *anxiety*, the elevated frontal EMG activity is a common finding (see e.g., Sainsbury and Gibson, 1954; Hazlett et al., 1994). Goldstein (1964) reported that the level effects (anxious versus non-anxious) were significant for the right forearm extensors and right masseter. There were abrupt breaks in frontalis EMG, as in trembling, in association with clinical anxiety (Malmo et al., 1951). Frindlund et al. (1986) investigated the motor irregularities in relation to anxiety. The authors found that the EMG level was higher in high than low-anxiety subjects, and concluded "the greater EMG levels in anxious subjects are due to a greater number of bursts of EMG activity associated with agitated movement."

Malmo and Malmo (2000) reported changes in EMG during *hallucinations* (perceptions in the absence of external stimuli), which are prominent among the core symptoms of schizophrenia. Innouye and Shimizu (1970) recorded EMGs from the speech muscles during verbal hallucinations in nine schizophrenic patients. There were increased EMG levels in most patients during verbal hallucinations. Cerny (1965) reported increased EMG levels in nine of 28 psychotics during hallucinations. McGuigan (1966) was interested in EMG immediately preceded hallucinations. His patient pressed a button upon hearing voices, and consistently showed increased amplitude of the chin EMG immediately before auditory hallucinations. During the same period, i.e., prior to hearing voices, there was whispering that could be heard on the tape. This a common finding reported by others, i.e., tongue and lip movements prior to hearing voices (but nor during hallucinations). Thus, the verbal hallucinations may be processed by neural mechanisms for language, but the muscle contractions generating speech appear to be gated out (see Gandevia 1994). According to Liberman et al (1967), verbal hallucinations depend upon supraspinal neural structures that control movements. There is indeed evidence that the central motor-speech mechanisms may be responsible for verbal hallucinations. In accord, Bick and Kinsbourne (1987) showed that *verbal hallucinations in schizophrenic patients ceased during opening the mouth wide, though other actions not involving speech muscles (e.g., a fist and holding it tight) did not.*

There are more evidence indicating that hallucinations are motoric in origin rather than being sensory. Silbersweig et al. (1995) could not find enhanced regional cerebral blood flow in the primary visual and auditory cortices during auditory verbal hallucinations, but there were enhanced blood flow in the motor regions of the brain. So, the neural mechanisms for hallucinations closely involve the motor system, but these may not be revealed by EMG, since the muscular contractions during speech appear to be gated out during hallucinations.

It was reported that the prevalence of involuntary movements in *schizophrenia* approaches 100% (Quinn et al., 2001), but these patients received prolonged exposure to antipsychotic medication. However, in numerous studies concerning schizophrenia, spontaneous movement abnormalities were reported to occur both in medicated and neuroleptic-free patients (see for a review, Walker, 1994). Cassidy et al. (1998) reported more spontaneous dyskinetic-like movements in individuals with schizotypal personality than subjects with schizoid personality or healthy controls. Recently, Walker et al. (cited in Neumann & Walker, 1999) reported an elevated rate of spontaneous involuntary movements in schizotypal personality disorder, which is seen in some relatives of schizophrenia patients with similar symptoms of schizophrenia. Moreover, Caliguiri and Lohr (1994) reported more manual force instability in neuroleptic-free schizophrenia patients with positive symptom ratings than comparison subjects. Vrtunski et al. (1986) studied response time and fine motor control during a classification task in schizophrenics and nonschizophrenics; the latter responded more quickly and exhibited a smoother and faster motor response on all tasks, compared to schizophrenics. The authors suggested: "the decisions about the abstract referential meaning of words and pictures produce greater cognitive loads in schizophrenics than in nonschizophrenics." Vrtunski et al (1989) also investigated several aspects of fine motor control in schizophrenics, and found that the motor steadiness prior to the button-press was reduced; the motor response was made with excessive force (hyperdynamia), and agonist-antagonist synchrony was impaired (more contralateral motor overflow consequent of increased force in the non-responding hand), suggesting an involuntary movement.

Neumann and Walker (199) concluded that

> "These and related findings suggest that the brain regions that give rise to schizophrenia and spectrum disorders may also play a role in motor regulation. Further, because motor dysfunction is known to precede the clinical onset of schizophrenia by many years (Walker et al., 1994), motor assessments may be promising, along with other indicators (Neumann and Walker, 1996), for identifying individuals at risk."

Accordingly, there are indices for the various syndromes of motor dysfunction. For instance, patients with Parkinson's disease show a pronounced increase in movement time, but not reaction time or involuntary movement (Ebmeir et al., 1992), whereas schizophrenia patients manifest increased reaction time and involuntary movement, but not movement time (Caliguri et al., 1993). Neumann and Walker (1999) studied the changes in an instrumental motor task (manual response forced-choice task) administered to the adult subjects with schizotypal personality disorder, and found that these subjects manifested a motor performance profile similar to that shown by schizophrenia patients, i.e., excessive force and force variability, and increased motor overflow. The findings appeared to be specific for schizotypal personality disorder, especially for the right-hand responses, indicating problems in left-brain functioning, which is frequently reported to be dysfunctional in schizophrenia (see Miller et al., 1995), as is for the schizotypal subjects (Mikhailova et al., 1996; Sailsbury et al., 1996). Interestingly enough,

> the heightened dopamine-receptor activation was reported to induce both movement abnormalities and schizophrenia-spectrum symptoms (see Walker, 1994).

The quintessence of schizophrenia is still puzzling the neuroscientists. However, there are many reports indicating a coupling of this mind disorder with the motor system. One of this, except the above mentioned motor symptoms, there is also a dysfunction of smooth pursuit eye movements accompanying this illness. The dysfunction in smooth pursuit eye movements is one of the co-familial traits, which have higher recurrence rates than schizophrenia itself. This psychomotor event, appearing only if the subject tracks a moving target, occurs in about 40 to 80% of schizophrenic patients and about 25 to 40% of their first degree relatives (see Holzman, 2000). In sum, many studies showed a high prevalence of discrete motor disturbances in schizophrenic patients. In this context, Tigges et al. (2000) studied the neurological soft signs, which are discrete motor and sensory disorders that cannot be linked to special cerebral lesions or dysfunction (see Tigges et al., 2000), in schizophrenic patients. This event was observed as early as in 1919 by Kraepelin in schizophrenics. This is seen more often in schizophrenic patients than in other psychiatric patients or healthy controls, independent from neuroleptic medication (Schroeder et al., 1992; Gupta et al., 1995). Moreover, the neurological soft signs are related to disorders of motor coordination and negative symptoms in schizophrenia (Heinrichs & Buchanan, 1988; Manschreck et al., 1990). Tiggers et al. (2000) found that the regularity of repetitive hand movements was considerably impaired in schizophrenics compared to the healthy controls, especially on the left side, indicating a right-hemisphere dysfunction in this disease. Their results were consistent with the findings of Walker et al. (1994), who found a predominance of motor abnormalities on the left side of the body in schizophrenics. These results indicated that a right-hemispheric brain damage, contrary to a left-hemisphere hypothesis (see Crow, 1990).

Another psychomotor disturbance, the obsessive compulsive disorder was found to be frequently occurred in schizophrenics (23.5%), as reported by Poyurovsky et al. (2001), who defined obsessions as intrusive, unwanted and repeated thoughts, and compulsions as the performance of repetitive goal-directed rituals clinically indistinguishable from schizophrenic mannerism or posturing. Porto et al. (1997) had found a much higher proportion (46%).

> "The meaning and relevance of the increased rates of neuromotoric deviation observed in patients with schizophrenia and their biological relatives remain unclear...Among high-risk offspring, an increased rate of neuromotoric deviation is very clearly associated with increased rates of current mental disorder.." (McNeil et al., 2003).

Deviations in the motor system (*ND: neuromotoric deviation)* was found among patients with schizophrenia, as compared both with normal controls and with psychiatric patients with other disorders (Woods et al., 1986; Heinrichs & Buchanan, 1988; Cantor-Graae et al., 1994; Ismail et al., 1998). However, The clinical and etiological significance of ND is unclear. Interestingly, in this context, there is a significant association between increased ND in schizophrenics and their global severity of illness (Ismail et al., 1998); This condition was also found in the mentally healthy first-degree biological relatives of schizophrenics (Ismail et al., 1998; Kinney et al., 1986; Rossi et al., 1990; Cantor-Graae et al., 1994; Egan et al., 2001).

Is the neuromotor deviation a general characteristic within families with schizophrenia? In other words, would it be an index for the personal risk for mental illness, *vs.* an individual's personal liability for mental illness. Some studies agree with this view: ND would be a sign for personal liability. Namely, an increased ND was observed during childhood in preschizophrenics (Walker & Lewine, 1990; Walker et al., 1994). Chronicity among schizophrenics was better predicted by ND than any other premorbid characteristics (Ricks & Berry, 1970, cited by McNeil et al., 2003). On the other hand, the development of schizophrenia, schizophrenia-spectrum disorders or schizotypal personality could be predicted using ND (see Hans et al., 1999). Neuromotoric items representing "overflow" (e.g., choreatic movements, tremor) were correlated with mental characteristics, such as language disorders and enuresis; an increase in ND was associated with an increase in rates of mental disorders (McNeil et al., 2003).

Depression

This is also a psychomotor disturbance. When depression occurs, movement generally lessens (slowing), or changes to a nonproductive agitation. In general, the psychomotor slowing is the main characteristic of depression. The cause of depression is still obscure. The clinical depression as also known as "depressive disorder" or "major depression" is characterized by loss of pleasure in almost all activities, loss of reactivity, depressed mood, weight loss, and marked psychomotor slowing or agitation among others (see Doris et al., 1999).

The most prominent bodily symptom is weight loss, which was shown to be related to the severity of depression: in patients with major depression, higher body weight is likely to be associated with less reduction in appetite and less pessimistic thoughts; in underweight women, the level of depression is higher than that in other weight categories (Berlin & Lavergne, 2003).

There are pharmacological interventions to treat depression, but there is not an adequate pharmacological therapy; antidepressants are often not beneficial; the patients often stop taking antidepressants generally within three weeks. The exercise therapy is used for several decades, and the literature on this subject is steadily growing. In general, the aerobic exercise was found to be beneficial in the treatment of depression (see e.g., Moore & Blumenthal, 1998; Dimeo et al., 2001; Dunn et al., 2001; Brosse et al., 2002; Neidig et al., 2003).

However, Ernst et al. (1998) performed systematic literature searches about complementary therapies in the treatment of depression, and concluded that scientific data to support the efficacy of complementary therapies is extremely limited. Furthermore, Lawlor and Hopket (2001) stated that *"the effectiveness of exercise in reducing symptoms of depression cannot be determined..."*

Haase and Tan (1965) studied the effects of amphetamine on the spinal motor system in cats. Stimulant drugs such as amphetamines were used in the therapy of depression, and to improve memory, attention, and thinking. Interestingly, Haase and Tan (1965) found that amphetamine increased the alpha- and gamma-motoneuronal activity in decerebrate and/or spinalized cats; the duration and frequency of the tonic alpha motoneurons increased considerably, but only in extensor system. This increase in extensor motoneuronal activity *was accompanied* by a decrease in flexor-motoneuronal activity. Furthermore, Tan and Henatsch (1969) studied the effects of the antidepressive agent imipramine upon the spinal motor system of decerebrate cats. The authors reported that, following imipramin injection, the discharge frequency of the extensor alpha motoneurones increased; the tonically discharging flexor motoneurones ceased firing; there was a regular and strong reduction in the spinal recurrent inhibition and presynaptic inhibition; since the affected systems are normally inhibiting the extensor motoneuronal system more strongly than the flexor motoneuronal system, the net result was a predominant increase in the extensor motor system. The authors suggested that

> "the enhanced motor activity favoring the postural extensor motoricity might be an important basis for the antidepressive actions of imipramine and related substances."

The two latter studies suggest that the psychomotor slowing in depression can be successfully treated if the extensor-system activity is increased, with or without using the pharmacological agents. Exercise increasing the tonic extensor-system activity may be a beneficial method for the treatment of depression, without using any medicine. As mentioned above, there are inconsistencies in the scientific literature concerning the effects of exercise on depression. They did not, however, study the extensor and flexor systems separately. *The above* experiments suggest that exercises especially increasing the extensor-system activity may be beneficial for the treatment of depression.

Psychomotor Theory; The Mind-Brain-Body Triad

Above I have presented some of the basic theories concerning the mind-body relations, and scientifically established facts about the psychomotor interactions. First of all, the above mentioned studies indicated that in psychomotor domain, not the mind-brain duality or unity, but *the mind-brain-body triad as a functional unit is essential in health and disease, since the mental actions (mind) do not end in the (brain), but further controls movements(body).*

The above presented studies suggest that

> "Psychic system is closely coupled with motor system; mental and motor events share the same neural substrate: the motoneuronal system; brain is the liaison between mind and body; This is the quintessence of the "Psychomotor Theory".

Accordingly, the motor and mental systems share the same motoneuronal domain within the central nervous system. Mental events emerge as an active mind from the central motoneuronal system, the output of which can induce movements in the body, and the output of the muscular activity feed-back to the central motoneuronal system, emerging the mind at the same time, consciously or unconsciously. The motor system is the nucleus, which coupled with mind quite tightly, so that any disturbance in this nucleus reflects as a mental disorder in the previously healthy persons. Above, I have presented examples about the mind-brain-body relations in health and disease. Because of the close relation between mental and motor events, the motoneuronal diseases are usually seen with mental disturbances. According to my theory, any pure mental disorder is unconceivable, since the mental events emerge only from the motoneuronal system; there is no independent mind. Therefore, our mind cannot be ill from itself. Therefore, mental disturbances may only originate from motoneuronal disorders; there may be no psychiatric disorder without an accompanying motor neuron disea*se. In* fact, the concepts about the neurological and psychiatric diseases are slowly changing.

Interestingly enough, Parkinson's disease, Alzheimer's disease, and motor neuron disease all share the same motoneuronal systems including the so-called "global neurons" (see Greenfield & Vaux, 2002). Normalizing these global neurons may be enough to treat all the symptoms of the motor neuron diseases. Accordingly, the psychomotor theory may open new strategies for the therapy of psychiatric disorders. For instance, it may be quite possible to treat depression, only increasing the extensor motoneuronal activity, as mentioned above. The motor system may be the key factor in understanding and improving our behavior in health and disease.

> "...an increased rate of neuromotoric deviation is very clearly associated with increased rates of current mental disorder.. (McNeil et al., 2003)."

> "The heightened dopamine-receptor activation was reported to induce both movement abnormalities and schizophrenia-spectrum symptoms (see Walker, 1994)."

> "These and related findings suggest that the brain regions that give rise to schizophrenia and spectrum disorders may also play a role in motor regulation. Further, because motor dysfunction is known to precede the clinical onset of schizophrenia by many years

(Walker et al., 1994), motor assessments may be promising, along with other indicators (Neumann and Walker, 1996), for identifying individuals at risk."

Sperry (1952) stated nearly half a century ago:

"The principal function of the nervous system is the coordinated innervation of the musculature. Its fundamental anatomical plan and working principles are understandable only on these terms (p. 298)… even the highest human cognitive activities, even those requiring no motor output, there are inevitably to be found certain critically essential motoric neural events.

Although Gold & Stoljar (1999) argued "The idea is not of course that neuroscience will explain everything about the mind; perhaps there are aspects of the mind we will never explain", the psychomotor theory will be important, in future, for the understanding and improving the human mind in health and disease.

SUMMARY

In this study I have outlined the grounds of a new theory, to explain the mind-brain-body triad in health and disease. This is the *psychomotor theory*. First, I have briefly analyzed the historical development of the relationship between mind and brain, which is being discussed since more than a few thousand years. The tight junctions between psychological and motor systems were subjected to a detailed analysis using examples in health and disease. The feedback circuits between mind, brain, and body were shown to occur within the mind-brain-body triad, in normal states, and psycho-neural diseases. It was stated that psychiatric signs and symptoms are coupled with motor disturbances; neurological diseases are coupled with psychological disturbances; changes in cortical and spinal motor-system activity may influence mind-brain-body triad, and *vice versa*. Accordingly, a psychomotor theory was created to explain the psychomotor coupling in health and disease, stating that, not the mind-brain duality or unity, but the mind-brain-body triad as a functional unit is essential in health and disease, since mind does not end in the brain, but further controls movements, in a reciprocal manner; mental and motor events share the same neural substrate, cortical and spinal motor neurons; mental events emerging from the motoneuronal system is strongly coupled with the unity of the mind-brain-body triad. So, the psychomotor theory rejects the mind-brain duality, instead, advances the unity of the psychomotor system, which will have important consequences in understanding and improving the human mind, brain, and body in health and disease.

REFERENCES

Abrahams, S., Goldstein, L.H., Al-Chalabi, A., Pickering, A., Morris, R.G., Passingham, R.E., Brooks, D.J., & Leigh, P.N.. (1997). Relation between cognitive dysfunction and Pseudobulbar palsy in amyotrophic lateral sclerosis. *Journal of Neurology, Neurosurgery, and Psychiatry*, 62, 464-472.

Andreasen, N.C., Paradiso, S., & O`Leary, D.S. (1998). "Cognitive dysmetria" as an integrative theory of schizophrenia: A dysfunction in cortical-subcortical-cerebellar circuitry? *Schizophneia Bulletin, 24,* 203-218.

Akshoomoff, N.A., & Courchesne, E. (1994). ERP evidence for a shifting attention deficit in patients with damage to the cerebellum. *Journal of Cognitive Neuroscience, 6,* 388-399.

Alain, H., Schuck, S., & Mauduit, N. (2000). Depression in Parkinson`s disease. *BMJ 320,* 1287-1288.

Bak, T.H., & Hodges, J.R. (2001). Motor neurone disease, dementia and aphasia: coincidence, Co-occurrence or continuum? *Journal of Neurology, 248* 260-270.

Barson, F.P., Kinsella, G.J., Ong, B., & Mathers, S.E. (2000). A neuropsychological investigation of dementia in motor neuron disease (MND). *Journal of the Neurological Sciences, 180,* 107-113.

Bartlett, F.C. (1958). *Thinking: An experimental and social study.* NY: Basic Books.

Bataille, S., Portalier, P., Coulon, P., Ternaux, J.P. (1998). Influence of acetylcholinesterase on embryonic spinal rat motoneurones growth in culture: a quantitative morphometric study. *European Journal of Neuroscience, 10,* 560-572.

Baum, E. (1995). Multiple personality disorder: A group movement therapy approach. In F. Levy (Ed.), *Dance and other expressive art therapies: When words are not enough* (pp. 83-92). New York: Routledge.

Berger, B.G. (1984). Running away from anxiety and depression: a female as well as male race. In: Sachs ML, Buffone G, editors. *Running as therapy: an integrated approach.* Lincoln (NE): Univ. of Nebraska Univ. Press.

Berlin, I., & Lavergne, F. (2003). Relationship between body-mass index and depressive Symptoms in patients with major depression. *European Psychiatry, 18,* 85-88.

Bick, P.A., & Kinsbourne, M. (1987). Auditory hallucinations and subvocal speech in schizophrenic patients. *Am. J. Psychiat., 144,* 222-225.

Blackburn, J. (2003). Trager psychophysical integration – an overview. *Journal of Bodywork and Movement Therapies, 7,* 233-239.

Brosse, A.L., Sheets, E.S., Lett, H.S., & Blumenthal, J.A. (2002). Exercise and the treatment of clinical depression in adults: recent findings and future directions. *Sports Med 32,* 741-760.

Butterwork, B. (1999). A head for figures. *Science, 284,* 928-929.

Caligiuri, M., Lohr, J.B., Panton, D., & Harris, J.M. (1993). Extrapyramidal motor abnormalities associated with late-life psychosis. *Schizophr. Bull., 19,* 747-754.

Caliguiri, M.P., & Lohr, J.B. (1994). A disturbance in the control of muscle force in Neuroleptic-naïve schizophrenic patients. *Biological Psychiatry, 35,* 104-111.

Cantor-Graae, E., McNeil, T.F., Rickler, K.C., Sjostrom, K., Rawlings, R., Higgins, E.S., and Hyde, T.M. (1994). Are neurological abnormalities in well discordant monozygotic co-twins of schizophrenic subjects the result of perinatal trauma? *American Journl of Psychiatry, 151,* 1194-1199.

Cassidy, S.L., Adami, H., Moran, M., Kunkel, R., & Thaker, G.V. (1998). Spontaneous Dyskinesia in subjects with schizophrenia spectrum personality. *American Journal of Psychiatry, 155,* 70-75.

Cerny, M. (1965). On neurophysiological mechanisms in verbal hallucinations: An electrophysiological study. *Activitas Nervosa Superior* (Prague) 7, 197-198.

Cohen, S.O., & Walco, G.A. (1999). Dance/movement therapy for children and adolescents with cancer. *Cancer OPract, 7,* 34-42.

Cooper, P.N., Jackson, M., Lennox, G., Lowe, J., & Mann, D.M. (1995). Tau, ubiquitin, and Alpha B-crystalin immunohistochemistry define the principal causes of degenerative Frontotemporal dementia. *Arch. Neurol., 52,* 1011-1015.

Crow, T.J. (1990). Temporal lobe asymmetries as the key to the etiology of schizophrenia. *Schizophrenia Bulletin,* 16, 433-443.

Davis, R.C. (1937). The relation of certain muscle action potentials to `mental work`.*Science series No.5.* Indiana University Publications, Indiana, pp. 5-29.

Dayi, E., Gungormus, M., & Okuyan, M. (2002). Predictability of hand skill and cognitive abilities from craniofacial width in right- and left-handed men and women: relation of skeletal structure to cerebral function. *International Journal of Neuroscience, 112,* 383-412.

Dehaene, S. (1997). *The number sense: How the mind creates mathematics.* Oxford: Oxford University Press.

DeLong, M.R. (1990). Primate models of movement disorders of basal ganglia origin. *Trends in the Neurosciences, 13,* 281-185.

Dimco, F., Bauer, M., Varahram, I., Proest, G., & Halter, U. (2001). Benefits from aerobic exercise in patients with major depression: a pilot study. *Br J Sports Med 35,* 114-117.

Doris, A., Ebmeier, K., & Shajahan, P. (1999). Depressive illness. *Lancet,* 354, 1369-1375.

Dunn, A.L., Trivedi, M.H., & O`Neal, H.A. (2001). Physical activity dose-response effects on outcomes of depression and anxiety. *Med Sci Sports Exerc 33,* 587-597.

Ebmeir, K.P., Potter, D.D., Cochrane, R.H. (1992). Event-related potentials, reaction time and cognitive performance in idiopathic Parkinson`s disease. *Biological Psychology,* 33, 73-89.

Eckstein, D., & Keeling, G. (1991). Principles of health from eastern disciplines are finding their way into Western workouts: East meets West. *IDEA Today, 10,* 47-50.

Egan, M.F., Hyde, T.M., Bonomo, J.H., Mattay, V.S., Bigelow, L.H., Goldberg, T.E., and Weinberger, D.R. (2001). Relative risk in neurological signs in siblings of patients with schizophrenia. *American Journal of Psychiatry, 158,* 1827-1834.

Ernst, E., Rand, J.I., & Stevinson, C. (1998). Complementary therapies for depression: an overview. *Arch Gen Psychiatry, 55,* 1026-1032.

Evans, J.B.T. (2003). In two minds: dual-process accounts of reasoning. *Trends in Cognitive Sciences, 7,* 454-459.

Fischer, K.W., & Bidell, T.R. (1998). Dynamic development of psychological structures in action and thought. In: Wm. Damon (Ed.), *Handbook of child psychology: Vol.1: Theoretical models of human development* (pp. 467-561). NY: Wiley.

Gandevia, S.C. (1994). Peripheral and central correlates of attempted voluntary movements (pp. 208-209). Commentary on Jeannerod, M. The representing brain: neural correlates of motor intention and imagery. *Behav. Brain Sci. 17,* 187-245.

Gardner, H. (1993). Frames of Mind: *The theory of multiple intelligences.* NY: Basic Books.

Gold, I., & Stoljar, D. (1999). A neuron doctrine in the philosophy of neuroscience. *Behavioral and Brain Science, 22,* 809-869.

Goldstein, I.B. (1964). Physiological responses in anxious women patients. *Arch. Gen. Psychiat. 10,* 382-388.

Greenfield, S., & Vaux, D.J. (2002). Parkinson`s disease, Alzheimer`s disease and motor neurone disease: identifying a common mechanism. *Neuroscience, 113,* 485-492.

Gupta, S., Adreasen, N.C., Arndt, S., Flaum, M., Schultz, S.K., Hubbard, W.C., & Smith, M.(1995). Neurological soft signs in neuroleptic-naïve and neuroleptic treated schizophrenic patients and in normal comparison subjects. *American Journal of Psychiatry, 152,* 191-196.

Haase, J., & Tan, U. (1965). Die excitatorischen Wirkungen von Desoxyephedrine (Pervitin) Auf die tonische spinalmotorik der Katze. *Naunyn-Schmiedeberg`s Arch. Exp. Path. Pharmak., 252,* 20-31.

Hans, S.L., Nuechterlein, K.H., Asarnow, R.F., Styr, B., & Auerbach, J.G. (1999). Neurobehavioral deficits at adoslescence in children at risk for schizophrenia: the Jerusalem infant development study. *Archive of General Psychiatry, 56,* 741-748.

Heinrichs, D.W., & Buchanan, R.W. (1988). Significance and meaning of neurological signs in schizophrenia. *American Journal of Psychiatry, 145,* 11-18.

Hazlett, R.L., McLeod, D.R., & Hoehn-Saric, R. (1994). Muscle tension in generalized anxiety disorder: elevated muscle tonus or agitated movement? *Psychophysiology, 31,* 189-195.

Hebb, D.O. (1980). *Essay on mind.* Hillsdale, N.J.: Lawrence Erlbaum.

Hinshaw, K.E. (1992). The effects of mental practice on motor skills performance: Critical evaluation and meta-analysis. *Imagination, Cognition, and Personality, 11,* 3-25.

Holton, J.L., Revesz, T., Crooks, R., & Scaravilli, F. (2002). Evidence for pathological involvement of the spinal cord in motor neuron disease-inclusion dementia. *Acta Neuropathologia, 103,* 221-227.

Holzman, P.S. (2000). Eye movements and the search for the essence of schizophrenia. *Brain Research Reviews, 31,* 350-356.

Inouye, T., & Shimizu, A. (1970). The electromyographic study of verbal hallucination. *J. Nerv. Ment. Dis., 151,* 415-422.

Ismail, B., Cantor-Graae, E., & McNeil, T.F. (1998). Neurological abnormalities in schizophrenic patients and their siblings. *American Journal of Psychiatry, 155,* 84-89.

Ito, M. (1993). Movement and thought: Identical control mechanisms by the cerebellum. *Trends in the Neurosciences, 16,* 448-450.

Ito, T., Hokezu, Y., Mori, T., Watanabe. O., & Nagamatsu, K. (2001). A case of motor Neuron disease with presenil dementia showing bilateral degeneration of the pyramidal Tract on cranial MRI. *Rinsho Shinkeigaku, 41,* 60-63.

Kern, D., & Baker, J. (1997). A comparison of a mind/body approach versus a conventional approach to aerobic dance. *Women`s Health Issue, 7,* 30-37.

Kinney, D.K., Woods, B.T., & Yurgelun-Todd, D. (1986), Neurologic abnormalities in schizophrenic patients and their families: II. Neurologic and psychiatric findings in relatives. *Arch. Gen. Psychiatry, 43,* 665-668.

Kraepelin, E. (1919). *Dementia Praecox and Paraphenia.* Livingstone, Edinburgh.

Laban, R. (1975). *Modern educational dance (3rd edition).* Boston: Plays, Inc.

Laban, R., & Lawrence, F.C. (1974). *Effort: Economy of human movement (2nd ed.).* Boston: Plays, Inc.

Leiner, H.C., Leiner, A.L., & Dow, R.S. (1986). Does the cerebellum contribute to mental skill? *Behavioral Neuroscience, 100,* 443-454.

Leiner, H.C., Leiner, A.L., & Dow, R.S. (1989). Reappraising the cerebellum: what does the hind brain contribute to the forebrain? *Behavioral Neuroscience, 103*, 998-1008.

Leste, A., & Rust, J. (1990). Effects of dance on anxiety. *American Journal of Dance Therapy, 12,* 19-26.

Liberman, A.M., Cooper, F.S., Shankweiler, D.P., & Studdert-Kennedy, M. (1967). Perception of the speech code. *Psychol. Rev. 74,* 431-461.

MacDonald, J. (1992). Dance? Of course I can! Dance movement therapy for people with learning difficulties. In H. Payne (Ed.), *Dance Movement Therapy: Theory and practice* (pp. 202-217). London: Routledge.

Malmo, R.B., & Malmo, H.P. (2000). On electromyographic (EMG) gradients and movement-related brain activity: significance for motor control, cognitive functions, and certain psychopathologies. *International Journal of Psychophysiology, 38*, 143-207.

Malmo, R.B., Shagass, C., & Davis, J.F. (1951). Electromyographic studies of muscle tension in psychiatric patients under stress. *J. Clin. Exp. Psychopathol. 12*, 45-66.

Manschreck, T.C., Keuthen, N.J., Schneyer, M.L., Celada, M.T., Laughery, J., & Collins, P. (1990). Abnormal involuntary movements and chronic schizophrenic disorders. *Biological Psychiatry, 27*, 150-158.

McDonald, W.M., Richard, I.H., & DeLong, M.R. (2003). Prevalence, etiology, and Treatment of depression in Parkinson`s diseas. *Biological Psychiatry, 54,* 363-375.

McGuigan, F.J. (1966). Covert oral behavior and auditory hallucinations. *Psychophysiology, 3*, 73-80.

McNeil, T.F., Cantor-Graae, E., & Blennov, G. (2003). Mental correlates of neuromotoric deviation in 6-year-olds at heightened risk for schizophrenia. *Schizophrenia Research, 60*, 219-228.

Middleton, F.A., & Strick, P.L. (1994). Anatomical evidence for cerebellar and basal ganglia involvement in higher cognitive function. *Science, 266*, 458-461.

Mikhailova, E.S., Viadimirova, T.V., Iznak, A.F., Tsusulkovskaya, E.J., and Sushko, N.V. (1996). Abnormal recognition of facial expression of emotions in depressed patients with major depression disorder and schzotypal personality disorder. *Biological Psychiatry, 40*, 697-705.

Miller, E.N., Fujioka, T.A.T., Chapman, L., & Chapman, J. (1995). Hemispheric asymmetries of function in patients with major affective disorders. *Journal of Psychiatric Research, 29*, 173-183.

Moore, K.A., & Blumenthal, J.A. (1998). Exercise training as an alternative treatment for depression among older adults. *Altern Ther Health Med 4*, 48-56.

Moretti, R., Torre, P., Antonello, R.M., De Masi, R., & Cazzato, G. (2001). Complex Cognitive disruption in frontal dementia related to motor neuron disease. *Perceptual and Motor Neuron Disease, 92,* 1213-1229.

Murray-Lane, M.B. (1995). Walls of addiction. In F. Levy (Ed.), *Dance and other expressive art therapies: When words are not enough* (pp. 93-100). New York: Routledge.

Neidig, J.L., Smith,B.A., & Brashers, D.F. (2003). Aerobic exercise training for depressive symptom management in adults living with HIV infection. *J Assoc Nurses AIDS Care, 14*, 30-40.

Neumann, C.S., & Walker, E.F. (1999). Motor dysfunction in schizotypal personality disorder. *Schizophrenia Research, 38*, 159-168.

Ogles, B.M., Lynn, S.J., Masters, K.S., Hoefel, T.D., & Marsden, K. (1994). Runner`s cognitive strategies and motivations: Absorption, fantasy style, and dissociative experiences. *Imagination, Cognition, and Personality, 13*, 163-174.

Paillard, J. (1955). *Reflexes et regulations d`origine proprioceptive chez l`homme*. Libraire Arnette, Paris, p. 293.

Portet, F., Cadilhac, C., Touchon, J., & Camu, W. (2001). Cognitive impairment in motor Neuron disease with bulbar onset. Amyotroph Lateral Scler *Other Motor Neuron Disord.* , *2*, 23-29.

Porto, L., Bermanzohn, P.C., Pollack, S., Morissey, R., & Siris, S.G. (1997). A profile of obsessive-compulsive symptoms in schizophrenia. *CNS Spectrums, 2,* 21-25.

A profile of obsessive-compulsive symptoms in schizophrenia. *CNS Spectrums, 2,* 21-25.

Poyurovsky, M., Hramenkov, S., Isakov, V., Rauchverger, B., Modai, I., Schneidman, M., Fuchs, C., & Weizman, A. (2001). Obsessive-compulsive disorder in hospitalized patients with chronic schizophrenia. *Psychiatry Research, 102*, 49-57.

Ranoux, D. (2000). Depression et maladie de Parkinson. *Encephale, 26*, 22-26.

Rossi, A., Cataldo, S., Di Michele, V., Manna, V., Ceccoli, S., Stratta, A., & Casachia, M. (1990). Neurological soft signs in schizophrenia. *Br. J. Psychiatry, 157*, 735-739.

Quinn, J., Meagher, D., Murphy, P., Kinsella, A., Mullaney, J., & Waddington, J.L.(2001). Vulnerability to involuntary movements over a life time trajectory of schizophrenia approaches 100%, in association with excessive (frontal) dysfunction. *Schizophrenia Research, 49*, 79-87.

Rose, S. (1995). Movement as metaphor: Treating chemical addiction. In F. Levy (Ed.), *Dance and other expressive art therapies: When words are not enough* (pp. 101-108). New York: Routledge.

Sailsbury, D.F., Voglmaier. M.M., Seidman, L.J., & MacCarley, R.W. (1996). Topographical abnormalities of P3 in schizotypal personality disorder. *Biological Psychiatry, 40*, 165-172.

Sainbury, P., & Gibson, J.G. (1954). Symptoms of anxiety and tension and the accompanying physiological changes in the muscular system. J. *Neurol. Neurosurg. Psychiatr. 17*, 216-224.

Saletu, B., Anderer, P., Saletu, M., Hauer, C., Lindeck-Pozza, L., & Saletu-Zyhlarz, G. (2002). EEG mapping, psychometric, and polysomnographic studies in restless leg syndrome (RLS) and periodic limb movement disorder (PLMD) patients as compared with normal subjects. *Sleep Medicine, 3,* S35-S42.

Schmidt, M.L., Zhukareva, V., Perl, D.P., Sheridan, S.K., Schuck, T., Lee, V., and Trojanowski, J.Q. Spinal cord neurofibrillary pathology in Alzheimer disease and Guam Parkinsonism-dementia complex. *J Neuropathol Exp Neurol 60*, 1075-1086.

Schroeder, J., Niethammer, R., Geider, F.J., Reitz, C., Binkert, M., Jauss, M., & Sauer, H. (1992). Neurological soft signs in schizophrenia. *Schizophrenia Research, 6,* 25-30.

Seitz, J.A. (2000). The bodily basis of thought. *New Ideas in Psychology, 18*, 23-40.

Silbersweig, D.A., Stern, E., Frith, C. et al. (1995). A functional neuroanatomy of Hallucinations in schizophrenia. *Nature, 378*, 176-179.

Sperry, R.W. (1952). Neurology and the mind-brain problem. *Am. Sci. 40,* 291-312.

Sudo, S., Fukutani, Y., Matsubara, R., Sasaki, K., Shiozawa, M., Wada, Y., Naiki, H., and Isaki, K. (2002). Motor neuron disease with dementia combined with degeneration of striatonigral and pallidoluysian system. *Acta Neuropathologia, 103,* 521-525.

Tan, U. (1989a). The Hoffmann reflex from the flexor pollicis longus of the thumb in left-handed subjects: spinal motor asymmetry and supraspinal facilitation to Cattell`s intelligence test. *Internatiopnal Journal of Neuroscience, 48,* 255-269.

Tan, U. (1989b). Right and left hand skill in left-handers: distribution, learning, and relation to nonverbal intelligence. *International Journal of Neuroscience, 44*, 235-249.

Tan, U. (1989c). Manual proficiency in Cattell`s Intelligence Test in left-handed male and female subjects. *International Journal of Neuroscience, 44*, 17-26.

Tan, U. (1990). Relation of hand skill to spatial reasoning in male and female left-handers with left- and right-hand writing. *International Journal of Neuroscience, 53*, 121-133.

Tan, U. (1991). The inverse relationship between nonverbal intelligence and the latency of the Hoffmann reflex from the right and left thenar muscles in right- and left-handed subjects. *International Journal of Neuroscience, 57,* 219-238.

Tan, U. (1996). Correlations between nonverbal intelligence and peripheral nerve conduction velocity in right-handed subjects: sex-related differences. *International Journal of Psychophysiology, 22,* 123-128.

Tan, U., & Gurgen, F. (1986). Modulation of spinal motor asymmetry by neuroleptic medication of schizophrenia patients. *International Journal of Neuroscience, 30,* 165-172.

Tan, U., & Henatsch, H.D. (1969). Wirkungen von imipramin auf die spinalmotorischen Extensor- und flexor-systeme der Katze. *Naunyn-Schmiedebergs Arch. Pharmak. Exp. Path., 262,* 337-357.

Tan, U., Okuyan, M., Albayrak, T., Akgun, A. (2003). Sex difference in verbal and spatial ability reconsidered in relation to body size, lung volume, and sex hormones. *Perceptual and Motor Skills, 96*, 1347-1360.

Trojanowski, J.Q., Ishihara, T., Higuchi, M., Yoshiyama, Y., Hong, M., Zhang. B., Forman, M.S., Zhukareva, V., & Lee, V.M.Y. (2002). Amyotrophic lateral sclerosis/ parkinsonism dementia complex: transgenic mice provide insights into mechanisms underlying a common taupathy in an ethnic minority on Guam. Experimental *Neurology, 176*, 1-11.

Uttal, W.R. (2001). *The New Phrenology,*Bradford Books, MIT Press.

Vrtunski, P.B., Simpson, D.M., Weiss, K.M., & Davis, G.C. (1986). Abnormalities of fine motor control in schizophrenia. *Psychiatry Research, 18*, 275-284.

Vrtunski, P.B., Simpson, D.M., & Meltzer, H.Y. (1989). Voluntary movement dysfunction in schizophrenics. *Biological Psychiatry, 25*, 529-539.

Walker, E. (1994). The developmentally moderated expression of the neuropathology underlying schizophrenia. *Schizophr. Bull. 20*, 453-480.

Walker, E.F., & Lewine, R.J. (1990). Prediction of adult-onset schizophrenia from childhood home-movies of the patients. *American Journal of Psychiatry, 147*, 1052-1056.

Walker, E.F., Savoie, T., & Davis, D. (1994). Neuromotor precursors of schizophrenia. *Schizophrenia Bulletin, 20*, 441-455.

Wallace, R.K., Orme-Johnson, D.W., Mills, P.J., & Dillbeck, M.C. (1984). Academic achievement and the paired Hoffman reflex in students practicing meditation. *International Journal of Neuroscience, 24*, 261-266.

Westbrook, B.K., & McKibben, H. (1989). Dance/movement therapy with groups of outpatients with Parkinson`s disease. *American Journal of Dance Therapy,* 11, 27-38.

Willingham, D.B. (1998). A neuropsychological theory of motor skill learning. *Psychological Review, 105*, 558-584.

Wilson, E.O. (1998). *The hand: How its use shapes the brain, language, and human culture.* NY: Random House.

Wilson, C.M., Brace, G.M., Munoz, D.G., He, B.P., & Strong, M.J. (2001). Cognitive impairment in sporadic ALS: a pathologic continuum underlying a multisystem disorder. *Neurology, 28*, 651-657.

Woods, B.T., Kinney, D.K., & Yurgelun-Todd, D. (1986). Neurologic abnormalities in schizophrenic patients and their families: 1. Comparison of schizophrenic, bipolar, and substance abuse patients and normal controls. *Arch. Gen. Psychiatry, 43*, 657-663.

Woolf, N.J. (1996). Global and serial neurons from a hierarchically arranged interface proposed to underlie memory and cognition. *Neuroscience, 74*, 625-651.

In: Depression and Dementia
Editor: Suptendra Nath Sarbadhikari, p. 55-83
ISBN 1-59454-114-0

Chapter 3

DEPRESSION, DEMENTIA AND DEXTERITY: IN QUEST OF A DENOMINATOR

Suptendra Nath Sarbadhikari
Associate Professor of Biomedical Engineering
Amrita Institute of Technology, Ettimadai, Coimbatore-641105, India
AND
Amrita Institute of Medical Sciences and Research Centre, Kochi-682026, India
Email: supten@amrita.edu , drsupten@yahoo.com

ABSTRACT

The cognitive organization of the human brain can be ascertained by electrophysiologic measures like EEG (electroencephalogram) and psychometric tests. Human cognition undergoes change with age as well as with various neuropsychiatric conditions. In younger age groups, the problem of dyslexia (reading and writing disability), in adolescents the problem of epilepsy, and in adults and geriatric people depression and/or dementia (e.g., Alzheimer's disease and Parkinsonism) are found in abundance. In this chapter the authors shall focus only on depression and dementia.

INTRODUCTION

Depression is not a homogeneous disorder. However, minor depression may be expressed as dysthymia (F34.1 of ICD-10 or 300.40 of DSM-IV), which is defined by: (A) depressed mood (or can be irritable mood in children and adolescents) for most of the day, more days than not, as indicated either by subjective account or observed by others, for at least two years (one year for children and adolescents); and, (B) presence, while depressed, of at least two: 1. poor appetite or over eating, 2. insomnia or hypersomnia, 3. low energy or fatigue, 4. low self esteem, 5. poor concentration or difficulty in making decision, 6. feelings of hopelessness.

Similarly, dementia can have varied etiology and may be defined as: (A) demonstrable evidence of impaired short- and long-term memory; (B) At least one of the following: 1. impairment in abstract thinking, 2. impaired judgment, 3. other disturbances of higher cortical functions like aphasia, apraxia, agnosia and "constructional difficulties", 4. personality change; (C) disturbance in A and B significantly interferes with work or usual social activities or relationships with others; (D) not occurring exclusively during the course of delirium; (E) either (1) or (2): 1. evidence from history, physical examination and laboratory tests of specific organic factor(s) judged to be etiologically related to the disturbance and 2. in the absence of such evidence, an etiologic organic factor can be presumed if the disturbance cannot be accounted for by any nonorganic mental disorder like Major depression accounting for cognitive impairment.

By dexterity, I am alluding to Cerebral or Hemispheric Lateralization (Handedness / Footedness / Sidedness). Laterality is the term used to describe ways in which the two hemispheres of the brain differ from each other in both anatomy and function. The rise in interest in hemispheric laterality really dates back to days of the earliest functional neuroanatomical research in the late 1800's. The classic view of laterality involved the theory that the left hemisphere is the dominant hemisphere for higher order or complex cognitive functions including the control of all language processing. In accordance with this classic view the right hemisphere is more "animal" like and controls more basic sensory-related functions [Walker 1980]. In contrast, the more contemporary view is that neither hemisphere is "dominant". Both play an important role in most complex cognitive tasks. Present theories are based on the idea that the two hemispheres seem to prefer a different processing styles. The division of labor between the two hemispheres is supposed to be increasing efficiency and enabling the brain to specialize on specific tasks. Left hemisphere (LH) is sequential, analytic and time dependent regardless of stimuli (speech, music, visual stimuli); and involved in verbal, analytic processing. Right hemisphere (RH) is synthetic, and forms holistic overall patterns in nonverbal and synthetic processing.

LH is also known as "categorical" while RH is called "representational". Further, Laterality is believed to be relative, not absolute. Cerebral side is not the most important anatomical characteristic, but just one of the important functional neuroanatomical characteristics. Many factors (including gender, genetics or 'nature' and environment or 'nurture') alter the more "normal" patterns of laterality. Many nonhuman animals also show cerebral laterality. One very obvious way to compare the hemispheres is to look at their anatomical asymmetries [Mandal *et al* 1996]. Many differences in structure size and other basic physiological differences have been found out, like, Frontal lobe is slightly longer and wider on the right, Occipital lobe is slightly larger (longer and wider) on the left and Parietal, spatial processing areas are larger on the right. Similarly, Planum temporale (part of the primary auditory cortex) is much larger in the left because of the asymmetrical location of the Sylvian fissure. Cytoarchitectonic asymmetries are found in the distribution of the gray versus white matter Even, Neurochemically, there is more dopamine in the left globus pallidus and more norepinephrine in the right thalamus. In all probability, the distributions for the various receptor subtypes are different, in diverse areas of the brain, for each neurotransmitter.

In the subsequent sections we shall elaborate more on the concepts of lateralization, relations between depression and lateralization, roles of lateralization in dementia, and finally try to ascertain some common features balancing the brain dynamics in various conditions of cognition and its impairment.

HEMISPHERIC LATERALIZATION

The brain asymmetry understood as an anatomical, functional or biochemical difference between both cerebral hemispheres is a phenomenon extensively studied, essentially from an anatomical and functional perspective. The molecules and physical particles of which living cells are constructed are themselves asymmetrical. In addition, asymmetry is characteristic of many single-celled organisms and of individual cells in more complex organisms. These observations among others, have led to the realization that despite its inherent beauty, bilateral symmetry is no more fundamental a property of biological systems than is bilateral asymmetry. In fact, growing evidence support the idea that the brain is intrinsically asymmetric, and that virtually all brain functions are organized, in more or less degree, in an asymmetrical fashion. In addition, it could be speculated that imbalances in established brain asymmetry (toward symmetry or toward increasing asymmetry, through nonlinear dynamics, as described by both Jelic and Jeong, in two chapters of this book) might lead to neuropathological deviations of brain functions. This asymmetrical organization is the result of evolutionary adaptation and evidences of brain asymmetries have been found not only in our ancestors but also in all stages of the brain evolution.

The intercellular communication is a necessary function of every pluricellular organism, which is mediated essentially by chemical messengers. Neuropeptides are a relatively recent class of neurotransmitters involved in a large variety of brain functions. After their release from neurones, neuropeptides are substrates rapidly inactivated or biotransformated by neuropeptide-degrading enzymes (neuropeptidases); therefore their study reflects the function of their substrates. The neurochemical basis underlying anatomical and/or functional asymmetries in the brain are not well understood, but some findings imply the existence of neurotransmitters or neuromodulators with a lateralized function. Researchers have investigated several brain asymmetries in neuropeptidase activities and postulated that this distribution may reflect putative lateralized functions of their susceptible endogenous substrates. The modes of action of the neurotransmitters also seem to be mostly nonlinear [Sarbadhikari 2004].

Electrophysiological and Behavioral Findings

Electroencephalograms (EEGs) reflect the electrical activity of the brain. Even when they are analyzed from healthy individuals, they manifest chaos in the nervous system [Sarbadhikari and Chakrabarty 2001]. EEGs are likely to be produced by a nonlinear system. The basis for this conjecture is that a nonlinear system with at least 3 degrees of freedom (or state variables) may exhibit chaotic behavior. As an example of chaotic activity, the waxing and waning of α-EEG activity in alert subjects may be considered. Albeit α-EEG activity closely resembles a sine wave, it is (i) certainly not periodic (*i.e.*, does not repeat itself after a period T), (ii) is bounded (*i.e.* amplitudes are generally confined up to 100 μV) and (iii) is too regular to qualify as a noise. Therefore, it is more likely to be chaotic.

The domain of EEG, with all of its related fields, covers clinical medicine, psychophysiology, neurophysiology, general electrophysiology and certain areas of basic EEG research. Now there seems to be a gap between the "classical EEG" and the "sophisticated, modern, 21st century oriented EEG". But, classical EEG has not become obsolete as long as this clinical method is carried out with proper technique, a good training background and some ingenuity. Evoked potentials (EP) or event-related potentials in EEG (ERPs, described in details by Idiman in his Chapter) changes are now seen in a broad view that practically integrates EEG and EP approaches. In the highest degrees of sophistication, these methods are now playing a major role in neurocognitive research – though in hot competition with fMRI (functional magnetic resonance imaging) and PET (positron emission tomography) scanning. It is now fair to state that the psychophysiologic orientation of Hans Berger (founder of human EEG) has successfully been revived and promises a better comprehension of neurocognitive functions. The general hemispheric differences in EEG are reviewed by Sarbadhikari and Chakrabarty [2001]. The specific changes in depression and dementia are described in Sections 3 and 4 of this chapter.

Behavioral tests are also known as psychometric tests. They may be defined as reading information from an object about events involving the person who owns it, usually by handling it or the art of measuring duration of mental processes or determining time relations of mental phenomena.

Hans Eysenck had proposed that the structural model of psychology has 3 dimensions which he called Extraversion, Neuroticism and Psychoticism, ***ENP*** for short. This was based on his 50 years of computerized psychometry work. Psychometry is the mathematical analysis of the correlations that appear in psychology tests such as the Weschler and Stanford-Binet IQ tests or the Minnesota Multiphasic Personality Inventory (MMPI). Raymond B. Cattell's psychometry work also supported this conclusion. The problem was that no one could explain why the personality structure should be 3 dimensional. Then Hammond [1994] pointed out that the human brain is actually cleaved by 3 orthogonal planes. Each of these cleavages causes one of the dimensions ENP. The "Sperrian Lateralization" causes Eysenck's ***N*** dimension. The ***E*** dimension is caused by the motor-sensory division across the Central Fissure.

It turns out that the 3-axis cleavage of the brain is not accidental. The entire human body has a 3-axis cleavage structure. The Medial, Lateral, and Transverse septa cleave the entire body 3 ways (the sagittal plane divides our body into left and right, frontal or coronal plane divides the body into anterior and posterior halves, while the horizontal plane divides us into upper and lower regions). The three cleavages of the brain are just a continuation of this. The body seems to be cleaved in three directions since space itself is 3-dimensional orthogonal. Because the body is a machine, it has to have 3-orthogonal degrees of freedom, and this is the origin of the 3-axis cleavage. Therefore, the effects of various factors on our body vary according to these planes.

The defining features of human lateralization are taken to be right-handedness, as a skewed but continuous distribution of preferences, and a greater involvement of the left hemisphere in species-specific vocalization, with right-hemisphere superiority in spatial perception and emotionality less well-marked characteristics [Walker 1980].

Various behavioral tests [Mandal *et al* 2000] confirm the presence of handedness, footedness and sidedness as pure left, pure right and mixed or clumsy. It is the last group that is prone to accidents much more than either pure right sided or left sided persons.

Gender Differences

Another interesting feature is the sex-difference of cerebral asymmetries in humans. Many lateralization studies demonstrate that males have more pronounced functional left-right differences than females. A significant part of these sex-effects could be explained by variations of steroids during the menstrual cycle that probably alter interhemispheric communication via the corpus callosum. Cognitive processes change in correlation with these hormonal alterations. These results show that human cerebral asymmetries are not completely determined by static neuromorphological wiring principles, but also have a 'dynamic' component.

Hampson and Moffat [1994] found that even when the salivary testosterone concentrations fall within the normal physiological range in both males and females, non-right handers of both sexes have significantly lower average testosterone concentrations than do right handers. In their sample, left handers or ambidextrous individuals tended to have lower, rather than higher, testosterone concentrations. However, this does suggest that some relationship between testosterone and hand preference may in fact be present, and it will be important to work out the mechanisms that account for the difference in free testosterone, as these may eventually shed light on the ontogeny or correlates of hand preference. It has also been found that due to lesion effects, women are more likely to have bilateral language representation, while, men are more likely to have "anterioralized" language representation. However, genuine 'ambidexters' are indeed very rare. Usually these people are mixed or 'clumsy' handed / sided.

Schizophrenia, a heterogeneous psychiatric abnormality, with substantial cognitive impairment, is expressed differently in men and women with respect to the age at onset, symptom expression, course of illness, and outcomes. The sex differences may have etiologic implications, as demonstrated by recent studies showing a small but significantly higher incidence of schizophrenia among men compared with women when stringent classification criteria are applied [Goldstein and Lewine 2000]. Brain abnormalities and the genetics of schizophrenia are also influenced by sex. Briefly, women show a superior premorbid adjustment, relative to men: their symptoms begin later in life, and outcome is usually superior (at least in the first 15 years after onset). They also show a second paramenopausal peak onset not seen in men.

Mood symptoms such as depression are more common in women, whereas apathy, flat affect, paucity of speech, and social isolation are more often seen in men, although this difference in symptoms is not always seen. Also, more brain structure impairment has been reported in men. Premenopausal women may respond at lower antipsychotic dosages than do men. Although the etiology of the sex differences is not entirely understood, hormone-gene interactions probably account for part of the variance.

Recent studies [Kulkarni 2001a,b] on the gender differences in the quality of life of people with schizophrenia have shown that women are more likely to present with affective symptoms as part of their psychosis presentation. Other differences include the finding that women have fewer negative symptoms (*i.e.*, anhedonia, apathy, alogia, and amotivational states) compared with men. This finding was also replicated in studies of first-episode psychosis patients. In many patients with established schizophrenia, the Global Assessment of Function (GAF) scores were significantly better in women, although overall they were only in the mild to moderate range of function. The gender difference in GAF scores may in fact reflect a difference in the premorbid functioning of patients, which may in turn be a product of the age difference. These data suggest that current treatment strategies are targeting key illness symptoms, but psychosocial rehabilitation measures to improve the patient's quality of life are either not being implemented or else are not effective. The cost of managing patients with schizophrenia showed that women were significantly more expensive to treat than men. This was mainly thought to be due to women receiving attention later than men, therefore being sicker and requiring longer inpatient stays. To study the relevance of gender on social functioning in schizophrenia, a sample of 200 schizophrenic (DSM-IV criteria) out-patients were followed-up [Usall *et al* 2002] during 2 years and were administered the following instruments: Positive and Negative Symptom Scale (PANSS), Disability Assessment Scale (DAS-sv), and GAF Scale. A regression model was created with DAS and GAF as dependent variables, and gender, PANSS, age of onset, duration of illness and marital status as independent variables. Separate regression models were then generated for females and males. It was observed that gender influenced significantly on DAS and GAF, with men showing worse functioning. In gender specific analyses, they found a significant influence of illness duration and Positive and Negative PANSS on social functioning in men, and of age at onset and Negative PANSS in women. In other words, gender had a significant influence on social functioning in schizophrenia, even after adjusting for the other independent variables.

A key hypothesis put forward to explain the earlier age at onset of schizophrenia by 5-10 years in men compared with women is the "estrogen protection hypothesis" [Castle *et al* 2000]. Broadly, this hypothesis proposes that women are protected against the early onset of severe schizophrenia by estrogen. Furthermore, researchers have suggested that women are vulnerable to relapses of established illness or their first-ever episode of schizophrenia in the perimenopausal period, when estrogen production diminishes. The hypothesis also encompasses early estrogen effects on the developing brain such that a structural effect of estrogen acting on brain maturation causes the delay of first-onset schizophrenia in females by raising the vulnerability threshold for schizophrenia. Following puberty, this putative structural effect is reinforced by a functional effect. Fading estrogen secretion around menopause causes women predisposed for schizophrenia, but who until then have been protected by estrogen, to fall ill with late-onset schizophrenia. The estrogen protection hypothesis rests on 3 main lines of work: epidemiologic studies, basic science studies using animal models, and clinical studies [Grigoriadis and Seeman 2002].

Epidemiologic data [Hafner *et al* 1998] reinforce the later age at onset of early schizophrenia in women and another peak of onset in women aged 50 years and older. Early animal studies showed that estradiol downregulated dopamine neurotransmission, while more recent studies [Fink 2001] have shown that estrogen induces a significant increase in serotonin receptors. In this way, the actions of estrogen on the serotonin receptor (5-HT_{2A}) and the dopamine receptor (D_2) mimic the actions of the new antipsychotic drugs, such as risperidone and olanzapine.

Clinical studies showed that the symptoms of schizophrenia varied with the menstrual cycle phase in 32 acutely unwell women. Riecher-Rössler [2001] found a significant excess of admissions to hospital during the premenstrual (*i.e.*, low-estrogen phase) compared with the high-estrogen phase. Grigoriadis and Seeman [2002] reported that neuroleptic dose requirements in psychotic women rise as they approach menopause. They attributed an increased vulnerability to psychosis in the postmenopausal period to the fall in circulating estrogen levels. Therefore, the 'female' hormone Estrogen is seen to exert some beneficial effect in schizophrenia through these four putative mechanisms: (i) blocking dopamine receptors, (ii) inhibiting cytokines, (iii) enhancing neuronal connections through NMDA, (iv) facilitating the action of serotonin.

Drug treatment available for women with schizophrenia includes a wide range of atypical and typical antipsychotic medications. Kinon [2001], presented data on hyperprolactinemia caused by antipsychotic drugs and the impact of high prolactin levels on the hypothalamic-pituitary-gonadal (HPG) axis. The study reported a decrease in the sex hormones that was significantly and inversely correlated with prolactin levels. Sex hormones play a major role through their effects on central brain neurotransmitters and may be an important key to the etiology of schizophrenia. The recognition of such hormonal influences during monthly cycles or at key lifetime hormonal events such as menopause in women may also lead to more effective treatments such as preventive ERT. Addition of estrogen to antipsychotic drug treatment may improve psychotic symptoms as well as assist with the management of hyperprolactinemia caused by some antipsychotic drugs.

Antipsychotic drugs are currently prescribed in standard doses, although women generally weigh much less than men and should be prescribed lower doses. Tailoring the dose of medication for weight and hormone effects would result in fewer side effects, better treatment adherence, and therefore better outcome in the longer term. Also, many women present with coexisting symptoms of depression or mania and psychosis. Hence, a tailored combination of antipsychotic drug plus mood-stabilizer may achieve better results for women with schizophrenia [McGorry 2001].

For dementia also, there appears to be some role of sex hormones. One such study [Ouyang *et al* 2001] has determined that estrogen receptor alpha subtype (ER alpha) genetic polymorphisms may affect the expression of ER alpha, and are associated with Alzheimer's disease.

Often depression and obesity coexist. Gustafson *et al* [2003] have also found a correlation between obesity and AD in women. They measured body-mass index (BMI) - the ratio of weight to height. Normal subjects score between 18.5 and 25. Elderly, demented women had an average BMI of 28, which borders on the obese. Each additional point raised the risk of Alzheimer's disease by 36%, the team found. Dementia affects 18 million people worldwide, and there is no cure. The chances of succumbing to Alzheimer's disease, the most common form of dementia, rise rapidly with age. Genetics also plays a part - those with an altered version of a key gene are 16 times more likely to develop the disease. Obesity is one of the few risk factors that you can do something about. Dietary factors may play a key role in preventing dementia, like some micronutrients may be related to Alzheimer's – a lower intake of vitamin E is linked to a higher risk of the disease. People should eat plenty of foods that provide vitamin E, such as vegetable oils and nuts. Morris *et al* [2002, 2003] also believe that dietary factors have some role in AD. Antioxidants like vitamins C and E (acting against ROS – Reactive Oxygen Species or 'aging factors'), and ω-3 fatty acids (commonly found in sea fish, making the Eskimos almost immune to cardiovascular disorders) have some preventive role in AD. Gustafson's study supports the idea that atherosclerosis, coronary heart disease and diabetes mellitus may contribute to Alzheimer's disease. Obesity raises the risk of developing these vascular disorders, and so may also contribute to the dementia process. Gustafson's team also monitored their subjects for signs of increased blood pressure and cardiovascular disease. They reckon that they have teased apart these factors, allowing them to focus on obesity alone. The significant link between large body size and dementia was found only in women as there were far fewer men in the study.

In men a decrease in dietary fat content and an increase in the degree of unsaturation of fatty acids reduce the serum concentrations of androstenedione, testosterone and free testosterone [Hamalainen *et al* 1984]. Further studies may be designed to find the effects of dietary factors affecting disorders of brain function, through lateralization.

In a study by Pennington *et al* [1985], six early treated children with phenylketonuria (PKU) were compared on the Halstead Neuropsychological Battery for Older Children with three groups of children with documented neurological disorders involving predominantly the left, the right, or bilateral dysfunction. The children with PKU had an overall level of neuropsychological impairment similar to that of the brain-damaged groups. The PKU group did not show a consistent pattern of lateralization, but there was some specificity to their deficits. The analyses showed that they were most similar to the right-hemisphere group. The children with PKU tended to show deficits consistently in two neuropsychological domains, conceptual and visuospatial skills, which would help explain their reported difficulty with mathematics. Further work is needed to test these results in a larger sample and to examine possible relationships with dietary compliance.

Children with early treated phenylketonuria (ETPKU), a disorder associated with developmental dopamine depletion, were tested [Craft *et al* 1992] with a visual orienting paradigm to determine the existence of lateralized deficits in specific attentional operations. Male ETPKU subjects showed a right visual field impairment in disengaging attention, indicating left hemisphere dysfunction, and overall slowed reaction times. Female ETPKU and normal subjects did not differ. The results suggest that for males, dopamine depletion disrupts left hemisphere function. This finding has important implications for disorders with suspected developmental dopamine abnormalities, and may also illustrate how sex differences in functional lateralization develop in the normal brain.

The purpose of the study by Bortolozzi *et al* [2003] was to determine whether the regional brain biogenic amine levels in adult rats were altered by pre- and post-natal exposure to 2,4-dichlorophenoxyacetic acid (2,4-D). Pregnant rats were daily orally exposed to 70 mg/kg per day of 2,4-D from gestation day (GD) 16 to post-partum day (PPD) 23. After weaning, the pups were assigned to one of two subgroups: T1 fed with untreated diet up to post-natal day (PND) 90 and T2 (maintained with 2,4-D diet up to PND 90). In addition, they wanted to know the effect of 2,4-D on lateralization in the monoamine systems of the basal ganglia of these adult rats and whether there was any correlation with the behavioral developmental pattern previously reported by them. In this study the content of noradrenaline (NA) was significantly increased in substantia nigra (SN) while it decreased in cerebellum in male and female rats of T2 group. The decreased dopamine (DA), 3,4-dihydroxyphenylacetic acid (DOPAC) and homovallinic acid (HVA) contents in cerebellum, midbrain, ventral tegmental area (VTA) and prefrontal cortex (PFc) showed an alteration in the mesocorticolimbic system. However, an increase of DA in SN and of DOPAC and HVA in nucleus accumbens (NAc) in both sexes and of DA and DOPAC (only in females) in striatum was detected. The contents of serotonin (5-hydroxytryptamine, 5-HT) were significantly increased in both sexes in PFc, striatum (St), midbrain, SN and cerebellum. Variations of any monoamine levels in NAc and VTA were determined. T1 rats were irreversibly altered: a diminution in DA and/or DOPAC levels in PFc, midbrain, VTA and cerebellum was determined. Indolamines of these rats were increased in both sexes in PFc and St. There was also a large increase in 5-HT levels in midbrain of male rats. Although no changes in the dopaminergic system with respect to their control values in any side of these brain structures were observed, DA and DOPAC levels were found to be decreased in the right side with respect to the left side in striata and accumbens nuclei in T2 female rats supporting the behavioral rotation previously registered by us in these rats. In addition, the increased 5-HT content detected in both the right and left striata observed in this study could be the answer to the behaviors observed and to the early alterations in dopamine in basal ganglia by 2,4-D in neonatal exposed rats, mediated by a serotonergic modulation on the dopaminergic system.

Similarly, how do dietary factors differentially influence people of the opposite sexes, also may be tested. Frank *et al* [2002] found that in (4501) US lady doctors, the average intake of fruit and vegetables was four servings per day, while the alcohol intake of those who consumed it at all averaged one drink per week. However, almost 60% claimed they were trying to lose weight, almost all were trying to get more exercise and 82% were trying to change their diet.

Multimodal Findings

The brain is intrinsically asymmetric and virtually all brain functions are organized in more or less degree, in an asymmetrical fashion. Imbalances in this established brain asymmetry might lead to neuropathological deviations of brain functions.

Complex bodily rhythms are ubiquitous in living organisms. These rhythms arise from stochastic, nonlinear and biological mechanisms interacting with a fluctuating environment. Disease often leads to alteration from normal to pathological rhythm [Glass 2001]. Mathematical and physical techniques combined with physiological and medical studies are transforming our understanding of the rhythms of life. Chaotic dynamics might be easier for the body to control than stochastic dynamics. There is a wide spectrum of dynamical behavior associated with both normal and pathological physiological functioning. Extremely regular dynamics are often associated with disease, including periodic (Cheyne – Stokes) breathing, certain abnormally rapid heart rhythms, cyclical blood diseases, epilepsy, neurological tics and tremors. However, regular periodicity can also reflect healthy dynamics – for example in the sleep-wake cycle and menstrual rhythms. Finally, irregular rhythms can also reflect disease. Cardiac dysrhythmias such as atrial fibrillation and frequent ectopy, and neurological disorders like post-anoxic myoclonus, are often highly irregular. The term 'dynamical disease' captures the notion that abnormal rhythms, which could be either more irregular or more regular than normal, arise owing to the modifications in physiological control systems that lead to bifurcations in the dynamics. What is more important in distinguishing health from disease is that there is a change in the dynamics from what is normal, rather than regularity or irregularity of dynamics.

Much of our understanding of functional (Sperrian, as mentioned in § 2a) lateralization comes from the study of both split-brain patients (having undergone commissurotomy or the surgical resection of Corpus Callosum – the tract that is mainly responsible for interhemispheric information exchange) and other brain damaged patients (such as people with unilateral lesions). The salient findings with split-brain patients are (a) Both hemispheres can do most cognitive tasks to some degree, (b) In general, one hemisphere is generally better then the other on most tasks, (c) RH does have some language ability, but the LH is definitely better at many aspects of language processing and (d) The RH seems to be better than the LH at various kinds of visual spatial processing.

Apart from commissurotomy, methods for looking at functional asymmetry in patients include: Wada technique, Single-cell recording work and fMRI (discussed by Subodh and Mandal in their Chapter).

The geophysical character of the earth impose a natural cyclic condition, such as the daily light-dark cycle, to which unavoidably all the biological systems, including human beings, must adapt and respond. As a result, virtually all the organisms have developed an internal system, not only capable of responding to the cyclic nature of environmental stimuli, but also capable of anticipating to that external rhythm with internal programs of metabolic, physiologic, endocrine or behavioral character. Therefore, environmental light generates important neuromorphological, behavioral, neurochemical and neuroendocrine changes. In this response is involved the central circadian oscillator of the endogenous rhythms: the suprachiasmatic nucleus of the anterior hypothalamus. This nucleus receives information of the environmental light-dark conditions through a direct connection with the retina. To investigate the environmental light-dark influence on brain function, Ramirez *et al* [2001] have studied the effect of different light-dark conditions on several neuropeptidase activities, in the left and right sides of the retina and the anterior hypothalamus, among other bilateral structures of the brain. They studied these activities under different light-dark conditions during a regular 12 h- 12 h, light-dark cycle under specific light-dark schedules and under the influence of standard and non standard light-dark conditions. Their results show the existence of laterality which depends on light (left predominance) or dark (in some cases right predominance) conditions. They have demonstrated conclusively that an external factor, such as the environmental light conditions, influences endogenous neurochemical change in the levels of neuropeptidase activity in the retina and hypothalamus. Specific environmental conditions, such as programmed rhythms of light and darkness, can determine the existence and the side (left or right predominance) of laterality in the same locations. The endogenous substrates of neuropeptidases play a functional role in the retina, and the hypothalamus. Therefore, changes in their activity levels under different environmental conditions may reflect modifications in the function that the enzyme's substrates exert in these locations.

Jell *et al* [1993] have shown that unilateral forced nostril breathing (UFNB) affects cerebral hemispheric dominance patterns. Left sided UFNB leads to RH stimulation and improvement of spatial skills. Similarly, right sided UFNB induces LH activity and enhances verbal skills.

There are various neurotransmitters in the brain and all of them act through a multitude of receptor subtypes. However, the same neurotransmitter acting on a particular subtype of receptor may actually cause the opposite effect of what it would have caused through another subtype of receptor. This phenomenon is exemplified in Figure 1.

It is quite likely that the distribution of these neurotransmitter receptor subtypes is also lateralized.

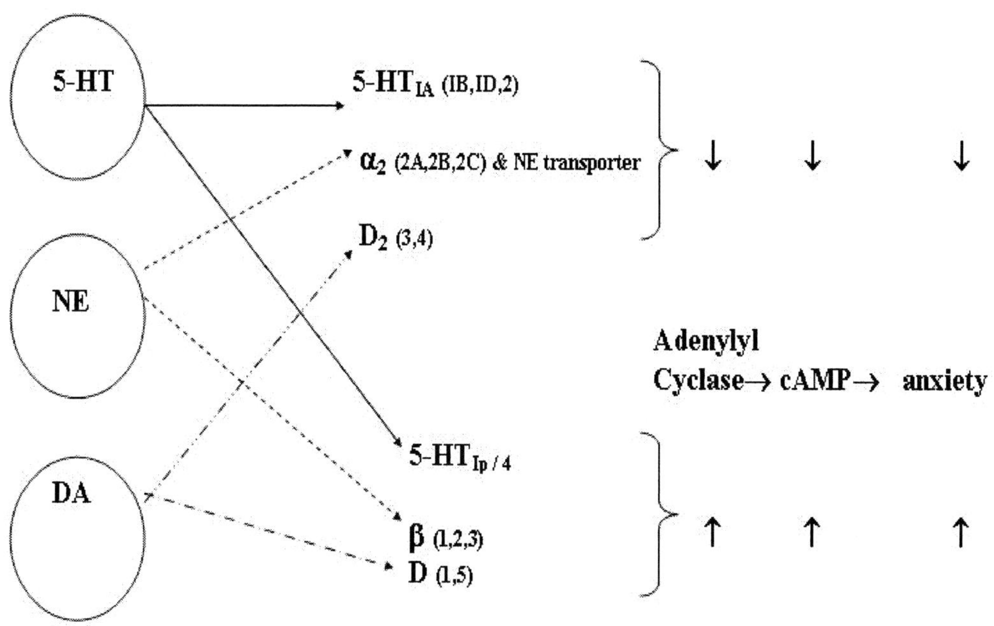

Fig. 1: Typical example of complementary action of some neurotransmitter receptor subtypes. Legend: DA: dopamine; NE: norepinephrine; 5HT: 5-hydroxy Tryptamine or serotonin

Adenosine is a neuromodulator in the nervous system and Adenosine A_{2A} receptors are abundant in the caudate-putamen and involved in the motor control in several species. Whether their distribution also follows the lateralization pattern of the brain or not has to be seen. Coming to neurotransmitter receptor subtype interaction, Adenosine and its analogues have been shown to induce "behavioral despair" in animal models believed to be relevant to depression. Recent data have shown that selective adenosine A_{2A} receptor antagonists (*e.g.*, SCH 58261, ZM241385, and KW6002) or genetic inactivation of the receptor has been effective in reversing signs of behavioral despair in the tail suspension and forced swim tests, two screening procedures predictive of antidepressant activity. A_{2A} antagonists have been active in the tail suspension test using either mice previously screened for having high immobility scores or mice that were selectively bred for their spontaneous "helplessness" in this test. At stimulant doses, caffeine, a nonselective A_1/A_{2A} receptor antagonist, has been effective in the forced swim test. El Yacoubi *et al* [2003] have hypothesized that the antidepressant-like effect of selective A_{2A} antagonists is linked to an interaction with dopaminergic transmission, possibly in the frontal cortex. In support of this idea, administration of the dopamine D_2 receptor antagonist haloperidol prevented antidepressant-like effects elicited by SCH 58261 in the forced swim test (putatively involving cortex), whereas it had no effect on stimulant motor effects of SCH 58261 (putatively linked to ventral striatum). The interaction profile of caffeine with haloperidol differed markedly from that of SCH 58261 in the forced swim and motor activity tests. Therefore, a clear-cut antidepressant- like effect could not be ascribed to caffeine. In conclusion, available data support the proposition that a selective blockade of the adenosine A_{2A} receptor may be an interesting target for the development of effective antidepressant agents. Further studies may be required to extrapolate these findings on the blueprint of lateralization in the brain. Initially this would necessitate mapping of the various adenosine receptor subtypes in different parts of the brain.

Mason and Just [2004] found that theoretical models of text processing, such as the Construction-Integration framework, pose fundamental questions about causal inference-making that are not easily addressed by behavioral studies. In particular, a common result concerning causal relatedness finds a different effect on text reading times than on memory for the text: whereas reading times increase linearly as causal relatedness decreases, memory for the text is best for events that are related by a moderate degree of causal relatedness and is poorer for low and high relatedness. Their fMRI study of the processing of two-sentence passages that varied in their degree of causal relatedness suggests that the inference process can be analyzed into two components, generation and integration, that are subserved by two cortical networks (a right hemisphere language network and a reasoning network). These two cortical networks, which are distinguishable from the classical left hemisphere language network, approximately correspond to the two functional relations observed in the behavioral results. Summarily, their results show how different parts of the brain may be differentially involved in the component processes of making inferences during the reading of narrative text. The relevant parts of the brain appear to be dynamically recruited as their involvement in text comprehension becomes needed. Bilateral DLPFC (dorsolateral prefrontal cortex) is involved whenever the generation of an inference is necessary to maintain coherence in the text. If an inference is successfully generated, the right hemisphere language network plays an active role in integrating that inference into the reader's internal representation of the text.

In the next section we shall discuss the effects of lateralization in depression.

Depression and Lateralization

Depression is a psychosomatic (psychobiosocial) disorder, which affects every aspect of human physiology. Yet under-diagnosis and under-treatment in general medical practice is all pervasive.

The theory of dynamical systems allows one to describe the change in a system's macroscopic behavior as a bifurcation in the underlying dynamics. From the example of depressive syndrome, the existence of a correspondence between clinical and electro-physiological dimensions and the association between clinical remission and brain dynamics reorganization (*i.e.*, bifurcation) can be shown. On the basis of experimental study, such results concerning the question of normality versus pathology in psychiatry and the relationship between mind and brain have been discussed by Melancon *et al*, [2000].

Interestingly, there is a greater right sided (non-dominant hemispheric) EEG abnormalities in depression due to impaired cerebral lateralization. So, females are more prone (because of earlier cerebral lateralization) and males are less predisposed to depression. Therapeutically too, better antidepressant results are obtained with nondominant unilateral electro convulsive shock.

Shagass *et al*, [1988] testing 'eyes open' and 'eyes closed' awake EEGs, in 12 leads, in different psychiatric patients, found that depressives, like the personality disorder group, had a low level of EEG activation. They had also performed time series analysis of amplitude, frequency and wave symmetry. Differences between eyes open and closed were adjusted for 'eyes closed' values to obtain measures of reactivity. These reactivity measures yielded the main difference between the unmedicated and non-patients. Depressives were more reactive. Reactivity differences were eliminated or reversed in medicated patients. The EEGs of unmedicated depressives were over-reactive and with medication, EEG reactivity declined.

Nyström *et al* [1986] had chosen 5-second epochs from 5-minute awake-EEG recordings and averaged to a total of 60-second recordings. In primary major depressive disorder (MDD), they found an increase in 'δ' amplitude and in retarded MDD, increased 'δ' and 'θ' amplitude along with EEG variability. In cases of recurrent unipolar MDD, a reduction of total alpha symmetry was found. Symmetry was measured by left / right ratio in amplitude values (mean amplitude = square root of power). The number of the former depressive episodes were positively correlated with 'β' amplitude and negatively correlated with EEG symmetry for 'δ'.

Usually mood or affect changes are due to: left sided activity leading to RH inhibition or negative valence, which, in turn, gives rise to sadness (more negative interpretation). On the other hand, right sided activity leads to LH stimulation or positive valence, causing positive/assertiveness (less negative interpretation). It is generally claimed that "affect" processing is a right hemisphere (RH) function. It is also claimed that RH dysfunction is characteristic of depressive illness. Both these claims are controversial and it has been found that the relationship between affect processing and affective illness, in terms of intra- and inter-hemispheric role play, is not straight forward. There is an exchange of information and action between the two hemispheres (inter-hemispheric, *i.e.*, between left and right; intra-hemispheric *i.e.*, between anterior and posterior; and also cross-hemispheric coupling *i.e.*, similarities among the left anterior and right posterior quadrants). Summarily, sad mood is a function of positive coupling (stimulation) of left posterior and right anterior areas and/or negative coupling (depression) of left anterior and right posterior areas of the brain [Mandal *et al* 1996].

Neuropsychological research provides a useful framework to study emotional problems, such as depression, and their correlates. Shenal *et al* [2003] review several prominent neuropsychological theories. Functional neuroanatomical systems of emotion and depression are reviewed, including those that describe cerebral asymmetries in emotional processing. Following the review, a model that is composed of three neuroanatomical divisions (left frontal, right frontal, and right posterior) and corresponding neuropsychological emotional sequelae within each quadrant is presented. It is proposed that dysfunction in any of these quadrants could lead to symptomatology consistent with a diagnosis of depression. The proposed model combines theories of arousal, lateralization, and functional cerebral space and lends itself to scientific methods of investigation. Accordingly, research, prevention, and treatment programs in accordance with the proposed model may promote an improved understanding of the neuropsychological mechanisms involved in depression.

Increased incidences of clinical pain complaints from patients with major depression, as well as increased experimental pain thresholds have been reported. The basis of this phenomenon remains unclear, as well as its relation to medication, clinical recovery, gender and lateralization of hemispheric function. Bar *et al* [2003] aimed to further elucidate heat pain perception in depression applying a testing battery including assessment (on both arms) of warmth perception, heat pain perception and heat pain tolerance, and the jaw opening reflex (duration of ES2 component) as a putative indicator of descending pain inhibition. The battery was applied to 20 patients and 20 age- and sex-matched controls. Patients were assessed: on admission (acutely depressed, off-medication), few days after admission (depressed, on medication), and after clinical recovery (mostly on medication), and controls at corresponding intervals. Significant elevated heat pain thresholds were found off and on medication in the acute stage (mainly in women) and after recovery on the right arm only. Elevated heat pain tolerance (on the right arm only) was seen in medicated patients in the acute and recovered stage. Significant prolongation of ES2 duration was only found in acutely depressed patients off medication. While confirming hypalgesia to heat pain in major depression, their findings demonstrate a close relation to gender and strong influence of lateralization after recovery. Altered pain processing at brain stem level might only partially be responsible for the observed finding.

Papo *et al* [2003] used event-related potentials (ERPs) to probe the effects of feedback in a hypothesis testing (HT) paradigm. Thirteen college students serially tested hypotheses concerning a hidden rule by judging its presence or absence in triplets of digits and revised them on the basis of an exogenous performance feedback. ERPs time-locked to performance feedback were then examined. The results showed differences between responses to positive and negative feedback at all cortical sites. Negative feedback, indicating incorrect performance, was associated to a negative deflection preceding a P300-like wave. Spatiotemporal principal component analysis (PCA) showed the interplay between early frontal components and later central and posterior ones. Lateralization of activity was selectively detectable at frontal sites, with a left frontal dominance for both positive and negative feedback. These results can be elaborated in terms of a proposed computational model of trial-to-trial feedback in HT in which the cognitive and emotive aspects of feedback are explicitly linked to putative mediating brain mechanisms. The properties of different feedback types and feedback-related deficits in depression are also discussed in their article.

In mice, lateralization as assessed by paw preference represents a behavioral trait linked to immune reactivity and stress susceptibility. Right-pawed mice are more reactive to stress than left-pawed animals when brain metabolism, activation of the corticoid axis, and depression of lymphoproliferation are studied. Since stress responses include cytokine production, Neveu and Merlot [2003] address the possibility that lateralization influences the production of cytokines – especially interleukin (IL)-1 – responsible for depression of lymphoproliferation and activation of the corticoid axis. Increased plasma IL-1 level that may be considered as a stress marker, was observed in right- but not in left-pawed mice submitted to a 4 h-restraint. Likewise, plasma levels were greater in right- than in left-pawed animals 2 h after the administration of a low dose of lipopolysaccharides (LPS). By contrast, there was no lateralization effect in restraint-induced plasma level of IL-6 or in the LPS-induced increase in plasma IL-10. Prazosin, an alpha1/alpha2 adrenoreceptor antagonist, drastically increased plasma IL-10 induced by LPS, reduced plasma levels of IL-1 and abolished the effect of lateralization observed after LPS alone. This suggests that alpha-adrenergic modulation of IL-1 production depends on lateralization through mechanisms that need further investigation.

Atchley *et al* [2003] examined hemispheric lateralization of emotion processing by comparing the performance of clinically depressed, previously depressed, and control individuals on a divided visual field task. Participants were asked to make affective valence judgments for each in a series of laterally presented person-descriptive adjectives. Study results suggest that the right cerebral hemisphere (RH) is preferentially sensitive to the affective context of language. Among targets presented to the RH, depressed and previously depressed participants were significantly faster and more accurate in their judgments of negative target words, while controls responded more quickly and accurately to positive target words. No such effects were observed for targets presented to the left hemisphere. It is hypothesized that affective sensitivity may result in differences in semantic network organization across individuals who vary in affective experience.

Lyoo *et al* [2003] investigated to detect differences in regional areas of the corpus callosum (CC) in subjects with early-onset minor depression (dysthymia or depressive personality disorder) and healthy comparison subjects. Based on previous reports that have suggested reduced frontal lobe volume and reduced hemispheric lateralization in the frontal regions of the brain in depression, they hypothesized that the area of the CC that interconnects the frontal regions of the brain, *i.e.*, the genu, will be smaller compared to that of healthy comparison subjects. Forty female subjects with early-onset dysthymia or depressive personality disorder, as defined by the Structured Clinical Interview for DSM-III-R and the Diagnostic Interview for Depressive Personality, respectively, and age- and gender-matched healthy comparison subjects (n = 42) were recruited (age: 21.4 +/- 2.1 and 20.9 +/- 2.8 years, respectively). All subjects were psychotropic medications-naive and right-handed. A 1.5T GE Sigma scanner was used to acquire 124 1.5-mm-thick contiguous coronal images. Midsagittal slice images were carefully selected from reconstructed magnetic resonance images both from native and stereotaxic space to measure seven regional areas of the CC. There were significant diagnosis by CC region interactions [$F(6,480) = 4.06$, $p <.001$; $F(6,480) = 3.30$, $p =.003$, native and stereotaxic space, respectively]. Early-onset minor depression subjects had a 9.9% (native space) and 6.9% (stereotaxic space) smaller genu of the CC compared to the healthy comparison subjects (the Newman-Keuls post hoc test, p =.005 and.019, native and stereotaxic space, respectively). Early-onset minor depression subjects also had a 7.8% smaller posterior midbody relative to the comparison subjects (the Newman-Keuls post hoc test, p =.033) only in the native space. Severity of current depressive symptoms or duration of illness did not correlate with the size of the genu or the posterior midbody parts of the CC. These results suggest frontal lobe structural, and possibly functional, abnormalities in the brain in young female adults with a milder spectrum of depression, *i.e.*, DSM-IV early-onset dysthymia or depressive personality disorder. The present findings point out the possible role of frontal lobe abnormality in pathophysiology of early-onset minor depression.

In general, 30%–50% of stroke patients [Berg *et al* 2003] develop major or minor depressive disorders. Although the mechanisms involved are likely complex, the nature of the depressive symptoms may be associated with the site of the lesion. Major depression has been found to occur more frequently in patients with left anterior lesions (frontal or basal ganglia), whereas minor depression has been associated with either right or left parieto-occipital lesions. Symptoms can be delayed months or years after an initial insult.

In the next section we shall try to analyze how dementia can be affected by lateralization.

DEMENTIA AND LATERALIZATION

Neuroimaging studies of memory have consistently shown that episodic retrieval is associated with right frontal activation, whereas semantic retrieval is associated with left frontal activation. Various hypotheses have been proposed to account for this lateralization in terms of underlying psychological processes. Alternatively, this lateralization may reflect the complexity of information retrieved: retrieval of complex, contextual information accompanying episodic retrieval invokes right-lateralized processes preferentially. This hypothesis was tested by manipulating the type and complexity of information retrieved. Initial increase in complexity of both episodic and semantic information was associated with right inferior frontal activation; further increase in complexity was associated with left dorsolateral activation. That implies that frontal activation during retrieval is a non-linear function of the complexity of retrieved information [Hunkin *et al* 2000].

Interestingly, in Alzheimer's disease, significant nonlinear changes in left hemisphere (O_1 lead of EEG) have been found in qEEG [Stam *et al* 1996].

The electrophysiological measures of MEG (Magnetoencephalography) consisting of 6 spectral band measures together with spectral edge frequency and spectral entropy, plus the time-domain-based entropy of amplitudes (ENA) and the nonlinear measures correlation dimension D2 and Lyapunov exponent L1 has been measured during cognitive tasks. The results indicate a pronounced task-dependent difference between the anterior and the posterior region, but no lateralization effects. Though the nonlinear measures ranged in the middle field compared to the number of significant contrasts, they were the only ones to be partially successful in discriminating the mental tasks from each other [Fell *et al* 2000].

The left cerebral hemisphere controls the production and comprehension of spoken and written language, and hand preference is associated with hemisphere dominance. The left hemisphere is dominant for righthanded individuals and most left-handed people. The right hemisphere is known to contribute to certain linguistic features such as affective prosody and emotional gesturing. The angular gyrus, located in the left temporal lobe, is part of the language system of the brain, which also includes Broca's area and Wernicke's area; damage to the angular gyrus gives rise to alexia and agraphia. Even if the angular gyrus is spared, it can still be isolated by lesions immediately subcortical to it or by lesions involving the mesial part of the occipital cortex and the splenium of the corpus callosum, which will result in alexia and agraphia.

A 67-year-old left-handed woman with a diagnosis of pseudodementia was being treated for depression with little benefit. Neuropsychological evaluations revealed features of angular gyrus syndrome, namely, agraphia, alexia, Gerstmann's syndrome and behavioural manifestations such as depression, poor memory, frustration and irritability. A computed tomographic scan showed a right occipito-temporal infarction, which had occurred 18 months earlier. The patient demonstrated aspects of language dysfunction associated with the syndrome and showed reversed lateralization of cerebral functions. Recognizing and distinguishing between angular gyrus syndrome and depression is important because the appropriate therapies differ. The use of the term pseudodementia can be misleading [Nagaratnam 2002].

Patterns of aberrant language due to lateralized frontal brain lesions have been described. Tallberg *et al* [2002] investigated the consequences of lateralized lesion for aspects of semantic range and relevance in speech of patients with frontotemporal degeneration. Demented patients with predominantly left (n=10) and right (n=4) brain degeneration as well as 5 healthy controls participated. Significant differences were found concerning semantic range and relevance in descriptions of emotionally loaded pictures within the demented group and between the demented group and the controls. The demented individuals' speech was less varied and relevant in contrast to the healthy individuals. The speech of the left hemispheric group was more relevant but also more stereotypic and unspecified than that of the right hemispheric group. The results are discussed in terms of impaired semantic retrieval and in relation to lateralization of lesion.

The staging of Alzheimer disease (AD) dementia could be improved by a neurometabolic analysis using magnetic resonance spectroscopy. To examine the correlation between regional cerebral metabolic alterations measured by proton magnetic resonance spectroscopy and neuropsychological dysfunctions in patients with early AD, Chantal *et al* [2002] designed a case-control study. A cohort of 14 patients with mild AD and 14 control subjects were paired for age and sex. Single-voxel proton magnetic resonance spectroscopic brain examination (60 minutes) and a comprehensive battery of psychometric tests (2 hours) were done to measure Metabolite ratios relative to unsuppressed water calculated for magnetic resonance spectroscopic metabolites (N-acetylaspartate, choline, creatine-phosphocreatine, and myo-inositol) in the medial temporal lobes (MTLs), parietotemporal cortices (PTCs), and frontal cortices of both hemispheres. Correlations were examined between metabolic changes in an area and psychometric scores of its known regional function: MTL and verbal memory, PTC and language and visuoconstructional abilities, and frontal cortices and executive functions. A significant reduction of N-acetylaspartate/water (H_2O) in the left MTL and of choline/H_2O in both MTLs, as well as a significant increase of myo-inositol/H_2O in the right PTC were observed. Metabolic alterations in the left MTL were correlated with a loss of verbal memory, in the left PTC with language impairment, and in the right PTC with a loss of visuoconstructional abilities in the group with AD. These findings are consistent with regional distribution of neuropathologic changes and cognitive symptoms characterizing early phases of AD, and with the pattern of lateralization of normal brain function.

Cerebral autosomal dominant arteriopathy with subcortical infarcts and leukoencephalopathy (CADASIL) is an inherited small-artery disease that clinically involves only the brain. Particularly early in the disease, patients can show substantial or complete recovery after individual strokes. Cortical functional reorganization may contribute to limiting disability with such ischemic injury. Reddy *et al* [2002] sought to test whether the extent of any functional changes in the motor cortex increases with greater brain axonal injury from CADASIL. Functional MRI (fMRI) was used to characterize cortical activation during a simple hand-tapping task. Disease-associated pathology in subcortical white matter was assessed with the use of conventional fluid-attenuated inversion recovery (FLAIR) MRI and MR spectroscopic imaging for measurement of N-acetyl aspartate decreases, a relatively specific measure of axonal injury. There was evidence for variable but substantial hyperintense white matter signal in all of the patients with FLAIR imaging. With the use of fMRI, the brain regions activated during motor tasks were similar for the 9 CADASIL patients and 7 controls, except that most (6 of 9) patients showed primary motor cortex activation both ipsilateral and contralateral to the hand moved, a finding in only 1 of 7 healthy controls. Ipsilateral motor cortex activation increased ($r=-0.77$, $P<0.05$) and motor cortex activation lateralization index decreased ($r=0.68$, $P<0.02$) with greater white matter injury (as assessed from decreases in the relative N-acetyl aspartate concentration) in a region of interest including descending motor fibers of the corticospinal pathway. The extent of functional reorganization of motor cortex increases with increasing axonal injury, consistent with an adaptive role for these changes. Increased functional recruitment of cortex ipsilateral to the limb moved therefore may contribute to limiting motor impairment from the subcortical injury of CADASIL.

The aim of the study by Kowalski *et al* [2001] was to analyze EEG changes in patients with Alzheimer disease (AD) and to determine how closely EEG reflects the progression of mental impairment in people with AD. Ninety-five patients with probable AD according to National Institute of Neurological and Communicative Disorders and Stroke/Alzheimer's Disease and Related Disorders Association criteria treated in their Clinic for Memory Disorders were selected for this study. Patients were divided into three subgroups with mild, marked, and severe dementia according to the results of psychometric scales. The EEG findings were classified using an eight-degree scale according to the background activity, presence and amount of theta and delta waves, focal changes, lateralization of focal changes, synchronization, and presence of sharp and spike waves. A significant correlation between the degree of EEG abnormalities and cognitive impairment was found. They did not observe any correlation between the presence of delta waves and the results of neuropsychological tests. Their study revealed an important diagnostic value of EEG in the estimation of the severity of dementia parallel to psychometric scales.

Neuropsychologists who serve as members of an epilepsy surgery team are often asked to provide information regarding localized cerebral dysfunction that may relate to the seizure focus in patients with intractable temporal lobe epilepsy (TLE). However, the rate at which neuropsychological (NP) assessment results correspond with the side of seizure focus (*i.e.*, left versus right) in TLE patients is unknown. The majority of literature in this area has focused on the ability of single NP tests to detect lateralized cognitive dysfunction in groups of TLE patients, with mixed findings and few consistent replications. The primary purpose of a study [Ogden-Epker and Cullum, 2001] was to examine the rate at which qualitative clinician interpretations of NP profiles agree with seizure lateralization as determined by a multidisciplinary surgery team in temporal lobectomy candidates. Quantitative analyses of single NP test scores and groups of test scores (*i.e.*, cognitive domain composite scores) were also conducted to examine their effectiveness in discriminating left from right TLE groups. Only four of the 19 NP test variables and three of the nine composite cognitive domain scores significantly differed between the groups. However, clinician interpretation of NP profiles agreed with the surgery conference team's determination of seizure laterality in two-thirds of cases. These findings suggest that qualitative aspects of NP performance play an important role in identifying lateralized cerebral dysfunction in TLE patients, and provide additional support for the use of NP assessment results in the selection of temporal lobectomy candidates.

Although evidence from primates suggests an important role for the anterior temporal cortex in social behavior, human research has to date concentrated almost solely on the orbitofrontal cortex and amygdala. By describing four cases of the temporal variant of frontotemporal dementia, Perry *et al* [2001] show how this degenerative condition provides an excellent model for investigating the role of the anterior temporal lobe, especially the right, in emotions, empathy and social behavior. Assessments of semantic memory, processing of emotional facial expression and emotional prosody were made, empathy was measured, and facial expressions of emotion were coded. Of the two right handers described, one subject with predominantly left temporal lobe atrophy had severe semantic impairment but normal performance on all emotional tasks. In contrast, the subject with right temporal lobe atrophy showed severely impaired recognition of emotion from faces and voices that was not due to semantic or perceptual difficulties. Empathy was lost, interpersonal skills were severely affected and facial expression of emotion was characterized by a fixed expression that was unresponsive to situations. Additionally, two left handers with right temporal lobe atrophy are described. One demonstrated the same pattern of hemispheric lateralization as the right handers and had emotional impairment. The other left hander showed the opposite pattern of deficits, suggesting a novel presentation of anomalous dominance with reversed hemispheric specialization of semantic memory and emotional processing.

Now that we have discussed, in some detail, the role of hemispheric lateralization with special reference to depression and dementia, let us try to put together the individual links onto a bigger canvas.

Commonalty between Depression, Dementia and Lateralization

Once it was verified that the human brain is mostly asymmetrically organized, it was an attempt to assign an anatomical and/or neurochemical substrate to the lateralized brain functions. The extensive research performed on this subject has not yet reached any coherent conclusion. Therefore, the teleological meaning of brain asymmetry, as a global concept, is not yet understood. Brain functions, evolutionary and with an unknown objective, have been developed predominantly in one hemisphere, such is the case of language. Hypothetically, specific brain functions, apparently symmetric or with a certain degree of asymmetry, might be processed asymmetrically or more asymmetrically, in response to external or internal stimuli. Brain functions, processed more or less asymmetrically could be under a universal operating system, which would consist in the reciprocal inhibition of homologue centers located in both hemispheres. The regulation of a large number of brain processes is based in a system of inhibitory-stimulatory feedback. This could explain the existence of neurochemical asymmetries, which arise, change the side of their predominance, or increase their degree of predominance under specific environmental conditions. This is an example, which connects the elegant geometrical order of nature with the biological plasticity that exists between the two brain hemispheres.

Two schools of thought in 'cognitive modeling', *viz*., connectionism and computationalism are currently vying for hegemony. At first glance the opposition seems incoherent, because connectionism is itself computational, but the form of computationalism that has been the prime candidate for encoding the "language of thought" has been symbolic computationalism, whereas connectionism is nonsymbolic or, as sometimes it has been hopefully dubbed as, "subsymbolic". Hybrid nonsymbolic/symbolic systems have been sketched in which the meanings of the symbols are grounded bottom-up in the system's capacity to discriminate and identify the objects they refer to. Neural nets are one possible mechanism for learning the invariants in the analog sensory projection on which successful categorization is based. "Categorical perception", in which similarity space is "warped" in the service of categorization, turns out to be exhibited by both people and nets, and may mediate the constraints exerted by the analog world of objects on the formal world of symbols.

On the other hand, to apply the tools of modern dynamical systems theory to models of cognition is a good approach. The use of the *DH* (dynamical hypothesis) framework provides a viable empirical alternative to the Computational Hypothesis. The investigators in the area of cognitive science currently only use the tip of the dynamical systems theory iceberg.

Indeed, it may be rather difficult to make use of much of dynamical systems theory in studying cognitive processes. These theories were originally developed as mathematical models and applied to highly controllable physical systems, *e.g.*, electrical circuits. Biological systems, on the other hand, contain large amount of noise and, more seriously, have a high degree of nonstationarity. Nonstationarity refers to the lack of constancy in the laws governing the evolution of the system. Many of the measures which are used to characterize dynamical systems and on which much of dynamical systems theory is based, require very large amounts of data. Cognitive systems, however, tend to move rapidly from one state to another, making it frequently impossible to collect the quantity of data required to appropriately apply dynamical systems theory. Despite theses shortcomings, an entirely new *modeling* paradigm in cognitive science may be possible with this method [French and Thomas 1998].

The most widely used method in the conventional category, for EEG analysis, has been computing the fast Fourier transform (FFT) or the "Power (density) spectrum". FFT analysis is in the frequency domain, and though not superior to time-domain representations, is far more informative than the conventional analog (paper) recording still preferred by many clinicians [Sarbadhikari & Pal, 2002]. So, the term qEEG (quantitative EEG) is often used to differentiate it from the analog records. In the case of nonlinear analysis of EEG, correlation dimension (D2) is the commonly applied measure [Sarbadhikari and Chakrabarty 2001]. Lamberts *et al* [2000] found experimentally, that for subjects presented with a higher mental load (like calculation), compared to a moderate mental load (like a less complex time estimation task), the D2 is found to be higher for calculation. On the other hand, during epileptic fits, D2 is rather low. So, D2 is a very sensitive indicator for analyzing electrical brain activity.

Bremner *et al*, [2003] had used positron emission tomography (PET) measurement of brain metabolism with 18fluorodeoxyglucose (18-FDG). The patients receiving selective serotonin reuptake inhibitors (SSRIs) who have a tryptophan depletion-induced return of depressive symptoms have an acute decrease in metabolism in orbitofrontal cortex, dorsolateral prefrontal cortex, and thalamus. Many patients with depression in remission while taking norepinephrine reuptake inhibitors (NRIs) (but not SSRIs) experience a return of depressive symptoms with depletion of norepinephrine and dopamine using alpha-methylparatyrosine (AMPT). A randomized, controlled, double-blind trial was undertaken, in which 18 patients recruited in 1997-2000 from the general community who had depression in remission while taking NRIs had PET imaging in a psychiatric research unit following AMPT and placebo administration. After initial medication with desipramine and follow-up until response, patients underwent active AMPT (five 1-g doses administered orally over 28 hours) and placebo (diphenhydramine hydrochloride, five 50- mg doses administered similarly) catecholamine depletion challenges in randomized order of assignment, after which PET imaging was performed on day 3 of each condition. Both study conditions were performed 1 week apart. AMPT-induced return of depressive symptoms was experienced by 11 of the 18 patients and led to decreased brain metabolism in a number of cortical areas, with the greatest magnitude of effects in orbitofrontal (P =.002) and dorsolateral prefrontal (P =.03) cortex and thalamus (P =.006). Increased resting metabolism in prefrontal and limbic areas predicted vulnerability to return of depressive symptoms. It may be inferred that different neurochemical systems that mediate depression may have effects on a common brain circuitry. Baseline metabolism in successfully treated depressed patients may predict vulnerability to future episodes of depression.

Albeit we are not dealing with schizophrenia directly, in this chapter, since it is also a cognitive disorder, let us cite an interesting recent story. Svenningsson *et al* [2003] suggest that a single molecule may underpin the psychotic symptoms of schizophrenia. Since both depression and dementia also are supposed to be caused by derangement of various neurotransmitter receptor subtype interactions, like in schizophrenia, it may well have a final common pathway for the different neurotransmitters. Schizophrenics experience disrupted thoughts and behavior, and sometimes delusions. Three main neurotransmitter systems are implicated. Different researchers tend to favor one molecule the others as the disease's root cause. Nobel Laureate in Medicine and Physiology in 2000, Paul Greengard and his team members have treated mice with the hallucinogenic drugs (i) amphetamine: acting on adrenergic system, or (ii) LSD (d-lysergic acid diethylamide): acting on serotonergic system, or (iii) PCP (Phencyclidine or angel dust): acting on dopaminergic system. Each drug specifically targets one of the suspect neurotransmitter systems, but has similar effects on brain and behavior. Each hallucinogen altered the same mystery brain protein, a novel pivotal signaling switch, ***DARPP-32*** (dopamine and cyclic AMP-regulated phosphoprotein, Mr32kDA). The team has found four specific residues in DARPP-32 that are phosphorylated by distinct protein kinases and dephosphorylated by distinct protein phosphatases. The DARPP-32 molecule itself can act either as an inhibitor of cyclic AMP-dependent protein kinase or as an inhibitor of protein phosphatase-1, depending upon the particular residue that is phosphorylated. This is the first known example of a molecule that can act either as a protein kinase or phosphatase inhibitor. The state of phosphorylation of DARPP-32, through control of protein kinase and phosphatase activities, regulates the state of phosphorylation and activity of virtually every known physiological effector, including a variety of ion pumps, ion channels, neurotransmitter receptors and transcription factors. Dopaminoceptive neurons integrate all information coming into the neostriatum and are the only efferent pathway out of the striatum. DARPP-32 provides a molecular mechanism by which all efferent information is integrated and converted into a meaningful physiological response. Animals, treated with all the three hallucinogens, developed schizophrenic symptoms – in mice, this involves repetitive grooming and nervousness. The cause of the neurotransmitter imbalance is still a mystery. But the finding suggests that all three chemicals might influence DARPP-32, in turn causing schizophrenia. Schizophrenia is a complex disease that affects the brain's chemistry and structure. How a molecular change like this translates into hallucinations and delusions has to be found out. The finding may aid the production of new schizophrenia therapies. Mice lacking DARPP-32 were immune to the drugs' psychotic effects. Current therapies damp down one neurotransmitter called dopamine. Delusions subside but attention and memory problems often persist, and serious adverse effects are common. Drugs that target DARPP-32 would affect several neurotransmitters. This might make them more effective with fewer side-effects. The finding may also lead to improved animal models of schizophrenia. Mice with abnormal DARPP-32 might better mimic the brain chemistry and behavior of human patients than drug-treated animals.

Molecules like DARPP-32 may soon be discovered for depression and dementia (at least some of the subtypes).

We know that abnormal levels of certain neurotransmitters underlie the various brain disorders since drugs to treat these conditions alter activity of these molecules. The report by

Tkachev *et al* [2003] backs the idea that a class of brain cells called oligodendrocytes, which help nerves to transmit electrical pulses, are probably even more important for the causation of schizophrenia. They found that oligodendrocyte genes are also dampened down in the brains of patients suffering bipolar disorder, in which patients swing from depression to elation. The investigators screened over 22,000 genes in the brains of patients with schizophrenia, bipolar disorder or neither. The altered genes might cut the number of oligodendrocytes born or kill off existing ones, so that they fail in their job of producing the fatty substance myelin, which coats nerve cells and helps them to send electrical signals. Whatever the mechanism, the loss of myelin might lead to schizophrenic or bipolar symptoms if the circuits controlling thoughts or memories are the ones affected. They have found that the cell machinery making energy is also affected in schizophrenics' brains. Oligodendrocytes, which consume lots of energy, may be starved of fuel. If true, then current antipsychotic drugs maybe treating just the symptoms of schizophrenia. New therapies might rescue myelin or even bump up energy production. Thus, these disorders share common causative and pathophysiological pathways through oligodendrocyte genes and myelin genes.

Just as the study mentioned above, by Bremner et al [2003], hints at a common brain circuitry for depression, we may boldly surmise that there is some common final pathway for multiple (apparently unrelated) disorders like cognitive and affective disorders [Sarbadhikari 2004]. A nonpharmacological intervention for various disorders including hypertension, diabetes mellitus, depression and AD, regular moderate physical exercise, also seems to affect the final common pathway in some manner [Sarbadhikari & Chakrabarty, 2001]. Neveu and Merlot [2003] suggest that alpha-adrenergic modulation of IL-1 production depends on lateralization through mechanisms that need further investigation. Horne [1993] had proposed that exercise reduces adrenergic responsiveness through lateralized modulation of the prefrontal cortex. Chantal *et al* [2002] found data consistent with regional distribution of neuropathologic (neurotransmitter and protein) changes and cognitive symptoms characterizing early phases of AD, and with the pattern of lateralization of normal brain function.

All these studies hint towards the final common pathway working through localized (anteriorized / posteriorized) and lateralized brain circuitry. However, all the missing links of the final common pathway are yet to be discovered.

Toro *et al* [1999] have reviewed and compared all therapies that have shown efficacy in depression and Parkinson's disease, although some are not in current use and others are at the experimental stage. They include pharmacological modification of neurotransmitter pathways, electroconvulsive therapy (ECT), sleep deprivation, psychosurgery, electrical stimulation through cerebral electrodes, and transcranial magnetic stimulation. Stemming from a pathophysiological model that stresses the brain as an open, complex, and nonlinear system, all therapies have been attributed a common mechanism of action. This report suggests that the therapeutic isomorphism is related to their ability to help the CNS (central nervous system) deactivate cortical-subcortical circuits that are dysfunctionally coupled. These circuits are self-organized among neurons of their informational subsystem (rapid conduction) and modulating subsystem (slow conduction). We can summarize these in the form of Figure 2.

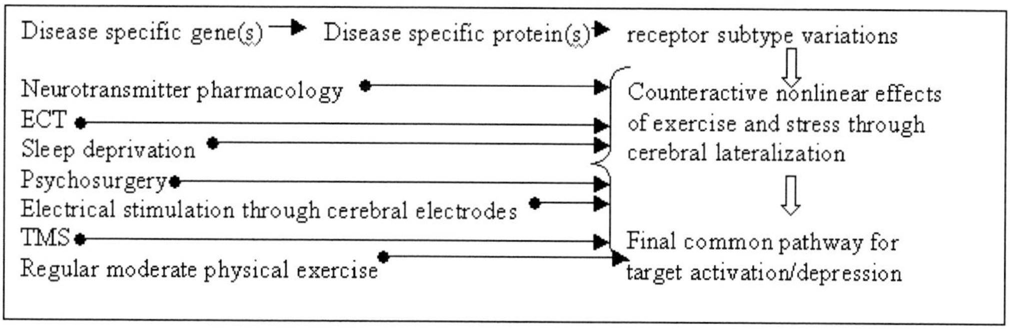

Figure 2: overview

Albeit the early 19th century European doctor Franz Joseph Gall's "phrenology" was ridiculed as "bumpology", he was the first to study fetal development and clinical psychology. He was also the first person to insist that organization of behavior was related to the organization of the brain. In 1820, the French physiologist and neurosurgeon Pierre Fluorens forwarded the belief that the brain 'functioned as a whole'; supported by the fact that normal work was possible despite excessive removal of the brain tissue. This view was challenged by Paul Broca, a neurosurgeon in Paris, in 1861, as he discovered the "speech center" (later named after him), by autopsy from a patient aphasic for thirty years. The contrary outlook was presented by a Michigan psychologist Marty Merrill in 1984, as a patient with "cortical blindness" was cured with the help of a new branch now known as "Behavioral Medicine ". In this way our knowledge about the brain and its functions are still being updated, the balance tilting in favor of one or the other concepts of "Generalization (Equipotentiality)-Regionalization-Lateralization" with time [Sarbadhikari 1995a]. However, it cannot be doubted that the function of the brain is multimodal and certainly nonlinear like most biological complex systems. Therefore, the role of lateralization is a very crucial factor for the causation, progress and amelioration of depression and dementia. Further multi-disciplinary studies will be able to establish the genetic-neurochemical-cellular receptor complex interactions leading to the manifestations of various conditions of mental health and disease.

Summary

The cognitive organization of the human brain can be ascertained by various measures like EEG (electroencephalogram) and psychometric tests. Human cognition undergoes change with age as well as with various neuropsychiatric conditions. In adults and geriatric people depression and/or dementia (e.g., Alzheimer's disease and Parkinsonism) are found in abundance. Depression is not a homogeneous disorder. However, minor depression may be expressed as dysthymia. Similarly, dementia can have varied etiology. By dexterity, I am alluding to Cerebral or Hemispheric Lateralization (Handedness / Footedness / Sidedness). Laterality is the term used to describe ways in which the two hemispheres of the brain differ from each other in both anatomy and function.

The brain asymmetry understood as an anatomical, functional or biochemical difference between both cerebral hemispheres is a phenomenon extensively studied, essentially from an anatomical and functional perspective. The molecules and physical particles of which living cells are constructed are themselves asymmetrical. In addition, asymmetry is characteristic of many single-celled organisms and of individual cells in more complex organisms. These observations among others, have led to the realization that despite its inherent beauty, bilateral symmetry is no more fundamental a property of biological systems than is bilateral asymmetry. In fact, growing evidence support the idea that the brain is intrinsically asymmetric, and that virtually all brain functions are organized, in more or less degree, in an asymmetrical fashion. In addition, it could be speculated that imbalances in established brain asymmetry (toward symmetry or toward increasing asymmetry, through nonlinear dynamics, as described by both Jelic and Jeong, in two chapters of this book) might lead to neuropathological deviations of brain functions. This asymmetrical organization is the result of evolutionary adaptation and evidences of brain asymmetries have been found not only in our ancestors but also in all stages of the brain evolution.

EEG reflects the electrical activity of the brain, during rest and mental work, as recorded from electrodes placed on the scalp. There are two contradictory conjectures for the generation of EEG signals. Conventionally it is believed that since the EEG is a very complex-looking, virtually unpredictable signal, it must be produced by a very complex linear system. However, the more recent view is that the EEG signal could be produced by a relatively simple, nonlinear system, which can be explained by the chaos theory. Researchers all around the world have been trying to study these changes so that the quality of life can be improved in patients with dementia and depression.

Another interesting feature is the sex-difference of cerebral asymmetries in humans. Many lateralization studies demonstrate that males have more pronounced functional left-right differences than females. A significant part of these sex-effects could be explained by variations of steroids during the menstrual cycle that probably alter interhemispheric communication via the corpus callosum. Cognitive processes change in correlation with these hormonal alterations. These results show that human cerebral asymmetries are not completely determined by static neuromorphological wiring principles, but also have a dynamic component.

The brain is intrinsically asymmetric and virtually all brain functions are organized in more or less degree, in an asymmetrical fashion. Imbalances in this established brain asymmetry might lead to neuropathological deviations of brain functions. Complex bodily rhythms are ubiquitous in living organisms. These rhythms arise from stochastic, nonlinear and biological mechanisms interacting with a fluctuating environment. Disease often leads to alteration from normal to pathological rhythm. Mathematical and physical techniques combined with physiological and medical studies are transforming our understanding of the rhythms of life. Chaotic dynamics might be easier for the body to control than stochastic dynamics.

Neuroimaging studies of memory have consistently shown that episodic retrieval is associated with right frontal activation, whereas semantic retrieval is associated with left frontal activation. Various hypotheses have been proposed to account for this lateralization in terms of underlying psychological processes. Alternatively, this lateralization may reflect the complexity of information retrieved: retrieval of complex, contextual information accompanying episodic retrieval invokes right-lateralized processes preferentially.

Many recent studies point towards nonlinear mechanisms working through localized (anteriorized / posteriorized) and lateralized brain circuitry, converging on some (yet to be finally deciphered) final common pathway, to produce various cognitive and affective disorders.

Albeit the early 19th century European doctor Franz Joseph Gall's "phrenology" was ridiculed as "bumpology", he was the first to study fetal development and clinical psychology. He was also the first person to insist that organization of behavior was related to the organization of the brain. In 1820, the French physiologist and neurosurgeon Pierre Fluorens forwarded the belief that the brain 'functioned as a whole'; supported by the fact that normal work was possible despite excessive removal of the brain tissue. This view was challenged by Paul Broca, a neurosurgeon in Paris, in 1861, as he discovered the "speech center" (later named after him), by autopsy from a patient aphasic for thirty years. The contrary outlook was presented by a Michigan psychologist Marty Merrill in 1984, as a patient with "cortical blindness" was cured with the help of a new branch now known as "Behavioral Medicine ". In this way our knowledge about the brain and its functions are still being updated, the balance tilting in favor of one or the other concepts of "Generalization-Regionalization-Lateralization" with time. However, it cannot be doubted that the function of the brain is multimodal and certainly nonlinear like most biological complex systems. Therefore, the role of lateralization is a very crucial factor for the causation, progress and amelioration of depression and dementia. Further studies will be able to establish the genetic-neurochemical-cellular receptor complex interactions leading to the manifestations of various conditions of mental health and disease.

REFERENCES

American Psychiatric Association, *Diagnostic and Statistical Manual of Mental Disorders,* Fourth Edition, (DSM-IV), APA, Washington DC, 1994

Anokhin A P, *et al,* Spatiotemporal organization of brain dynamics and intelligence: an EEG study in adolescents, *Int J Psychophysiol* 1999 Sep; 33(3):259-73

Atchley RA, Ilardi SS, Enloe A, Hemispheric asymmetry in the processing of emotional content in word meanings: the effect of current and past depression, *Brain Lang.* 2003; 84: 105-19

Bar KJ, Greiner W, Letsch A, Kobele R, Sauer H, Influence of gender and hemispheric lateralization on heat pain perception in major depression, *J Psychiatr Res.* 2003; 37: 345-53

Berg A, *et al,* Poststroke depression: an 18-month follow-up, *Stroke.* 2003; 34: 138-43

Bortolozzi A, Duffard R, de Duffard AM, Asymmetrical development of the monoamine systems in 2,4-dichlorophenoxyacetic acid treated rats, *Neurotoxicology.*, 2003; 24: 149-157.

Bremner JD, *et al,* Regional brain metabolic correlates of alpha-methylparatyrosine-induced depressive symptoms: implications for the neural circuitry of depression, *JAMA,* 2003, 289(23): 3125-34.

Castle D, McGrath J, Kulkarni J, eds. *Women and Schizophrenia.* Cambridge, UK: Cambridge University Press; 2000.

Chantal S, Labelle M, Bouchard RW, Braun CM, Boulanger Y; Correlation of regional proton magnetic resonance spectroscopic metabolic changes with cognitive deficits in mild Alzheimer disease, *Arch Neurol.* 2002; 59: 955-62

Craft S, Gourovitch ML, Dowton SB, Swanson JM, Bonforte S, Lateralized deficits in visual attention in males with developmental dopamine depletion, *Neuropsychologia*., 1992; 30: 341-351.

de Rotrou J, Moulin F, Critical review of psychometric tests, *Therapie* 1993 May-; 48: 195-9

Ehlers C L, Chaos and complexity — Can it help us understand mood and behavior? *Arch. Gen. Psychiatry*, 1995, 52: 960-964.

El Yacoubi M, Costentin J, Vaugeois JM, Adenosine A_{2A} receptors and depression, *Neurology*. 2003; 61(11 Suppl 6): S82-S87

Fell J, Roschke J, Grozinger M, Hinrichs H, Heinze H, Alterations of continuous MEG measures during mental activities. *Neuropsychobiology* 2000;42:99-106

Fink G. Oestrogen-serotonin link: effects on mood, mental state and memory. *Presentation at 1st World Congress on Women's Mental Health;* March 27-31, 2001; Berlin, Germany.

Frank E, Wright EH, Serdula MK, Elon LK, Baldwin G; Personal and professional nutrition-related practices of US female physicians; *Am J Clin Nutr*. 2002, 75: 326-32.

French, R. M & Thomas, E. The Dynamical Hypothesis: One Battle Behind. (Commentary), *TheBehavior and Brain Sciences,* 1998, *21*(5): 640-641

French, R. M & Thomas, E. The Dynamical Hypothesis: One Battle Behind. (Commentary), *TheBehavior and Brain Sciences,* 1998, *21*(5): 640-641

Goldstein JM, Lewine RRJ. Overview of sex differences in schizophrenia: where have we been and where do we go from here? In: Castle D, McGrath J, Kulkarni J, eds. *Women and Schizophrenia*. Cambridge, UK: Cambridge University Press; 2000.

Grigoriadis S, Seeman MV, The role of estrogen in schizophrenia: implications for schizophrenia practice guidelines for women, *Can J Psychiatry*. 2002, 47: 437-42

Gustafson, D. *et al*. An 18-Year Follow-Up of Overweight and Risk of Alzheimer's Disease. *Archives of Internal Medicine*, 2003, 163, 1524 - 1524.

Hafner H, Maurer K, Loffler W, *et al,* The ABC Schizophrenia Study: a preliminary overview of the results. *Soc Psychiatry Psychiatr Epidemiol.* 1998; 33: 380-386.

Hamalainen E, Adlercreutz H, Puska P, Pietinen P; Diet and serum sex hormones in healthy men. *J Steroid Biochem,* 1984, 20: 459-464.

Hammond G, The Cartesian Theory: Unification of Eysenck and Gray, *New Ideas In Psychology*, 1994, 12: 153-167

Hampson, E. & Moffat, S.D. (1994) Is testosterone related to spatial cognition and hand preference in humans? *Brain and Cognition* 26: 258 - 262

Harnad, S., Connecting Object to Symbol in Modeling Cognition. In, Clark A and Lutz R, Eds, *Connectionism in Context,* Springer Verlag, 1992: 75-90

Horne JA, Human Sleep, Sleep Loss and Behavior, Implications for the Prefrontal Cortex and Psychiatric Disorders, *Brit. J Psychiatry*, 1993, 162:413 – 419.

Hunkin NM, Mayes AR, Williams SC, Gregory LJ, Nunn JA, Nicholas AK, Brammer MJ, Bullmore ET, Does frontal lobe activation during retrieval reflect complexity of retrieved information? *Neuroreport* 2000;11:557-561

Jell SA and Shannahoff Khalsa DS, The effects of unilateral forced nostril breathing on cognitive performance, *Intern. J Neurosci.*, 1993, 73: 61 – 68

Jelles B, Strijers RL, Hooijer C, Jonker C, Stam CJ, Jonkman EJ; Nonlinear EEG analysis in early Alzheimer's disease, *Acta Neurol Scand* 1999 Dec; 100(6):360-8

Jeong J, Chae JH, Kim SY, Han SH.; Nonlinear dynamic analysis of the EEG in patients with Alzheimer's disease and vascular dementia, *J Clin Neurophysiol* 2001 Jan;18(1):58-67

Jeong J, Chae JH, Kim SY, Han SH.; Nonlinear dynamic analysis of the EEG in patients with Alzheimer's disease and vascular dementia, *J Clin Neurophysiol* 2001 Jan;18(1):58-67

Kinon B. Prevalence of hyperprolactinemia in a large cohort of schizophrenic patients treated with conventional antipsychotic drugs or risperidone [abstr S185]. *Archives of Women's Mental Health.* 2001; 3 (Suppl 2): 41.

Kowalski JW, Gawel M, Pfeffer A, Barcikowska M, The diagnostic value of EEG in Alzheimer disease: correlation with the severity of mental impairment, *J Clin Neurophysiol.* 2001; 18: 570-5

Kulkarni J. Clinical adjunctive trials of estrogen in women with schizophrenia. *Presentation at 1st World Congress on Women's Mental Health;* March 27-31, 2001a; Berlin, Germany.

Kulkarni J. Gender differences in the quality of life of people with schizophrenia. *Presentation at 1st World Congress on Women's Mental Health*; March 27-31, 2001b; Berlin, Germany.

Lamberts J *et al*, Correlation dimension of the human electroencephalogram corresponds with cognitive load, *Neuropsychobiology*, 2000, 41: 149-153.

Lamberts J *et al*, Correlation dimension of the human electroencephalogram corresponds with cognitive load, *Neuropsychobiology*, 2000, 41: 149-153.

Liebovitch L S, *Fractals and chaos simplified for the life sciences*, Oxford University Press, New York, 1998

Lyoo IK, Kwon JS, Lee SJ, Han MH, Chang CG, Seo CS, Lee SI, Renshaw PF; Decrease in genu of the corpus callosum in medication-naive, early-onset dysthymia and depressive personality disorder, *Biol Psychiatry.* 2002; 52: 1134-43.

Mandal M.K., Asthana H.S., Pandey R & Sarbadhikari S. ; Cerebral Laterality in Affect and Affective Illness : A Review, *J. Psychology*, 1996, 130(4): 447 – 459

Mandal, M.K., Bulman-Fleming, B., & Tiwari, G; Eds, *Side bias — A Neuropsychological Perspective.* Kluwer Intl. Publishers, The Netherlands, 2000.

Mason RA and Just MA, How the Brain Processes Causal Inferences in Text: A Theoretical Account of Generation and Integration Component Processes Utilizing Both Cerebral Hemispheres, *Psychological Science*, 2004, 15: 1-7.

Mason RA and Just MA, How the brain processes causal inferences in text: A theoretical account of generation and integration component processes utilizing both cerebral hemispheres, *Psychological Science*, 2004, 15: 1–10

McGorry P. Early psychosis – gender aspects of treatment. *Presentation at 1st World Congress on Women's Mental Health*; March 27-31, 2001; Berlin, Germany.

Melancon G, Joanette Y & Belair J; Chaos, Brain & Cognition: Toward a nonlinear order ?, *Brain & Cognition*, 2000, 42: 33-36.

Morris MC, Evans DA, Bienias JL, *et al,* Fish consumption and ω-3 fatty acids and risk of incident Alzheimer's disease. *Arch Neurol.* 2003; 60: 940-946.

Morris MC, Evans DA, Bienias JL, *et al,* Dietary intake of antioxidant nutrients and the risk of incident Alzheimer's disease in a biracial community study. *JAMA.* 2002; 287: 3230-3237.

Nagaratnam N, Phan TA, Barnett C, Ibrahim N, Angular gyrus syndrome mimicking depressive pseudodementia, *J Psychiatry Neurosci.* 2002, 27: 364-8

Nagaratnam N, Phan TA, Barnett C, Ibrahim N, Angular gyrus syndrome mimicking depressive pseudodementia, *J Psychiatry Neurosci.* 2002; 27: 364-8

Neveu PJ, Merlot E; Cytokine stress responses depend on lateralization in mice, *Stress*. 2003; 6: 5-9

Nouguier-Soule J, Nouguier J, Bicakova-Rocher A, Gorceix A, Reinberg A, Utilization of a self-contained psychometry-oriented device, for study of affective and cognitive function of a subject, *Encephale* 1999, 25:110-7

Nyström C, Matousek M & Hällström T,Relationships between EEG and clinical characteristics in major depressive disorder, *Acta Psychiatr. Scand.*,1986,73: 390 – 394

Ogden-Epker M, Cullum CM, Quantitative and qualitative interpretation of neuropsychological data in the assessment of temporal lobectomy candidates, *Clin Neuropsychol.* 2001; 15: 183-95

Ouyang WC, Wang YC, Hong CJ, Tsai SJ, Estrogen receptor alpha gene polymorphism in schizophrenia: frequency, age at onset, symptomatology and prognosis. *Psychiatr Genet.* 2001, 11: 95-8

Papo D, Baudonniere PM, Hugueville L, Caverni JP, Feedback in hypothesis testing: an ERP study, *J Cogn Neurosci*. 2003; 15: 508-22

Pennington BF, van Doorninck WJ, McCabe LL, McCabe ER, Neuropsychological deficits in early treated phenylketonuric children, *Am J Ment Defic*. 1985; 89: 467-474.

Perry RJ, Rosen HR, Kramer JH, Beer JS, Levenson RL, Miller BL, Hemispheric dominance for emotions, empathy and social behaviour: evidence from right and left handers with frontotemporal dementia, *Neurocase*. 2001; 7: 145-60

Ramirez M, Arechaga G, Martinez JM, Prieto I, Ramirez-Exposito MJ, Sanchez B, Alba F, Environmental light-darkness conditions induce changes in brain and peripheral pyroglutamyl-peptidase I activity, *Neurochem Res.* 2001; 26: 463-8

Reddy H, De Stefano N, Mortilla M, Federico A, Matthews PM, Functional reorganization of motor cortex increases with greater axonal injury from CADASIL, *Stroke*. 2002; 33: 502-8

Riecher-Rossler A. Oestrogens and schizophrenia -- a brief overview. *Presentation at 1st World Congress on Women's Mental Health*; March 27-31, 2001; Berlin, Germany.

Rossi EL, The Feigenbaum scenario as a model of the limits of conscious information processing, *Biosystems* 1998; 46: 113-22

Sarbadhikari SN, Balancing the Brain Activity: Putative links between Epileptic, Cognitive and Affective Disorders, In Benjamin SM, Ed, *Focus on Epilepsy Research*, Nova Science Publishers, Hauppauge, USA, 2004: 309 – 367.

Sarbadhikari S.N. & Pal S.K.; Automated Techniques for identifying depression from EEG, In, Leondes C T, Ed, *Handbook of Computational Methods in Biomaterials, Biotechnology & Biomedical systems*, Kluwer Academic Publishers, 2002, Vol. 4, Chapter 3: 51–81.

Sarbadhikari S.N. & Chakrabarty K, Chaos in the brain: a short review alluding to epilepsy, depression, exercise and lateralization, *Med. Eng. Phys*, 2001, 23(7): 445–455.

Sarbadhikari SN. Neural network aided analysis of electrophysiological signals from brain of an animal model of depression subjected to chronic physical exercise. *Ph D Thesis,* Banaras Hindu University, India 1995a:1-2

Sarbadhikari S N, Medical Informatics – Are the doctors ready? *J. Indian Med. Assoc.*, 1995b, 93: 165 – 166.

Sarbadhikari S.N. A neural network confirms that exercise reverses EEG changes in depressed rats, *Med. Eng. Phys.*, 1995c, 17: 579-582.

Schellenberg R, Todorova A, Wedekind W, Schober F, Dimpfel W, Pathophysiology and psychopharmacology of dementia--a new study design. 2. Cyclandelate treatment – a placebo-controlled double-blind clinical trial, *Neuropsychobiology* 1997; 35: 132-42

Shagass C, Roemer RA & Josiassen RC, Some quantitative EEG findings in unmedicated and medicated major depressives, *Neuropsychobiology*, 1988, 19: 169 – 175.

Shenal BV, Harrison DW, Demaree HA, The neuropsychology of depression: a literature review and preliminary model, *Neuropsychol Rev.* 2003; 13: 33-42

Stam CJ, Jelles B, Achtereekte HA, van Birgelen JH, Slaets JP, Diagnostic usefulness of linear and nonlinear quantitative EEG analysis in Alzheimer's disease. *Clin Electroencephalogr* 1996, 27:69-77

Svenningsson, P. *et al.* Diverse psychotomimetics act through a common signalling pathway. *Science*, 302, 1412 - 1415, (2003).

Tallberg IM, Persson H, Wangmar L, Wahlund LO, Almkvist O, Semantic range and relevance of emotive utterances in patients with frontotemporal degeneration, *Brain Lang.* 2002; 82: 146-58

Tkachev D, *et al*, Oligodendrocyte dysfunction in schizophrenia and bipolar disorder, *Lancet*, 2003, 362: 798 – 805.

Toro MG, Ruiz JS, Talavera JA, Blanco C, Chaos theories and therapeutic commonalities among depression, Parkinson's disease, and cardiac arrhythmias. *Compr Psychiatry* 1999 40:238-244.

Usall J, *et al*, Influence of gender on social outcome in schizophrenia, *Acta Psychiatr Scand.* 2002, 106: 337-42.

Walker SF, Lateralization of functions in the vertebrate brain: A review, *Brit. J Psychol.*, 1980, 71: 329 – 367.

WHO, *International Statistical Classification of Diseases and Related Health Problems*, Tenth revision, (ICD-10), World Health Organization, Geneva, 1992

Zanetti O, Vallotti B, Frisoni GB, Geroldi C, Bianchetti A, Pasqualetti P, Trabucchi M; Insight in dementia: when does it occur? Evidence for a nonlinear relationship between insight and cognitive status, *J Gerontol B Psychol Sci Soc Sci* 1999 Mar; 54(2):P100-6

In: Depression and Dementia
Editor: Suptendra Nath Sarbadhikari, p. 85-95
ISBN 1-59454-114-0

Chapter 4

BIOMARKER EPIDEMIOLOGY OF DEPRESSION – POPULATION BASED EVIDENCES OF NEUROCHEMICAL AND GENETIC ABNORMALITIES

Amit Chakrabarti
Associate Professor
Department of Pharmacology
Sikkim Manipal Institute of Medical Sciences
5th Mile. Tadong
Gangtok – 737 102
Sikkim, India
Tel: +91-3592-270598
Fax: +91-3592-231147
e-mail: amitchakrabarti@hotmail.com,
amitchakrabarti@sancharnet.in

ABSTRACT

Depression is associated with significant morbidity and mortality spread over a wide age range. Diagnosis and estimation of prevalence of depression in the community are carried out by Diagnostic and Statistical Manual of Mental Disorders, fourth edition (DSM-IV) and International Statistical Classification of Diseases and Related Health Problems, 10th revision (ICD-10) based diagnostic criteria. However, these diagnostic tools are not adequate for estimation of susceptibility and vulnerability of a subset of population depression, so that preventive interventions could be initiated at an early age. A more accurate prediction of susceptibility to depression can be carried out by correlation of life events with biomarker epidemiologic observations, which can estimate presence of certain biochemical and genetic alterations in the susceptible individuals detectable before the onset of the disease. Population based studies have demonstrated that life events like stress and child abuse are associated with markedly elevated rates of major depression (MDD) in child, adolescent and adult cohorts. Studies have also demonstrated that stress early in life can alter the development of multiple neurotransmitter systems and promote structural and functional alterations in brain regions similar to those seen in adults with depression. Clinical studies, also, suggest that long-term neurobiological changes associated with early stress can be modified by familial / genetic factors, the quality of the subsequent care giving environment, and appropriate pharmacological interventions. There is compelling evidence that the serotonergic system, involved in depression, is partly under genetic control and further unknown genetic factors mediate the risk for suicidal behavior independently of the genetic factors responsible for the hereditary factors of MDD associated with suicide. This review will examine currently available neurochemical and genetic evidences and their possible correlation with life events from population based studies, which could be useful in screening for susceptibility to depression.

Key Words: Depression, Epidemiology, Prevalence, Biomarker, Genetic, Screening

INTRODUCTION

Depression has important public health impact because of its chronic and disabling nature. Based on findings of the National Institute of Mental Health (NIMH) supported 1981 Epidemiologic Catchment Area (ECA) Study in the United States, one of the largest community-based surveys on mental health, lifetime prevalence of any affective disorder in the age range of 18 – 54 years has been estimated 9.3% [1]. Lifetime prevalence of a major depressive episode in the same age group is 7.2% [1]. These figures outline the burden of depression in the community resulting in staggering health care costs and loss of productivity.

Prevention and treatment are the two main approaches to limit public health consequences of mental health disorders. Effective treatment depends on valid and reliable diagnostic criteria. Updated editions of ICD and DSM have provided effective means for diagnosis of mental health disorders. Better diagnosis has helped in improving standards of treatment over the years. However, prevention of depression needs valid and reliable screening criteria. If susceptibility to depression can be estimated more precisely, it will lead to better directed preventive efforts. Better prevention will lead to fewer requirements for treatment. This will not only reduce burden of the disease in the community, but also will save health care costs. Advances in epidemiologic methods have helped in better understanding of natural history of depression and thereby proper identification of risk factors. Natural history and risk factors are two key components in screening for susceptibility to depression. However, estimating susceptibility can be made more objective by incorporating biochemical and genetic predictors. Addition of these parameters to life events may evolve in to a better screening method for susceptibility to depression.

Biomarker epidemiology is a comparatively newer advance in epidemiology [2]. This branch of epidemiology helps in trait analysis by identifying biomarkers in population based studies. Biomarkers could be any biologic compound present / absent / altered in the susceptible population as a marker of susceptibility to a particular disease. It could also be represented by alterations in the genetic constituency when the term genetic epidemiology is more appropriately used. Depression is associated with neurobiological and genetic changes. It will be possible to make more valid and reliable diagnosis of susceptibility to depression when key life events identified from natural history and risk factors are corroborated with biomarker evidences of trait to susceptibility.

This review will examine recent evidences of neurobiological and genetic linkages to depression in population based studies and delineate any correlation between them and life events.

NATURAL HISTORY OF DEPRESSION

The 1981 ECA study and the 1991 National Comorbidity Survey (NCS) [3] conducted at various sites in the US had been the two largest community based surveys to estimate the prevalence and distribution of mental diseases in the community. Both ECA and NCS have demonstrated a maximum lifetime prevalence of major depression among males below the age of 45 years and onset of incidence as early as in the age of 15 years. The same age trend has been observed in females, although the prevalence of major depression has been higher in females (Odds ratio 1.36, 95% Confidence interval 1.01 – 1.84, $p<0.05$) [3] than in males.

Race and ethnicity did not seem to exert a significance influence on incidence of depression. Evidences suggest that cultural, social and religious customs account for variations in the presentation of depression across cultures. Feelings of guilt and suicide rates vary across cultures and depression may be underdiagnosed [4]. This observation gives a clue that prevalence of depression could be influenced by cultural differences and differences in risk factors across the countries. Income inequality was significantly associated with depression among older Americans. Those living in counties with higher income inequality were more depressed, independent of their demographic characteristics and physical health [5].

Women are more vulnerable to depression and a number of epidemiological studies conducted in different countries examined risk factors of depression in women. To investigate the social and cultural risk factors of postnatal depression using ethnographically informed epidemiological methods a total of 959 women were assessed at their first ante-partum visit (baseline), in the third trimester, immediately after delivery, and 3 months postpartum. Six domains of risk factors were examined. The dependent variable was postnatal depression (as defined by the Edinburgh Postnatal Depression Scale) at 3 months postpartum. Conflict with mother-in-law, marital dissatisfaction, past depression and antenatal depression independently predicted the occurrence of postnatal depression [6].

To examine the relation between birth weights and risk of depression a cohort of 5187 participants at age 16 years in the 1970 British Cohort Study completed the 12-item General Health Questionnaire to assess psychological distress. At age 26 years 8292 participants completed the Malaise Inventory to assess depression and provided information about a history of depression. Women whose birth weight was </=3 kg had an increased risk of depression at age 26 years compared with those who weighed >3.5 kg. Birth weight was not associated with a reported history of depression at age 16 years. In men there were no associations between any measurement and the full range of birth weight but, compared with men of normal birth weight, those born weighing </=2.5 kg were more likely to be depressed at age 16 years and to report a history of depression at age 26 years [7].

Significant studies on natural history and risk factors of depression have come from Iran and Pakistan, providing insights on influence of cultures on risk factors. In a mental health survey conducted in Iran prevalence of depression increased with age and was higher in the married, widowed, divorced, unemployed and retired people. Prevalence rates were comparable with international studies. There was a wide regional difference in the country, and women were found to be at greater risk [8]. In Pakistan 8.66% (1248) out of 14,400 patients of psychiatric disorders presented with postpartum disorders. 60% out of these 1248 had post partum psychoses while the rest had postpartum depression. The majority of our patients with postpartum depression were young (20 – 31 years), illiterate (80%), having past history of psychoses / depression (70%), housewives (95%), from rural areas (65%), highly religious (60%), poor (90%), with husband away for job (70%), primipara (80%) and with a live baby born (70%). Significantly a number of stressors were identified in 65% of subjects [9].

Neurochemical Predictors of Depression

Recent research into depression has focused on the involvement of long term intracellular processes, leading to abnormal neuronal mechanisms. Accumulating evidence suggests that brain serotonin (5-HT) pathways play an important role in the neurobiology of depression. Several promising hypotheses regarding etiopathogenesis of depression have been formulated recently. These hypotheses are based largely on evidences of dysregulation of the hypothalamic-pituitary-adrenal (HPA) axis and hippocampus and implicate corticotrophin releasing factor (CRF), glucocorticoids and brain derived neurotrophic factor. Recent work has looked beyond hippocampus to other brain areas that are also likely to be involved. For example, nucleus accumbens, amygdala, and certain hypothalamic nuclei are critical in regulating motivation, eating, sleeping, energy level, circadian rhythm, and responses to rewarding and aversive stimuli, which are all abnormal in depressed patients.

Of late there have been a few path breaking studies regarding identification of neurochemical markers for trait analysis of depression. In light of the postulated role of thyrotropin releasing hormone (TRH) as an endogenous antidepressant, 56 refractory mood-disordered patients and 34 healthy adult control subjects underwent lumbar puncture for cerebrospinal fluid (CSF) TRH analysis. By two way analysis of variance (ANOVA), there was no difference between CSF TRH in patients (as a group or by diagnostic subtype) and control subjects ($n = 90$, $F = 0.91$, $df = 2.84$, $p = 0.41$). There was, however, a CSF TRH gender difference (females, 2.95 pg/ml; males, 3.98 pg/ml; $n = 90$, $F = 4.11$, $df = 1.84$, $p < 0.05$). A post hoc t-test revealed the greatest gender difference in the bipolar group ($t = 2.52$, $p < 0.02$) [11]. Growth hormone (GH) has also been studied as a marker for depression. Decreased growth hormone (GH) response to pharmacologic stimulation has been found in children and adolescents during an episode of major depressive disorder and after recovery. Similarly the authors sought to examine whether GH secretion is similarly altered in children and adolescents who had never experienced depression but were at high risk of developing depression. Selected subjects were 8 through 16 years of age and selected for high- and low-risk status according to familial loading for mood disorders. 64 high-risk and 55 low-risk healthy subjects participated in the study, which assessed the following GH measures.

(1) GH before growth hormone releasing hormone (GHRH) infusion, every 15 minutes for 30 minutes
(2) GH response after intravenous infusion of GHRH (0.1 ug / kg), every 15 minutes for 90 minutes

(3) Nocturnal GH every 20 minutes from 9 pm until morning awakening

After stimulation with GHRH, the high-risk subjects secreted significantly less GH compared with the low-risk healthy controls (effect sizes for mean and peak GH, 0.52 ($p = 0.007$) and 0.40 ($p = 0.04$), respectively). In contrast, there were no between-group differences in the pre-GHRH and nocturnal GH secretion levels. Significantly exposure to recent stressors was not associated with GH secretion [15]. Taken together with previous evidence of decreased GH after GHRH infusion in acutely depressed and recovered children, these results indicate that the decreased GH response found in high-risk subjects may represent a trait marker for depression in children and adolescents.

The prevalence of depression increases with age, as does the prevalence of higher levels of the cytokine interleukin-6 (IL-6). This analysis was performed to determine the association between increased levels of this cytokine and depression in a population based sample. The association between IL-6 and other biologic variables with self-report depression was examined in 1686 persons aged 70 years and older in the third in-person survey wave (1991) of the Duke Established Population for Epidemiologic Studies of the Elderly (EPESE). Bivariate associations were established by the Spearman correlation, adjusted for age. A stepwise linear logistic regression model was used to derive a final model. Depression was correlated with IL-6 ($p = 0.011$), α-1-globulin ($p = 0.023$), α-2-globulin ($p = 0.002$), and β-globulin ($p = 0.012$). After controlling for age, race, and gender, IL-6 levels remained the only biologic variable significantly associated with depression ($p = 0.035$). These results are compatible with the hypothesis of cytokine (IL-6) stimulation in geriatric depression as part of an overall immunoendocrine dysregulation [16]. Another significant study examined the association between rheumatic fever and psychiatric illnesses in children using biomarker approach. An immunological marker associated with rheumatic fever (monoclonal antibody D8/17) has been reported to be elevated in several neuropsychiatric disorders, most frequently tics and obsessive compulsive disorder (OCD). This association was examined in a community sample of children previously identified as being D8/17 positive or negative. It was hypothesized that D8/17 positivity would predict increased rates of tics and OCD. Possible associations with other disorders, e.g., chorea--hyperactivity, anxiety, and depression, also were explored. In a 2- to 5-year follow-up of 240 of these children (108 positive and 132 negative), structured psychiatric interviews and rating scales were administered to the child and main caretaker. Assessments were conducted and scored blind to the child's D8/17 status. No association was seen between D8/17 positivity and tics or OCD and the study failed to provide support for the generalized use of D8/17 as a marker of susceptibility to psychiatric disorders in children in a community sample [12]. There is some evidence that major depression is accompanied by activation of the inflammatory response system (IRS). There is also evidence that pro-inflammatory cytokines and induction of IRS activation are associated with behavioural disturbances in experimental animals. One study was to examine possible immunological differences between major depression, somatization and healthy controls. IRS variables of interleukin-6 (IL-6), interleukin 1 receptor antagonist (IL-1RA), plasma soluble interleukin-6 receptor (IL-6R), soluble suppressor / cytotoxic antigen (CD8), leukemia inhibitory factor (LIF-R), and Clara cell protein (CC16), an endogenous anticytokine were measured in patients with major depression ($n = 36$), somatization syndrome ($n = 37$), major depression & somatization ($n = 40$) and healthy controls ($n=37$). Of significant findings serum CD8 & IL-6 concentrations were significantly increased and serum CC16 concentrations were significantly reduced, in patients with major depression. Results indicated an activation of the IRS in depression with signs of T cell activation (increased CD8), monocytic activation (IL-1RA) and a lowered anti-inflammatory capacity of the serum (lower CC16) [13].

Thyroperoxidase antibodies (TPOAbs) have also been investigated during pregnancy as a possible marker for depression in the first year postpartum, particularly in relation to thyroid dysfunction and other determinants of depression. A cohort of 310 unselected women (residing in the Kempen Region, southeastern Netherlands) was visited at 12 and 32 week's gestation and at 4, 12, 20, 28 and 36 weeks postpartum. At each visit, TSH, free thyroxine and TPOAb testing was performed, determinants associated with depression were asked for, and depression was assessed (according to the Research Diagnostic Criteria). Multiple logistic regression was performed to determine independent risk factors for depression in gestation and / or postpartum depression. 41 women (14.1%) had TPOAbs at one or more time points and 117 women (40.1%) had depression at one or more time points postpartum. The multiple logistic regression analysis showed that TPOAbs were independently associated with depression at 12 weeks gestation and at 4 and 12 weeks postpartum (Odds ratio, 95% Confidence interval: 2.4 (1.1 – 6.0), 3.8 (1.3 – 7.3) and 3.6 (1.2 – 7.1) respectively). The authors concluded that the presence of TPOAbs during gestation is associated with the occurrence of subsequent depression during the postpartum period and as such can be regarded as a marker for depression [14]. There was another study investigating plasma folate levels in a Chinese population sample. However, the study failed to elicit a correlation between plasma folate level and depression [17].

Genetic Evidences of Depression

A neurobiologic understanding of depression also requires identification of the genes that make individuals vulnerable or resistant to the syndrome. Although genetic epidemiological studies of bipolar (BP) illness are consistent with a heritable component, inherited risk factors remain unknown. In one study the localization of BP susceptibility loci was investigated through linkage strategies, including a genome wide search. The linkage study included 22 BP families comprising almost 400 persons, 173 of whom have been diagnosed as having BP I, schizoaffective, BP II with major depression, or recurrent unipolar illness. Using an autosomal dominant disease model with 85% or 50% age dependent penetrance, and a recessive model with 85% penetrance, linkage analyses were performed assuming a narrow (BP and schizoaffective) or a broad (BP, schizoaffective, or unipolar) definition of the BP spectrum. Affected sibling pairs and affected pedigree member analyses were also performed. Linkage analysis of 310 DNA markers on chromosomes 1, 5p, 6, 8, 10q, 11q, and 12 to 18 was carried out. None of the loci examined disclosed compelling evidence for linkage. Analysis by multilocus affected pedigree member method in the pericentromeric chromosome 18 region disclosed statistically significant evidence ($p < 0.0001$) for a BP susceptibility gene in this region. Multilocus analysis by affected sibling pair method also disclosed evidence for linkage ($p < 0.00008$). Findings from this study implied that in BP susceptibility gene exists near the centromere of chromosome 18. Confirmation of this finding (by independent investigators studying different pedigrees) has been published, suggesting that a valid BP disease linkage may have been discovered [18].

There are different diagnostic variants of depression. Manic depression is a severe cyclic mental illness that can be unipolar or bipolar and has a lifetime risk of approximately 7 per 1,000 in most populations. Families with multiple cases of manic depression have been described that are compatible with both autosomal dominant and X-linked modes of genetic transmission. Psychoactive antidepressant and stimulant drugs that help to ameliorate depression and mania are thought to act by affecting catecholamine neurotransmitter systems such as adrenaline, noradrenaline and 5-HT. Mutations affecting the tyrosine hydroxylase (TH) gene, which encodes the rate limiting enzyme for the synthesis of these three neurotransmitters, might therefore be responsible for causing the manic depressive phenotype. In a genetic study involving three Icelandic kindreds among whom it appeared that a single autosomal dominant disease allele is segregating, there were 44 cases among 73 individuals at risk. Genetic linkage studies were carried out using clones encoding tyrosine hydroxylase in the variable portion of the Harvey-ras-1 (HRAS1) locus and the variable region of the insulin gene (INS). All three markers are closely linked on chromosome 11 and were used to observe the segregation of restriction fragment length polymorphisms (RFLPs) in the three affected kindreds. No evidence for linkage to these markers in any of the three families was found. In contrast, Ginns et. al., [21] found linkage between manic depression and HRAS1 in a single large Amish kindred. The authors concluded that there is genetic heterogeneity of linkage in manic depression. Therefore, mutations at different loci are responsible for the manic depressive phenotype in the Amish and in Iceland [19].

Attempts were made to follow up results of a previous linkage study, which suggested that a locus modifying susceptibility to bipolar and related unipolar affective disorder might be present in the pericentromeric region of the short arm of chromosome 18. 23 multiply affected pedigrees collected from Iceland and the UK were genotyped using three highly polymorphic microsatellite markers at D18S37, D18S40 and D18S44 which span the region implicated. Analysis allowing for heterogeneity did not suggest that any subgroup of the families was linked. Model free linkage analysis using extended relative pair analysis and MFLINK also failed to detect any evidence for linkage. The study concluded that there is no support for the presence of a locus-modifying genetic susceptibility to bipolar affective disorder in the pericentromeric region of chromosome 18q11. Further analyses in independent samples should help to reveal whether these negative results are due to locus heterogeneity or whether the original results were false-positive [20].

Bipolar affective disorder (BPAD; manic depressive illness) is characterized by episodes of mania and / or hypomania interspersed with periods of depression. Compelling evidence supports a significant genetic component in the susceptibility to develop BPAD. To date, however, linkage studies have attempted only to identify chromosomal loci that cause or increase the risk of developing BPAD. To determine whether there could be protective alleles that prevent or reduce the risk of developing BPAD, similar to what is observed in other genetic disorders, a mental health wellness (absence of any psychiatric disorder) as the phenotype was used in a genome wide linkage scan of several large multigeneration Old Order Amish community in Pennsylvania, USA pedigrees exhibiting an extremely high incidence of BPAD. A strong evidence was detected for a locus on chromosome 4p at D4S2949 and suggestive evidence for a locus on chromosome 4q at D4S397 that are linked to mental health wellness. These findings are consistent with the hypothesis that certain alleles could prevent or modify the clinical manifestations of BPAD and perhaps other related affective disorders [21].

Another study was carried out to in a Korean population to verify the relationship between major depression and cytotoxic T lymphocyte antigen-4 (CTLA-4), which is related to immunological function such as T-cell regulation. Among the Korean patients diagnosed with major depression according to DSM-IV, 77 patients without neurological illness, hormonal disorder, or comorbid mental illness were selected. The stored data on 149 normal Koreans from the Catholic Hemopoietic Stem Cell Bank of Korea, were used as a control group. The data of the Korean control group were compared with those of the studies of different ethnic groups. There were significant differences in frequencies of CTLA-4 allele (Chi square = 56.472, df = 1, p = 0.001) and genotype (Chi square = 46.132, df = 2, p = 0.001) between the Korean population and the Caucasian population. However, there were no significant differences between the Korean and the Japanese population. There were no significant differences in genotype frequencies of CTLA-4*G/G, CTLA-4*G/A, and CTLA-4*A/A between the patients with major depression and the control group in the Korean population (48.1% vs. 46.3%, 41.6% vs 39.6%, 10.3% vs. 14.1%, respectively). There were no significant differences in allelic frequencies of CTLA-4*G and CTLA-4*A between the patients with major depression and the control group in the Korean population (68.8% vs. 66.1%, 31.2% vs. 33.9%, respectively). Although the present study produced negative results for the association of exon 1 polymorphism of CTLA-4 gene with major depression in the Korean population, further systematic research, including diverse clinical variables, would be necessary [22].

In a Finish study population the X-chromosomal region was further analyzed using a denser marker map and monitored X-chromosomal haplotypes in a study sample of 41 Finnish bipolar families. Only a fraction of the families provided any evidence of linkage to this region, suggesting that a relatively rare gene predisposing to bipolar disorder (BPD) is enriched in this linked pedigree. The genome wide scan for BPD predisposing loci in this large pedigree indicated that this particular X-chromosomal region provides the best evidence of linkage genome wide, suggesting an X-chromosomal gene with a major role for the genetic predisposition of BPD in this family [23].

Influence of Life Events on Biomarker Predictors in Depression

Of late a number of gene environment interaction studies and studies on role of stress in early childhood on development of depression in adult life have tried to highlight interaction of biomarker abnormalities with life events.

One study aimed to separate genetic from environmental factors in the etiology of depression spectrum disease, a type of major depression characterized by families in which male relatives are alcoholic and females are depressed. The genetic etiology hypothesis of depression spectrum disease proposes that an alcoholic genetic diathesis predisposes to depression in females but alcoholism, not depression, in males. The study examined 197 adult offspring (95 male and 102 female) of alcoholic biological parents and used logistic regression models to determine the contribution to major depression in male and female adoptees that could be explained by the genetic alcoholic diathesis combined with an environmental factor that was characterized by psychiatrically or behaviorally disturbed adoptive parents. Results showed that major depression in females was predicted by an alcoholic diathesis only when combined with the disturbed adoptive parent variable. The same regression model failed to predict depression in males. Other possible environmental confounding factors contributing to an increased chance of depression were found in females – fetal alcohol exposure, age at the time of adoption, and a family with an adopted sibling who had a psychiatric problem. These variables did not diminish the significance of the prediction of depression with the alcohol genetic diathesis and disturbed parent model. This study demonstrated that a genetic factor is present for which alcoholism is at least a marker, and, which exerts its effect in women as a gene environment interaction leading to major depression. This finding suggests that an important etiologic factor in depression spectrum disease is gene environment interaction [24].

Early stress is associated with long term alterations in brain circuits and systems that mediate the stress response. Early stressors have lasting effects on the HPA axis and norepinephrine systems. Other brain systems that are involved include benzodiazepine, opiate, dopaminergic and various neuropeptide systems. These neurochemical systems modulate function in brain regions, including the hippocampus, amygdala and prefrontal cortex. Long term alterations in these brain regions are hypothesized to play a role in the pathogenesis of depression and related psychiatric disorders after childhood abuse [25]. The first stage of the this proposed cascade involves the stress induced programming of the glucocorticoid, noradrenergic and vasopressin oxytocin stress response systems to augment stress responses. These neurotransmitters then produce effects on neurogenesis, synaptic overproduction & pruning and myelination during specific sensitive periods. Major consequences of these include reduced size of the mid-portions of the corpus callosum, attenuated development of the left neocortex, hippocampus and amygdala along with abnormal frontotemporal electrical activity and reduced functional activity of the cerebellar vermis. These alterations, in turn, provide the neurobiological framework through which early abuse increases the risk of depression.

CONCLUSION

Effective prevention of depression requires concerted knowledge about biochemical changes and life events effecting those changes. To date there are compelling evidences that stress in early life is a major trigger of depression in late childhood and early adulthood. Moreover, early life stress sets a chain of events, which result in neurobiological changes including structural alterations in the brain. These neurobiological changes are manifested as biomarkers, which may provide evidence to susceptibility to depression. So far, hormone markers and various immunologic markers have been proposed as putative markers of trait analysis in depression. These markers have also shown age and sex specificity, e.g., GH markers for childhood depression, thyroid markers for postpartum depression and immunologic markers for depression in the elderly.

Evidences are also emerging that some of these markers could be under genetic influence particularly, immunologic markers, which provide direction to an interesting interaction between life events, biomarkers and genetic predispositions. A further advance in this direction will be to find out any correlation between risk factors, biomarker and genetic changes providing an objective evidence in assessing susceptibility to depression.

REFERENCES

[1] Eaton WW, Kramer M, Anthony JC, Dryman A, Shapiro S, Locke BZ. The incidence of specific DIS/DSM-III mental disorders. Data from the NIMH Epidemiologic Catchment Area Program. *Acta Psychiatr Scand* 1989;79:163.

[2] Menninger JA, Baron AE, Conigrave KM, Whitfield JB, Saunders JB, Helander A, Eriksson CJ, Grant B, Hoffman PL, Tabakoff B. Platelet adenylyl cyclase activity as a trait marker of alcohol dependence. WHO / ISBRA Collaborative Study Investigators. International Society for Biomedical Research on Alcoholism. *Alcohol Clin Exp Res* 2000;24:810.

[3] Blazer DG, Kessler RC, McGonagle KA, Swartz MS. The prevalence and distribution of major depression in national community sample: The National Comorbidity Survey. *Am J Psychiatry* 1994;151:979.

[4] Bhugra D, Mastrogianni A. Globalisation and mental disorders. Overview with relation to depression. *Br J Psychiatry* 2004;184:10.

[5] Muramatsu N. County-level income inequality and depression among older Americans. *Health Serv Res* 2003;38:1863.

[6] Lee DT, Yip AS, Leung TY, Chung TK. Ethnoepidemiology of postnatal depression. Prospective multivariate study of sociocultural risk factors in a Chinese population in Hong Kong. *Br J Psychiatry* 2004;184:34.

[7] Gale CR, Martyn CN. Birth weight and later risk of depression in a national birth cohort. *Br J Psychiatry* 2004;184:28.

[8] Noorbala AA, Bagheri Yazdi SA, Yasamy MT, Mohammad K. Mental health survey of the adult population in Iran. *Br J Psychiatry* 2004;184:70.

[9] Irfan N, Badar A. Determinants and pattern of postpartum psychological disorders in Hazara division of Pakistan. *J Ayub Med Coll Abbottabad* 2003;15:19.

[10] Nestler EJ, Barrot M, DiLeone RJ, Eisch AJ, Gold SJ, Monteggia LM. Neurobiology of depression. *Neuron* 2002;34:13.

[11] Frye MA, Gary KA, Marangell LB, George MS, Callahan AM, Little JT, Huggins T, Cora-Locatelli G, Osuch EA, Winokur A, Post RM. CSF thyrotropin releasing hormone gender difference: implications for neurobiology and treatment of depression. *J Neuropsychiatry Clin Neurosci* 1999;11:349.

[12] Inoff-Germain G, Rodriguez RS, Torres-Alcantara S, Diaz-Jimenez MJ, Swedo SE, Rapoport JL. An immunological marker (D8/17) associated with rheumatic fever as a predictor of childhood psychiatric disorders in a community sample. *J Child Psychol Psychiatry* 2003;44:782.

[13] Rief W, Pilger F, Ihle D, Bosmans E, Egyed B, Maes M. Immunological differences between patients with major depression and somatization syndrome. *Psychiatry Res* 2001;105:165.

[14] Kuijpens JL, Vader HL, Drexhage HA, Wiersinga WM, van Son MJ, Pop VJ. Thyroid peroxidase antibodies during gestation are a marker for subsequent depression postpartum. *Eur J Endocrinol* 2001;145:579.

[15] Birmaher B, Dahl RE, Williamson DE, Perel JM, Brent DA, Axelson DA, Kaufman J, Dorn LD, Stull S, Rao U, Ryan ND. Growth hormone secretion in children and

adolescents at high risk for major depressive disorder. *Arch Gen Psychiatry* 2000;57:867.

[16] Dentino AN, Pieper CF, Rao MK, Currie MS, Harris T, Blazer DG, Cohen HJ. Association of interleukin-6 and other biologic variables with depression in older people living in the community. *J Am Geriatr Soc* 1999;47:6.

[17] Lee S, Wing YK, Fong S. A controlled study of folate levels in Chinese inpatients with major depression in Hong Kong. *J Affect Disord* 1998;49:73.

[18] Berrettini WH, Ferraro TN, Goldin LR, Detera-Wadleigh SD, Choi H, Muniec D, Guroff JJ, Kazuba DM, Nurnberger JI Jr, Hsieh WT, Hoehe MR, Gershon ES. A linkage study of bipolar illness. *Arch Gen Psychiatry* 1997;54:27.

[19] Hodgkinson S, Sherrington R, Gurling H, Marchbanks R, Reeders S, Mallet J, McInnis M, Petursson H, Brynjolfsson J. Molecular genetic evidence for heterogeneity in manic depression. *Nature* 1987;325:805.

[20] Kalsi G, Smyth C, Brynjolfsson J, Sherrington RS, O'Neill J, Curtis D, Rifkin L, Murphy P, Petursson H, Gurling HM. Linkage analysis of manic depression (bipolar affective disorder) in Icelandic and British kindreds using markers on the short arm of chromosome 18. *Hum Hered* 1997;47:268.

[21] Ginns EI, St Jean P, Philibert RA, Galdzicka M, Damschroder-Williams P, Thiel B, et. al. A genome-wide search for chromosomal loci linked to mental health wellness in relatives at high risk for bipolar affective disorder among the Old Order Amish. *Proc Natl Acad Sci U S A* 1998;95:15531.

[22] Jun TY, Pae CU, Chae JH, Bahk WM, Kim KS. Polymorphism of CTLA-4 gene for major depression in the Korean population. *Psychiatry Clin Neurosci* 2001;55:533.

[23] Ekholm JM, Pekkarinen P, Pajukanta P, Kieseppa T, Partonen T, Paunio T, Varilo T, Perola M, Lonnqvist J, Peltonen L. Bipolar disorder susceptibility region on Xq24-q27.1 in Finnish families. *Mol Psychiatry* 2002;7:453.

[24] Cadoret RJ, Winokur G, Langbehn D, Troughton E, Yates WR, Stewart MA. Depression spectrum disease, I: The role of gene-environment interaction. *Am J Psychiatry* 1996;153:892.

[25] Bremner JD. Long-term effects of childhood abuse on brain and neurobiology. *Child Adolesc Psychiatr Clin N A* 2003;12:271.

In: Depression and Dementia
Editor: Suptendra Nath Sarbadhikari, p. 97-152
ISBN 1-59454-114-0

Chapter 5

SELECTIVE NEURONAL VULNERABILITY, BLOOD-BRAIN BARRIER DISRUPTION AND HEAT SHOCK PROTEIN EXPRESSION IN STRESS INDUCED NEURODEGENERATION

Hari Shanker Sharma*
Laboratory of Cerebrovascular Research, Department of Surgical Sciences, Anesthesiology and Intensive Care, University Hospital, Uppsala University, SE-75185 Uppsala, Sweden

ABSTRACT

Stress depending on its magnitude and severity alters neurochemical transmission in the central nervous system (CNS) and induces breakdown of the blood-brain barrier (BBB) leading to Alzheimer's diseases and related neurodegenerative disorders. Expression of heat shock proteins (HSPs) in the CNS is another common finding in stressful situations. Thus, a possible inter-relationship between breakdown of the BBB, HSP expression and neuronal damage appears quite likely. In this review, the functional significance and clinical relevance of the BBB breakdown, HSP expression and selective neuronal injury in stress are discussed based on recent data and our own investigations.

Key words: Stress, psychological stimuli, Alzheimer's disease, fluid microenvironment of the brain, blood-brain barrier, microvascular permeability, heat shock protein, heat stress, cell injury

---

* Address for Correspondence and Reprint requests: Hari Shanker Sharma, Dr Med Sci, Frödingsgatan 12:28, SE-75421 Uppsala, Sweden, Phone & Fax: +46-18-243899, E. mail: sharma@surgsci.uu.se

INTRODUCTION

Stress influences brain function by activating or inhibiting a group of neurones or system within the CNS (Sapolsky 1992). Overexcitation/inhibition of nerve cells during prolonged stress may lead to brain pathology and/or neurodegeneration either directly or through indirect mechanisms involving several hormones and neurotransmitters (Sapolsky 1996b; Sharma and Dey 1988; Sharma et al., 1998a; Sharma 1999; Sharma and Westman 2000). Inadequate handling of stress often results in chronic systemic diseases, e.g., hypertension, affective disorders, viz., depression, post-traumatic stress disorders and neurodegeneration including Alzheimer's disease (McEwen and Stellar 1993; Luine et al., 1994; Kathol et al., 1989; Charney et al., 1993; Landfield and Eldridge 1991; see Herman and Cullinan 1997).

In recent years, our understanding on the stress-induced CNS disorders has been increased. However, the role of microvascular barriers in stress induced brain dysfunction is not well known. Since, the blood-brain barrier (BBB) maintains the fluid microenvironment of the brain (Rapoport 1976; Bradbury 1979; Bradbury 1990), a possibility exits that alteration in the microvascular barriers will result in the abnormal brain function.

Abnormal expression of heat shock proteins (HSPs) occurs at the time of increased BBB permeability in stress (Sharma et al., 1995). This suggests that cellular injury signals are able to induce HSP expression. However, the functional significance of this finding is still unclear. We have undertaken a series of investigations in stress induced BBB disruption in relation to HSPs expression and their modification with drugs (Sharma et al., 1992a-f). It appears that expression of HSP represents important cellular events in neuronal dysfunction.

This review is focused on the functional significance of the BBB dysfunction in stress in relation to HSP expression and brain pathology. In addition, pharmacological modification of BBB and HSP expression in relation to cell injury in the brain are also discussed.

Information-Processing System and Brain Dysfunction in Stress

Nerve cells are equipped with a stimulus-response information processing system (IPS). The nerve cells can exert short- or long-lasting changes in its phenotype depending on the magnitude and severity of the stress response. The early responses that last from milliseconds to minutes are caused by several neurotransmitters and growth factors (the first messengers) acting on the cell surface receptors to activate the second messenger systems. The second messenger systems through specific protein kinases induce phosphorylation of specific neuronal proteins leading to alteration in the structure and function of the nerve cells (Garthwaite 1991; Bronstein et al., 1993; Hughes and Dragunow 1995).

The major depressive illnesses, affective disorders and other neurodegenerative diseases e.g., Alzheimer's disease, dementia, schizophrenia etc., represent life time exposure to stress. Severe stress reaction and/or continued exposure to stress induces alarm reactions and adverse brain function. Further prolongation of stress with same intensity is able to induce pathological changes in the brain as seen during neurodegenerative diseases (Selye 1976; Sharma 1982; Sharma et al., 1998a,c; Sharma 1999; 200b).

There are reasons to believe that disruption of the BBB is one of the most important factors in stress induced alterations in the IPS and subsequent brain dysfunction (Fig. 1). Foot-electroshock, electrical or chemical induced seizures or training in water maze is associated with BBB breakdown within a very short exposure period (Rapoport 1976; Sharma 1982; Sharma et al., 1991a). However, restriction of movement, e.g., restraint or immobilization, peripheral nerve lesion or denucleation of one eye requires prolonged exposure to exhibit BBB disruption (Sharma 1982; Sharma and Dey 1986a; Bradbury 1990). Interestingly, degeneration of noradrenergic neurones (information underload), or stimulation of locus coeruleus (information overload) is associated with the increased water permeability in the brain.

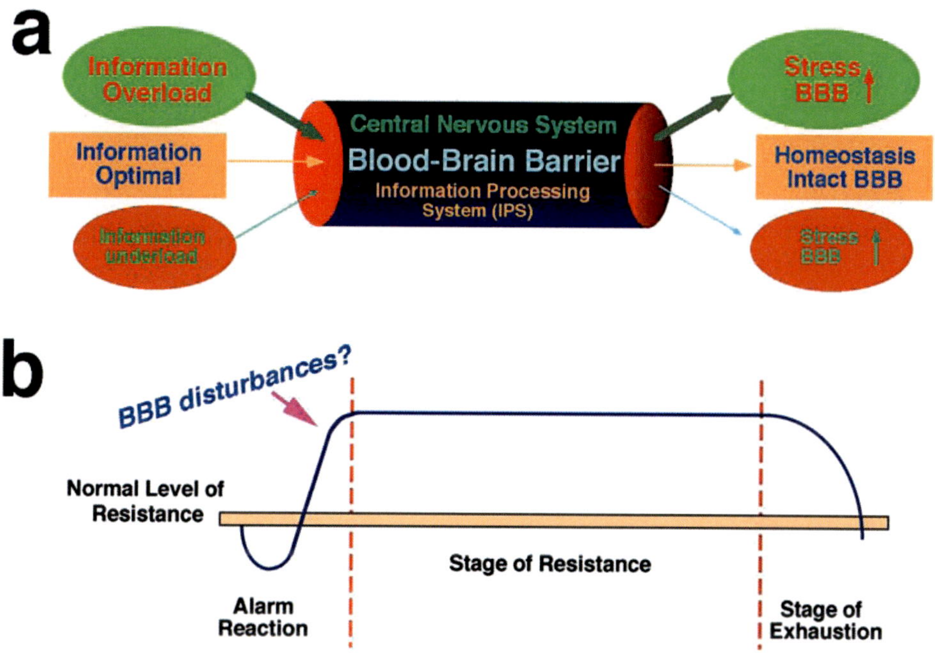

Fig. 1. Stress influences information processing system (IPS) and the blood-brain barrier (BBB) function. a. An overload or underload of information due to stress is often inadequately handled by the IPS of the CNS resulting in BBB dysfunction(for details see Sharma 2004). b. Stress effects are divided into 3 stages, e.g., the initial alarm reaction with symptoms followed by stage of adaptation exhibiting no apparent symptoms. Finally the stage of exhaustion in which the symptoms re-appear leading to death. The BBB disruption is common during alarm reaction that may set the stage for disease of adaptation and exhaustion leading to death. Modified after Sharma 1982; 1999; 2004.

CNS Pathways in Stress

The CNS pathways of stress include the hypothalamus, prefrontal cortex, hippocampus, amygdala and bed nucleus of the stria terminalis (see Herman and Cullinam 1997). The ascending serotonergic and noradrenergic system emanating from the brain stem also influences stress induced activation of the hypothalamic-pituitary-adrenal (HPA) axis directly as well as indirectly via the limbic system (HPA; Cullinan et al., 1995, Abercrombie and Jacobs 1987; Smith et al., 1991; see Herman and Cullinan 1997).

Stress is able to influence brain and behaviour and may precipitate in psychiatric illnesses or brain damage (Sapolsky 1992). Hippocampus is particularly vulnerable to stress-induced brain damage that mimics age-relate memory impairment. Specific cell damage in the CA 3 and CA4 subfields in the hippocampus are common following acute or chronic stress (Uno et al., 1989; Sharma et al., 1994a,b;1998a; Sharma 1999).

Acute or repeated stress, stroke, brain injury, ischemia, and ageing induce profound hippocampal damage (Sapolosky 1992) and results in a reversible atrophy of dendrites particularly in the CA3 region (McEwen 1999; Magarinos et al., 1996). Repeated stress causes reversible synaptogenesis in the CA1 region as well (Gazzaley et al., 1996) besides atrophy of dendrites in the CA3 area (Popov et al., 1992 for details see Sharma 2004).

The information generated by external or internal stimuli in stress are carried out directly through first messengers and indirectly via second messengers to the nerve cells that interacts with the cellular DNA to alter the gene expression (Hughes and Dragunow 1995. Production of specific mRNAs and the associated proteins are able to modify the phenotype of the cell. A brief survey over stress induced gene expression is sumarrised in Table 1. It is interesting to note that most of the stressors that are able to induce gene expression in the CNS are known to cause dysfunction of the BBB (see below). However, it is still unclear whether specific stressors activate particular sets of neurons or induce selective gene expression in certain areas of the brain or spinal cord.

Neurotrophic Factors and Stress

Neurotrophic factors act as intracellular messengers and induce gene expression in the target neurones (see Lindvall et al., 1994). Several members of the neurotrophic factors, e.g., brain derived nerve growth factor (BDNF), neurotrophin-3 (NT-3) and neurotrophin-4 (NT-4) are present in the adult brain to provide trophic support and enhance neuronal survival following CNS insults (see Sharma 2004). Exogenous administration of neurotrophic factors induces neurite outgrowth and branching (Patel and McNamara 1995; Sharma et al., 1997a; 1998d,e; 2000b,c; Sharma 2000b; 2003).

It appears that stress downregulates the expression or function of neurotrophic factors leading to neurodegenerative disorders. Acute immobilization stress for 2 h decreases the BDNF mRNA in the hippocampus of adult rats that is most pronounced in the dentate gyrus followed by CA3 and CA1 hippocampal pyramidal neurones (Smith et al., 1995a). Maternal separation in the rats on the postnatal day 12 and 20 is responsible for reduction in BDNF expression in hippocampus within 24 h. Repeated stress decreased the BDNF mRNA in the amygdala as well (Smith et al., 1995b). This effect of stress on BDNF expression in hippocampus and in the hypothalamus is most pronounced in the young rats (age 10-12 weeks) compared to the aged animal (age 2 years) (Smith and Cizza 1996).

Long-term treatment with antidepressants or electroconvulsive seizures prevents the stress-induced decrease in the BDNF expression (Nibuya et al., 1995). It appears that downregulation of BDNF expression in stress will influence neuronal communication and the signal transduction mechanisms in the brain. A reduction in the BDNF expression in chronic stress or ageing increases selective vulnerability of the neurons to injury.

Table 1. Stress induced immediate early gene expression (IEG) and blood-brain barrier (BBB) disruption

Stressors	IEG Protein/ mRNA	Time-interval	Brain regions	BBB disruption
Sensory stimulation	c-*fos*,	transient	spinal dorsal horn neurons	n.d.
Noxious/non-noxious, Olfactory and visual (gentle hair brushing, joint manipulation), Chemical or heat	c-Fos		post-synaptic neurones of dorsal horn	n.d.
stimulation of cutaneous sensory afferents	Fos	transient	superficial layers of Rexed's laminae I and II of the dorsal horn and layers III to V	n.d.
Noxious stimulation with hot water of the hind paw	c-*fos*, c-*jun*, *zif*-268 mRNAs c-*fos*, *jun*-B mRNAs	transient	neurones in Rexed's laminae I and II, V and X, superficial layers of dorsal horn neurons	
Repeated squeezing of rat planter surface of rat hind paw	c-Jun		Rexed's laminae I and III neurons	n.d.
Exposure to odours	c-*fos* mRNA		olfactory bulb	n.d.
Visual stimuli	*krox*-24 mRNA, *krox*-24,c-*fos*, *jun*-B		visual cortex	n.d.
Mono-ocular visual deprivation	*krox*-24 mRNA		monkey visual cortex	Yes?
Light stimulus	Fos Li		retinal neurons, SCN, hypothalamus	n.d.
Photic stimulation in night	Fos Li, c-fos, zif-268, *jun*-B, *jun*-D, c-*jun* mRNAs		hypothalamus, visual cortex	
Stressful situations	c-*fos*, c-*jun*, *jun*-B	transient	central amygdaloid nucleus, PVN	
Immobilization	Fos Li			Yes
Capsaicin administration,	*jun*-D		PVN	n.d.
Ear clipping	c-*fos* mRNA		mouse brain	
Isotonic saline injection	c-*fos* mRNA *fos*-B, *jun*-B, c-*jun*, *zif*-268, *fra*-1	transient	PVN, amygdaloid nucleus, hippocampus, neocortex 1 h after brain neurons	No
Sleep	c-*fos*, *zif*-268 mRNAs		lateral dorsal tegmental, pedunculopontine	n.d.?
deprivation	Fos Li, *jun*-B reticular formation		tegmental nuclei, LC, dorsal raphé, pontine	

Table 1. Continued

Stressors	IEG Protein/ mRNA	Time-interval	Brain regions	BBB disruption
Cardiovascular dysfunction Low blood pressure by stimulation of aortic depressor nerve or removal of blood	Fos	transient	nucleus tractus solitarius, area postrema	n.d.
			venterolateral medulla, nucleus ambiguus, medullary reticular formation, parabrachial nucleus, LC, supraoptic nucleus, inferior olive, subfornical organ, organ vasculosum hypothalamus, central nucleus of amygdala, bed nucleus of stria terminalis, islands of Calleja nucleus	n.d.?
			tractus solitarius, paratrigeminal nucleus	n.d.

Compiled from various sources; Hughes and Dragunow 1995; Sharma et al., 1998a,c; 2000; Sharma and Westman 2000; Sharma 2004;

? = more investigation needed; Transient = within 8 h, persistent = more than 24 h up to 72 h; IEG = immediate early genes; n.d = not done, Li=Like

Immunosupression in Stress

Stress-induced immune suppression appears to be important in causing brain dysfunction. Wide variety of stressors influences several aspects of immune function (see Maier et al., 1998) Activation of sympathetic nervous system together with the HPA axis in stress influences immune function, viz., lymphocyte proliferation (Lysle et al., 1988) or release of nitric oxide (NO) in response to mitogenic stimulation (Coussons-Read et al., 1994; Maier et al., 1998) in animals and in humans (see Sharma 2004).

Activated macrophages during stressful situations release proinflammatory cytokines, such as interleukin-1 (IL-1), tumour necrosis factor (TNF) and interleukin-6 (IL-6) (Blalock 1984; Dunn 1993; Gatti and Bartfai 1993; Kluger 1991). These cytokines modulate neural activity through specific receptors present in the brain (Watkins et al., 1995). This interaction between cytokines and brain are bidirectional and results in hormonal and autonomic changes causing peripheral responses leading to immune suppression (Watkins et al., 1995).

Cerebral Microcirculation and Metabolism in Stress

Stress influences cerebral circulation is apparent from the findings that 5 to 15 min immobilization elevates regional cerebral blood flow (CBF) in several regions (Ohata et al., 1981). Increased CBF and metabolism for oxygen consumption following immobilization stress is blocked by diazepam (Carlsson et al., 1975; 1976a,b). This indicates that anxiety plays important role in stress induced alterations in cerebral circulation and metabolism. Behavioural arousal in stress is mediated thorough noradrenergic neurones that innervate cortex and hippocampus (as above; Corrodi et al., 1971; Otake et al., 2002). Lesion of locus coeruleus prevents the increased turnover of the noradrenaline in the cortex supports this idea (Korf et al., 1973). However, long-term stress induces local ischemia impairing cerebral circulation and metabolism causing neuronal dysfunction.

Blood-Brain Barrier: A Gateway to Neurological Diseases and Brain Pathology

The breakdown of the BBB occurs in wide variety of neurological and psychiatric diseases. However, it is uncertain whether the breakdown of the BBB in different diseases is instrumental for brain damage (Table 2). Research carried out in our laboratory since last 25 years suggest that opening of the BBB is mainly associated with neuronal damage in several regions that exhibit overexpression of neuronal, glial and stress specific proteins. A direct relationship between opening of the BBB, neuronal damage and expression of stress proteins, e.g., HSPs are still not clearly understood. Since, pharmacological blockade of barrier breakdown results in neuroprotection, there are reasons to believe that the BBB functions as a gateway to various neurological diseases involving brain pathology.

Structural Basis of the Blood-Brain Barrier

The BBB resides mainly within the endothelial cells of cerebral capillaries that are connected with tight junctions and exhibit high electrical resistance (about 2000 Ohm x cm^2) (see Crone and Olesen 1982; Olesen 1989). The brain endothelial cells normally do not contain vesicles for transendothelial transport and are surrounded by basal lamina and glial cells (Fig. 2). These characteristics allow the permeability properties of cerebral capillaries very similar to that of an extended plasma membrane.

Transport of nutrients, ions and hormones that are essentials for brain functions is regulated across the BBB through specific transport system, e.g., molecule transporters, receptors, ionic pumps, and enzymes located within the endothelial cells (see Sharma et al., 1998d; Sharma 2004; 2004a).

The BBB remains tight in normal conditions to the wide variety of tracers ranging from 5 A° to about 85 A° (stoke radius) comprising about 500 kD to 150,000 kD (molecular weight). However, the integrity of the BBB is compromised under wide variety of experimental and in pathological conditions (Table 2). Upregulation of vesicular profiles within the endothelial cell cytoplasm and/or increased permeability of the endothelial cell membrane pay important roles in tracer transfer. In some cases, the tight junctions are also disrupted.

Table 2. Blood-brain barrier (BBB) dysfunction in neurodegenerative, stress and other diseases inflicting brain damage

Disease/conditions	BBB breakdown	Possible mechanisms
Neurodegeneration		
Alzheimer's disease, brain tumors, neoplasms, Schizophrenia, Dementia, ischemia, infarction, peripheral nerve lesion, leukemia	Serum proteins HRP Microperoxidase Lanthanum radiotracers	vesicular transport endothelial cell permeability
Vascular diseases		
hypertension[a] (mechanical, chemical or metabolic) hypotension, carotid artery occlusion, air embolism, gas embolism, atherosclerosis, periarteritis nodosa, thromboangitis obliterans, diabetic vasculitis	radiotracers, Evans blue HRP Lanthanum	widening of tight junctions[a] endothelial cell permeability vesicular transport
hypertensive encephalopathy, intracranial hypertension, hypovolaemic shock, hypervolaemia	HRP, Evans blue, radiotracers	widening of tight junctions[a]. vesicular transport, endothelial cell permeability?
Autoimmune diseases		
Viral encephalitis, experimental allergic encephalomyelitis, polyneuritis, multiple sclerosis	HRP, Evans blue, radiotracers	widening of tight junctions? vesicular transport,
Stressful situations		
immobilization[b], forced swimming[b], heat exposure[b], seizures, training in water maze, adrenalectomy, electroconvulsive shock, morphine withdrawal/dependence?	HRP, Evans blue Radiotracers Lanthanum	endothelial cell permeability vesicular transport widening of tight junctions?
Electromagnetic radiation		
Mobile telephony	Evans blue, HRP	vesicular transport
Microwave radiation	Evans blue, HRP, sucrose	endothelial cell permeability

Compiled from various sources, a = known to occur, b = authors own investigations, ? = not shown yet

Modified after Sharma 2004

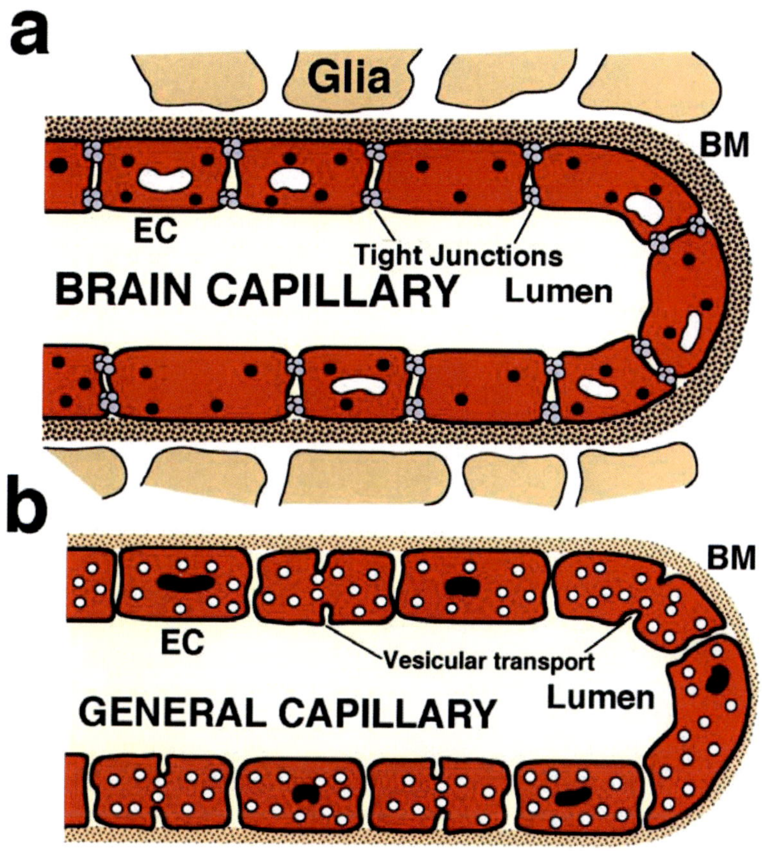

Fig. 2. Diagrammatic representation of the blood-brain barrier (BBB). The cerebral capillaries are different from non-cerebral capillaries. The endothelial cells (E) of cerebral capillaries are connected with tight junctions and do not contain microvesicles for vesicular transport as compared to the non cerebral capillary. The endothelial cells (E) in the brain are surrounded by thick basement membrane (B) and glial cells (G). The permeability of the BBB is thus very similar to that of an extended plasma membrane under normal conditions (Modified after Sharma 2004).

Blood-Brain Barrier in Stressful Situations and Neuronal Injury

Increased permeability of the BBB in stressful conditions is mainly based on the experiments done by Sharma and his group (Sharma and Dey 1981; Sharma 1982). These investigations showed that prolonged immobilisation, forced swimming and hyperthermia are able to induce breakdown of the BBB to protein tracers in specific brain regions (Sharma and Dey 1984, 1986a,b, Sharma et al., 1991, 1992a,b, 1994). These early studies formed the basis of selective vulnerability of the BBB in specific brain regions by different stressors. However, whether breakdown of the BBB in specific brain regions is associated with selective neuronal injury or damage is not well known and requires further investigation.

Neurochemical Basis of BBB Dysfunction in Stress

The increased permeability of the BBB in various stressful conditions was further shown by Sharma and his group to be well correlated with the elevation of plasma and brain serotonin (Sharma and Dey 1981; 1984). Since the amine is involved in several neurological and psychiatric diseases, the experimental studies in stress provided an important link between BBB breakdown, circulating vasoactive substances and neurological diseases. Furthermore, these observations opened a new avenue for research suggesting a neurochemical basis of the BBB dysfunction mediated thorough various neurotransmitter receptors and second messanger systems.

Table 3. BBB dysfunction and brain edema caused by various neurochemicals and vasoactive agents

Chemical mediators	BBB permeability tracers	Vasogenic edema
Bradykinin	Na^{+}-Fluroscein	Yes
Arachidonic acid	Na^{+}-Fluorescein FITC-dextran EBA	Yes
Free radicals	EBA, Na-fluorescein	Yes
Leukotrienes	EBA, Na-fluorescein	?
Cytokines	Na-fluorescien	Yes?
Histamine	EBA, Na-fluorescein FITC-dextran, HRP	Yes
Serotonin[a]	EBA, HRP, La^{++}	Yes
Endothelin	^{51}Cr, ^{45}Ca	?
Nitric oxide[a]	MEAP, EBA	Yes
Dynorphin[a]	EBA, La^{++}	Yes
protamine	Lanthanum,	?
norepinephrine		
5-HTP[b]	microperoxidase	Yes/?
prostaglandins	radiotracers	?
glutamate	radiotracers	Yes?
L-NAME	radiotracers	?
cAMP		?
dibutyric cAMP		?
adrenaline	EBA, Iodine	?
6-OHDA	EBA, Iodine	?
indomethacin	EBA, HRP	Yes?
bicuculline	various tracers	?
angiotensin	EBA, Iodine, HRP	Yes?
amphetamine	various tracers	?
metaramine	EBA, radiotracers	?
pentylenetetrazol	various tracers	?

Compiled from various sources, a = authors own investigations: Modifed after Sharma 2004, b = unpublished observation

Crone and Olesen group in Denmark using isolated frog microvessels meticulously showed that the electrical resistance of the pial vessels closely correlates with the tightness of the barrier (see Olesen 1989). Application of various vasoactive substances decreases the electrical resistance of the pial vessels reflecting the increased BBB permeability. The breakdown of the BBB appears to be receptor mediated and intracellular accumulation of Ca^{2+}.

Recently, several investigators examined the influence of different vasoactive substances on the BBB function by applying different neurochemicals on both luminal or abluminal sides of the cerebral microvessels (Table 3). Most of the compounds that open the BBB are also contribute to vasogenic edema formation. Since edema is one of the common complication of many brain diseases and brain pathology, it appears that leakage of endogenous plasma proteins plays important roles in neuronal injury.

However, in vivo situations, no single chemical compound is solely responsible to influence BBB function. A wide variety of neurochemicals may work synergistically or antagonistically on the cerebral microvessels to influence the BBB function in both experimental and in clinical situations.

Structural Basis of BBB Breakdown

Electron microscopy of the cerebral endothelium suggests that breakdown of the BBB in several experimental conditions is mainly due to an increase in the transendothelial transport and/or increased cell membrane permeability to tracers. Opening of the tight junctions are also seen in some experimental conditions, e.g., hyperosmotic shrinkage of the cerebral endothelium or increase in transmural pressure within the cerebral microvessels due to hypertension (Fig. 3). However, the permeability of endothelial cell membrane is also increased in these conditions (see Rapoport 1976; Bradbury 1990; Sharma and Westman 2004).

Leakage of Endogenous Serum Proteins and Neuronal Injury

Leakage of serum proteins in the brain microenvironment results in DNA fragmentation and cell death as soon as within 4 h (Matz et al., 2001a,b; Morita-Fujimura et al., 1999; Loberg and Torvik 1991). Oxidative stress triggers cytochrome c release that induces DNA fragmentation and cell death (Matz et al., 2001; Sugawara et al., 1999). However, cytochrome c induced DNA fragmentation or cell deaths are still complex and require further investigation (Saas et al., 1999). In contrast to DNA fragmentation, induction of HSP 70 in neurons indicates sublethal injury (States et al., 1996). However, HSP induction does not correlate well with the intracellular accumulation of Evans blue during subarachnoid haemorrhage (Matz et al., 2001a.b). Thus the relationship between breakdown of the BBB, oxidative stress, neuronal injury and HSP expression requires further studies.

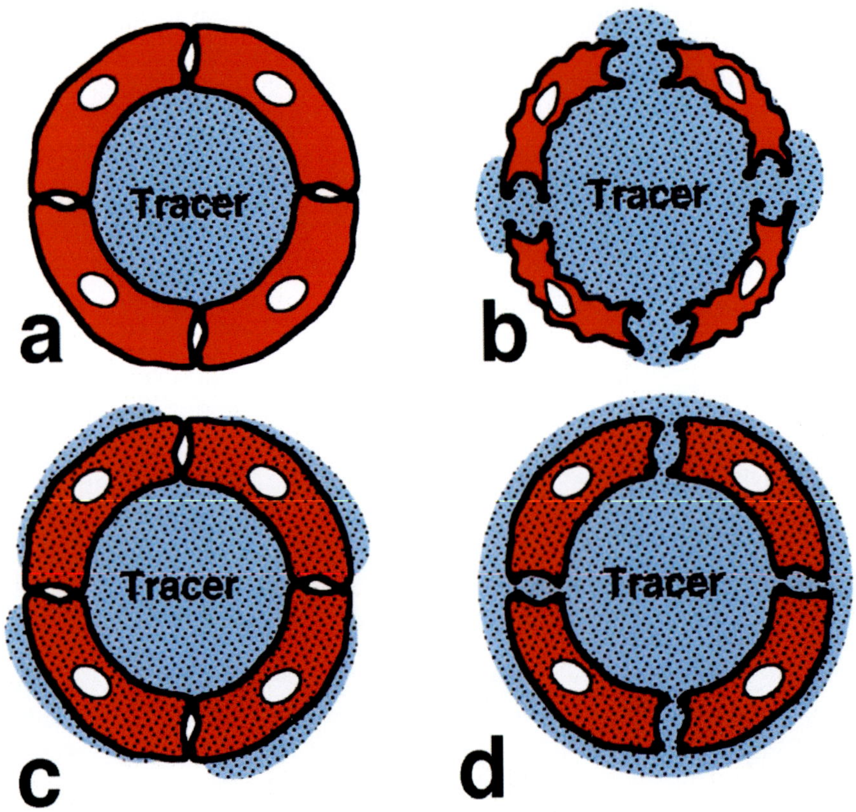

Fig. 3. Leakage of tracers across the blood-brain barrier (BBB). a. Tracers are mainly confined within the lumen of the normal cerebral capillary. b. Widening of tight junctions occur during osmotic opening of the BBB caused by infusion of hyperosmolar electrolytes and non-electrolytes. c. Increased endothelial cell membrane permeability and/or stimulation of vesicular transport without widening of the tight junctions are seen in several experimental and clinical conditions involving acute or chronic brain diseases, neurodegeneration and traumatic injuries. d. Widening of tight junction and increase in vasicular transport and/or endothelial cell membrane permeability is commin in acutre or chronic hypertension and vasular brain diseases. (Modified after Sharma 2004).

STRESS PROTEINS AND NEURODEGENERATION

The term "heat shock proteins" is derived from the fact that subjection of Drosophila melanogaster to heat shock (≈ 5 ° C above the normal body temperature) induces synthesis of the new class of proteins, that are normally not presents in normal tissues (Tissiéres et al., 1974). Expression of HSP 72 kD was first seen in the cell culture experiments when the medium was accidentally heated from 37° C to 45° C (see Craig 1985; Welch 1992). This abnormal expression of proteins was thus termed as "heat shock proteins (HSP)" that is also referred to as "stress proteins" (Sharma et al., 1992a; Ciocca et al., 1993; Blake et al., 1994; Marcuccilli and Miller 1994; Sharma et al., 1995; Marcuccilli et al., 1996; Sharma and Westman 1997; Snocekx et al., 2001; Kingsley et al., 2003), However, the term "heat shock proteins (HSPs)" is preferred by most workers and is still used widely (see Tables 4 and 5)

Table 4. Factors influencing synthesis of various heat shock proteins subtypes

Stimuli	Type of HSP synthesis
Stressors	HSP 100, HSP 90, HSP 70, HSP 60, HSP 27
heat stress[a]	
heat shock	
cold shock	
immobilization[a]	
UV radiation	
amino acid analogues	
arsenite	
cocaine, morphine, other chemicals	
drugs	
Physiological stimuli	HSP 90, HSP 70, HSP 60, HSP 27
hormones	
growth factors	
cell cycle	
immunomodulators	
Food restriction/Ageing?	
Pathological conditions	HSP 90, HSP 70, HSP 72, HSP 32, HSP 27
Trauma[a]	
ischemia	
hypoxia	
infarction	
infections	
glucose starvation	
anoxia	
Cardiovascular pathologies	
Atherosclerosis	
Oxidative stress	
Alzheimer's Disease	

a = authors own investigations; compiled from various sources; Modified after Westman and Sharma 1998; Sharma and Westman 2004

A mild heat shock induces greater tolerance to normally lethal temperatures (thermotolerance, Marcuccilli and Miller 1994; Westman and Sharma 1998) indicating that induction of HSPs is protective in nature (Marcuccilli and Miller 1994; Sharma et al., 1995; Marcuccilli et al., 1996; Sharma and Westman 1997; Snocekx et al., 2001). Injection of HSP antibodies into the oocyte before subjecting them to light stress decreases the cell survival supports this idea (Brown et al., 1989; Gonzalez et al., 1989; Li et al., 1992; Marcuccilli and Miller 1994). Furthermore, pretreatment with mild heat to initiate HSP induction significantly attenuated irradiation induced damage is in the line of the above hypothesis (see Welch 1992; Westman and Sharma 1998).

Table 5. Intracellular localisation and possible function of various heat shock protein (HSP) subtypes.

HSP type	localisation	possible function
The small HSP family	Nucleus[a]	cell survival
HSP 27	cytoplasm	maintenance
		stress resistance
HSP 32	endoplasmic reticulum membrane	heme degradation
Ubiquitin	cytoplasm	protein degradation
HSP 70 family		protein maturation
HSC 70	cytoplasm	protein translocation
HSP 70[b]	nucleus	unknown, inducible?
	nucleolus	
GRP 78	endoplasmic reticulum	secretory proteins
GRP 75	mitochondria	protein translocation
HSP 90 family		
HSP 90	cytoplasm	protein maturation
HSP 90 a (86 kDa)		
HSP 90 b (84 kDa)	steroid receptors	inactive receptor
GRP 94	endoplasmic reticulum	protein folding, secretory proteins
HSP 110	nucleus, cytoplasm	thermotolerance
HSP 100	nucleolus[a]	

Modified after Westman and Sharma 1998

a = incorporated after stress only; b = expression occurs after stress only; HSP = heat shock protein; HSC = heat shock cognate; GRP = glucose related protein; compiled from various sources.

However, HSPs participate in several cellular functions and are also considered as markers of cell injury. An increased threat to the cell survival may also induce HSP expression (Welch 1992; Lindquist 1996; Marcuccilli et al., 1996). This indicates that induction of HSP is beneficial in nature. It may be that mild heat treatment increases the cell adaptability to stress and consequently increases the threshold for cell damage.

The HSPs comprise four general molecular weight classes: 95-100 kD, 80-90 kD, 70-75 kD and 20-30 kD, with minor variations (Craig 1985; Lindquist 1986; Lindquist and Craig 1988; Kaufmann 1992; Welch 1992). HSP 32 is hemeoxygenase-1 (HO-1) that is often seen co-expressed following several forms of brain or spinal cord injuries (for details; Mautes et al., 2000) (see Tables 4 and 5).

Various forms of CNS insults induce profound cellular stress and cause BBB breakdown resulting in vasogenic brain edema and cell injury (Sharma 1982; Sharma and Dey 1987; Sharma and Cervós-Navarro 1990; Sharma et al., 1997a-c; 1998a; Sharma 1999). However, the consequences of BBB disruption and induction HSP is largely unknown (Craig 1985; Welch 1992; Marcuccilli and Miller 1994; Sharma et al., 2000a; Sharma and Hoopes 2003) (Table 4).

Since cellular injury signals are able to induce HSP and expression, overproduction of HSP could be either beneficial or harmful in nature. Thus, studies using neuroprotective drugs on expression of HSP and BBB breakdown will further clarify this point.

HSPs and Apoptosis

There are indications that induction of HSP influences apoptosis and cell death. The programmed cell death (PCD), commonly known as "apoptosis" appears to be a promising approach for therapy by pharmacological agents to attenuate cell death in several neurodegenerative diseases (see LeBlanc 2003). One of the key elements in the apoptosis is known as "caspases" (Shi 2002; Ranger et al., 2001) that are activated by autoproteolytic processing and oligomerization and are identified by the length of their proarm or by substrate specificity (Van de Craen et al., 1999). Initiation of a cell death signal activates the long proarm caspases (caspases-2,8,9 or 10) that triggers apoptosis. Activation of short proarm caspases (caspase 3.6.7) induces irreversible cell damage leading to cell death. Proinflammatory cytokines could also be influences by other caspases (caspase-1,4,5,11 and 14) causing apoptosis (Kidd et al., 2000).

The activity of caspases is inhibited by HSPS and other natural inhibitors of apoptosis protein (IAP) (Shi 2002; Stennicke et al., 2002); calpains, phosphoinositides, B-cell lymphoma 2 (Bcl-2) proteins, and proteases (see LeBlanc 2003). However the functional significance of these findings is still not well known.

HSP 70 and P53 Tumour Suppresser

Overexpression of HSP 70 and HSP 90 occurs in several tumour cells (see Helmbrecht et al., 2000; Jolly and Morimoto 2000) that is correlated with metastasis and poor prognosis (Ciocca et al., 1993; Vargas-Roig 1998; see Zylicz et al., 2001). Inhibitors of HSP 70 with antisense HSP 70 cDNA inhibits tumour cell proliferation and induction of apoptosis (Jaattela et al., 1998; Volloch and Sherman 1999). HSP 70 negatively regulate various stages of the p53 dependent or independent apoptotic pathways (Beere et al., 2000; Mosser et al., 2000, Nylandsted et al., 2000). Treatment of cells expressing mutant p53 with antibiotics results in an increase in p53 ubiquitylation and proteosome mediated degradation (Whitesell et al., 1998). Interestingly, antibiotic treatment also reduces the levels of HSP 90 bound to p53 and increase p53 translocation into the cell nucleus (Whitesell et al., 1998) indicating an interaction between HSP and p53 in cellular regulation (see Zylicz et al., 2001).

HSP in Heat Stress Induced Hyperthermia

HSP expression in the brain as well as in other organs occurs after whole body hyperthermia (WBH; Minowada and Welch 1995). WBH in rats up to 42° C for 15 min using a water bath temperature of 56° C resulted in profound upregulation of HSP in neurons (Xia et al., 1998; Abe et al., 1991; Nowak et al., 1990). In another experimental set up of WBH, HSP expression in the perikarya of neurones in the layer IV to X in the gray matter of the spinal cord occurs 2 h after heat exposure and lasted up to 8 h. The HSP expression is not seen in the glial cells or within the white matter (Xia et al., 1998). On the other hand, upregulation of HSP in the rabbit spinal cord in the glial cells and in fiber tracts but not in neurons is seen after D-lysergic acid diethylamide (LSD) induced hyperthermia (Manzerra and Brown,1992). This suggests that drug induced hyperthermia is not comparable to the WBH with regard to HSP expression (Sharma and Westman 2004).

HSP in Alzheimer's Disease

The HSPs are molecular chaperones involved in protecting the cells from various stressors. Abnormal expression of antioxidant enzymes and HSPs has been shown in Alzheimer's disease (AD) brains (Pappolla et al., 1996). Abnormal patterns of HSP expression are seen the cerebral cortex, hippocampus and in the choroid plexus in AD (Anthony et al., 2003). Thus, it appears that expression of HSPs is closely related to the amyloid precursor protein (APP) in brain of patients with AD. A significant increase in HSP 70 expression in temporal cortex of patients with AD is in line with this idea (Pappolla et al., 1996; Yoo et al., 1999; Clarimon et al., 2003).

Based on these observations, Ahlemeyer and Krieglstein (2003) suggested the possible use of Ginkgo biloba extract (EGb 761, see below) that is neuroprotective due to its antioxidant properties (see Sharma and Westman 2004) for the treatment in AD patients with mild and moderate dementia. However, use of antioxidant compounds in AD and related neurodegenerative diseases with regard to HSP expression and the BBB permeability (Sharma et al., 1999; 2000; 2003) require further investigation.

Blood-Brain Barrier in Alzheimer's Disease

Alzheimer's disease (AD) is considered as one of the most severe long-term stress induced neurodegenerative diseases. There are reasons to believe that extravasation of endogenous serum proteins plays important role in the pathogenesis of AD. AD is the most common cause of dementia and loss of cognitive functions in old age (Alzheimer 1907; Farkas and Luiten 2001; de la Torre 2002; Zlokovic 2002). Wide range of pathophysiological changes in the cerebrovascular endothelium and in brain parenchyma is responsible for severe cognitive dysfunction in AD (Kalaria 1999). Deposition of amyloid-β-peptide (ABP) in the brain during normal aging is accelerated in patients with AD (Wisniewski et al., 1997; Zlokovic 2002). Thus, ABP that represents the main constituents of brain parenchyma and vascular amyloid is primarily responsible for the pathological changes in the brain in AD (Selkoe, 1998; Younkin 1998; Roses 1998; Strittmatter 2001).

Interestingly, changes in spinal cord pathology or deposition of ABP in spinal cord parenchyma or microvessels are not investigated so far in AD. It would be interesting to see whether AD patients also exhibit selective pathology and deposition of ABP in the spinal cord, a feature that requires additional investigation.

Amyloid-β-Peptide and Alzheimer's Disease

ABP exists in multiple isoforms. ABP extracted from senile plaques contains mainly ABP1-40 and ABP1-42 isoforms (Masters et al., 1985). On the other hand, vascular amyloid contains predominantly ABP1-39 and ABP1-40 (Prelli et al., 1988). Another form of ABP is a soluble isoform of the peptide (sABP) present in the blood, cerebrospinal fluid (CSF) and brain that is mainly characterised as ABP1-40 (Seubert et al., 1992; Shoji et al., 1996; Vigo-Pelfrey et al., 1993; Tabaton et al., 1994; Kuo et al., 1996).

There are several theories to explain ABP deposits in the brain parenchyma or vessel walls leading to the pathology of AD. Most data favour the neuronal origin theory, which suggests that sABP is a precursor of ABP deposits (Busciglio et al., 1993). An increase in sABP in AD precedes amyloid plaque formation (Teller et al., 1996).

Since ABP is continuously produced in the brain, a possibility exists that an efficient clearance mechanism(s) is present across the BBB to prevent its accumulation and subsequent aggregation in the brain. It is likely that cerebrovascular degeneration and breakdown of the BBB in AD may also influence ABP transport across the cerebromicrovessels.

Cerebrovascular Pathology and the BBB in AD

Post-mortem studies of brain in AD patients show clear vascular lesions (Table 6) comprising pathological reactions in the endothelial cells, vascular smooth muscle cells, haemorrhages and infarction (Kalaria 1996; Vinters 1987). Deposition of ABP around the large arterial vessels and the cerebral capillaries is prominent. These pathological observations suggest that the permeability of the BBB in AD is altered (Mattila et al., 1994).

Table 6. Cerebrovascular lesions in AD

Pathology	Occurrence %(about 300 ases)
Degeneration	100 %
Extravasation of serum proteins	>80 %
Cerebral amyloid angiopathy	>90 %
Intracerebral haemorrhages	>10 %
Cerebral and cortical infarcts	>30 %

Data from Premkumar et al., 1996; Kalaria 1999

Changes in Vascular Enzymes and Proteins in AD

That the BBB function is compromised in AD is evident from the biochemical or immunohistochemical studies showing profound alterations in specific markers for the BBB function (Table 7). Thus, the metabolic rate for glucose consumption is much lowered in AD compared to the age-matched controls and can be confirmed by loss of glucose transporter 1 (GLUT 1) activity in the cerebral endothelial cells of AD patients (Kalaria and Harik 1989; Frey 1998; Mielke and Heiss 1998). Expression of GLUT 1 is limited to the cerebral endothelium connected with tight junctions. A loss of GLUT1 immunoreactivity suggests altered BBB function.

Additional evidences that BBB permeability is altered in AD is based on the observations of changes in key protein functions associated with BBB transport. Thus, γ-glutamyl transferase, alkaline phosphatase, acetylcholinesterase and butrylcholinesterase show a moderate loss in the brain microvessels in the brains of AD (See Kalaria 1996). However, no changes in the angiotensin converting enzyme activity in the endothelial cells of the AD brain was observed. A reduction in acetylcholinesterase and butrylcholinesterase in the cerebral microvessels of AD brain suggest that a defect or local breakdown of the BBB is possible. These local changes are likely to be involved in ABP deposition around the microvessels.

Similarly, the intracellular adhesion molecule (ICAM-1) that is often upregulated in several inflammatory diseases (see Engelhardt et al., 2004) is increased in both the capillaries as well as in neocortical extracts from the brains of AD subjects (see Kalaria 1998). These observations support the idea that activation of cerebral endothelium occurs in AD brain that can be instrumental for increased permeability to the circulating cells and thus reflects an alteration in the BBB function.

Table 7 Changes in BBB-related enzymes in AD

Enzymes	Alteration
GLUT1	Decrease
Na+/K+ ATPase	Decrease
Angiotensin converting enzyme	no change
Alkaline phosphatase	Loss
γ-glutamyl transpeptidase	Loss
acetylcholinesterase	Loss
butrylcholinesterase	Loss
alpha actin	Loss
carnitine acetyltransferase	Loss
Collagen proteins	Increase
Glucose 6 phosphate	increase
ABP	Accumulation
ICAM-1	increased

Data modified from Kalaria 1998.

Leakage of Endogenous Serum Proteins in AD

Leakage of endogenous serum proteins in the brains is often associated with the BBB breakdown (Rapoport 1976). Since these proteins are not produced by the brain cellular components, a leakage of these proteins derived from circulation may support the idea of a breakdown of the BBB in AD. An increased immunoreactivity of albumin and IgG in the amyloid plaques and neurofibrillary tangles were first reported in the brains from AD patients about 20 years ago by Wisniewski and Kozlowski (1982). However, it has been suggested that similar endogenous serum protein extravasation can be seen during aging (Munoz et al., 1997) and no differences can be assigned between aged-controls and patients with AD (Hachinski and Munoz 1997; Kalaria 1992). Thus, these observations may suggest a close interaction and/or communication of an immunological link between the brain parenchyma and the circulation in AD.

Increased Serum Proteins in the CSF in AD

There are clear indications of BBB disturbances in dementia (Frisoni et al., 1994) and evidences also support a role of BBB dysfunction in the pathogenesis of AD (Hardy et al.,

1986; Kalaria 1992; Frisoni et al., 1994). An increased CSF and serum albumin ratio indicates impairment of the BBB function (Bradbury 1990). Increased CSF: serum albumin ratios have been reported in AD patients, especially those exhibited peripheral vascular diseases (Blennow et al., 1990; Hampel et al., 1995; Zlokovic 2002; de la Torre 2002). It seems likely that patients exhibiting hypertension may have leakage of serum proteins in the brain. Thus, a communication between blood and brain exists in AD, which seems to be instrumental in initiating the cascade of amyloid deposition and encephalopathy.

Pathology of the Endothelial Cell and Basal Lamina in AD

The cerebral microvessels and basal lamina often show marked pathological changes in the brains of AD patients that may be independent of amyloid deposition (Table 8) (Kalaria 1996; Kalaria and Pax 1995; Kalaria and Hedera 1995). Thus, selective degeneration of endothelial cells, smooth muscle cells and basal lamina occurs in the brains of AD patients (for review see Kalaria 1998). Although, in most vascular profiles a close correlation between deposition of ABP and endothelial cell degeneration is seen, no apparent relationship is found between degenerated microvessels and neurofibrillary tangles or the damaged pyramidal neurones (Kalaria 1996). These observations suggest that local change in cerebral perfusion and oxygen tension could contribute to these pathological alterations (Schiebel et al., 1987).

Although, the microvascular pathology together with deposition of ABP suggests a breakdown of the BBB function in AD, a clear functional link between BBB abnormalities in AD is still lacking. A focal or transient opening of the BBB over a protracted period is partially responsible for the vascular pathologies seen in the patients of AD. Alternatively, an opening of the BBB may be helpful in the molecular mechanisms of neuronal growth and repair (Kalaria 1992; 2000), a feature that is still being investigated in several laboratories.

Table 8. Pathological changes in the endothelial cells and related structures in AD

Cell type	Pathology	References
Vascular Smooth muscle cells	Degeneration	Degeneration Perry et al., 1998
	focal constriction	Miyakawa et al.,1998
Cerebral endothelium	necrosis degeneration	Kalaria and Hedera 1995
	decrease in mitochondria, increase in pinocytosis; loss of tight junctions	Claudio 1996; Stewart et al., 1992;
Basal lamina	degeneration; accumulation of collagen	Perlmutter et al., 1994; Kalaria and Pax 1995;
Intracerebral capillaries	deformed; collapsed	Kalaria et al., 1996

Data modified after Kalaria 1998

Infusion of β-Amyloid (1-42) Peptide Impairs BBB Function in Animal Models

There is an experimental link between ABP and disruption of the BBB in rats (Janscó et al., 1998). An intracarotid injection of β-amyloid (1-42) results its accumulation in the brain parenchyma (Maness et al., 1994; Martel et al., 1996). This observation suggests that circulating ABP in plasma may somehow be responsible for brain deposition of the peptide (Seubert et al., 1992). It seems likely that infusion of ABP induces alterations in the BBB function. Infusion of high concentrations of ABP (10^{-4} to 10^{-5} M) at a rate of 200 µl/min into the internal carotid artery of rats resulted in a marked extravasation of Evans blue into the ipsilateral half of the brain (Janscós et al., 1998). In this study, the authors also found sporadic extravasation in the contralateral side. This observation suggests that ABP has the capacity to induce breakdown of the BBB even in small doses that may leak into the general circulation during infusion into the one internal carotid artery.

The increase in the BBB permeability to Evans blue was seen in animals 30 to 240 min after ABP infusion. Interestingly, the authors found a pronounced loss of lectin binding sites within the luminal surface of the endothelium (Janscós et al., 1998). This suggests that the ABP is capable to alter the endothelial cell membrane structure resulting in the loss of lectin binding sites. A similar decrease in lectin binding is previously reported in heat stress, a condition that is associated with massive breakdown of the BBB permeability and degeneration of cerebral endothelium (Sharma et al., 1998a; Sharma 1999).

These observations suggest that ABP can induce a direct damage of the cerebral endothelium resulting in breakdown of the BBB permeability indicating that alterations in the brain microvasculature significantly contribute to the pathogenesis of AD.

Role of Nitric Oxide in Degenerative Changes in Brains of AD

Nitric oxide (NO) is recently considered as one of the most important factors in neurodegeneration (see Sharma and Alm 2004). The NO is produced by different isoforms of nitric oxide synthase (NOS) can be highly neurotoxic, particularly when generated in excess following cytokine dependent transcriptional upregulation of inducible isoform (iNOS) (London et al., 1996; Meda et al., 1995; Xia et al., 1998; Sharma et al., 1998b). There are reports that NO induces neurotoxicity in the vicinity of senile neuritic plaques and thus participates in the pathogenesis of AD (Wallace et al., 1997).

Haas et al. (2002) using frozen postmortem specimens from the frontal and parietal cortex of 20 severely demented AD patients examined inducible NOS (iNOS) expression as well as the rate limiting enzyme argininosuccinate-synthase (ASS), responsible of recycling of L-citruline to L-arginine) (Hass et al., 2002). The authors reported a 4-fold increase in iNOS mRNA transcripts using PCR techniques in the cortex of AD patients compared to normal controls. Similarly, the enzyme ASS was found to be 3-fold elevated in the cortex of ADS patients in comparison with control groups (Haas et al., 2002).

In cell culture experiments, these authors examined the effects of synthetic ABP (1-40) or ABP (1-42) in rat primary cortical cells on NOS production (Haas et al., 2002). A massive upregulation of iNOS was seen 24 h after stimulation that declined after 48 h in this experimental set-up. On the other hand, elevation of ASS was present even 48 h after stimulation. Interestingly, stimulation with ABP (1-42) resulted in significantly higher iNOS and ASS mRNAs compared to the ABP (1-40) induced stimulation at all the time points (Haas et al., 2002).

To find out the probable mechanisms of NOS stimulation, these authors measured inflammatory cytokines (Haas et al., 2002). The results showed a significant elevation of IL-1β, IL-6 and TNF-α in the culture supernatant of ABP stimulated cells compared to the unstimulated cells.

These observations suggest that mRNA levels of the enzyme iNOS and ASS are elevated in the cortex of AD patients and indicates a positive role of NO in the vascular pathology and the neurodegeneration in AD brains. Since NO is involved in the breakdown of the BBB in several animal models (see Sharma and Alm 2004) alteration in BBB function in the brains of AD patients is quite likely.

To characterize the involvement of NO in AD, Lüth et al (2001) examined endothelial isoforms of NOS (eNOS) in Human brains of AD. The eNOS expression is present in the astrocytic processes on the pial surface and in endothelial cells of the blood vessels in both AD and in control brains. However, the number of eNOS immunostained astrocytes and the endothelial cells in the deeper layers of the cortex is significantly increased in the AD brains (Lüth et al., 2001). The authors showed a strong expression of eNOS compared to iNOS in the brains of AD (Lüth et al., 2000) indicating that endothelial cell functions are somehow influenced by AD. Alternatively, the NO production from the endothelial cells is much more intense than NO induced by iNOS expression in other cells types.

Human BBB Receptors for ABP 1-40

It appears that ABP is the key factor for the pathology of AD due to its neurotoxicity, directly inducing oxidative stress and/ or indirectly by activating microglia (Mattson and Rydel 1996; Yan et al., 1996; El Khoury et al., 1996). The cytotoxic effects of ABP are mediated through the pathological "chaperone" proteins in the brain (Wisniewski et al., 1997).

A soluble monomeric form of ABP (sABP) is present in the brain parenchyma (Tabaton et al., 1994), cerebrospinal fluid (CSF) and in circulation (Seubert et al., 1992; Shoji et al., 1992). In cell culture studies, 60 % of plaques are labelled with ABP1-42 while only 30 % of all plaques contain ABP1-40 (Prior et al., 1996). About 90 % release of ABP in cell culture come from the 40 amino acid peptide ABP1-40 that is predominant form of cerebrovascular amyloid (Suzuki ct al., 1994; Castano ct al., 1996). Thc longcr 42-rcsiduc pcptidc ABP 1-42 accounts for only 10 % of secreted ABP, but is the major constituent of senile plaque (Masters et al., 1985).

The origin of ABP deposition in the cerebral vasculature or in brain parenchyma is still uncertain. It is likely that ABP is produced locally in the brain (neuronal theory) or can gain access into the brain from circulation (vascular theory) by breaching the BBB (Zlokovic 1997). A receptor mediated transcytosis can play important role in transport of several peptides and proteins across the cerebral endothelium (Banks et al., 1991). Thus, it may be that circulating sABP1-40 is transported from blood to brain through specific receptor mediated effects (Zlokovic 1997).

According to the neuronal theory (as mentioned above), the soluble form of ABP (sABP) is a precursor of ABP deposits. A decreased clearance of ABP from brain and CSF is the main cause of ABP deposition in AD (Rosenberg 2000). Since ABP is continuously synthesized in the brain, a possibility exists that an efficient clearance mechanism(s) exists at the BBB to prevent its accumulation and subsequent deposition in the brain (Shibata et al., 2000).

Etiology of AD

Contribution of vascular factors to the etiology of AD has become a rapidly expanding subject for research in the last decade (see Farkas and Luiten 2001). Several vascular pathophysiology such as atherosclerosis, hypertension and disturbed brain perfusion is recognised as potential risk factors in AD (de la Torre 1999; Farkas et al., 2000). A decreased global or cortical CBF is supposed to be one of the main contributing factors to dementia and decline in cognitive functions in AD (Kobari et al., 2000; Farkas et al., 2000).

Microvascular Pathology in AD

Microvascular abnormalities in AD include atrophic thin vessels, glomerular loop formation, fragmentation along with twisted or tortuous vessels (Buée et al., 1997). At the ultrastructural levels, distorted abluminal surface of the terminal arterioles and capillaries with loss of vascular smooth muscle in the AD brain is quite frequent (Hashimura et al., 1991; Kimura et al., 1991). The smooth muscle cells exhibit degeneration and focal constriction, the astrocytic end-feet is often swollen and the pericytes display severe atrophy in AD brains (Miyakawa et al., 1988). The endothelial cells are swollen and contain irregular shaped nuclei (Hashimura et al., 1991). The basal lamina is thickened and shows local disruption (Yamashita et al., 1991). The perivascular plexus often disappeared (Scheibel et al., 1989).

Epidemiological and clinico-pathologic cases suggest that overlaps between AD and cerebrovascular lesions amplify the AD pathology, exacerbate cognitive decline and induce neuronal damage and dementia. The microvascular changes associated with regional metabolic and BBB dysfunction further contributes to the neuronal damage (Jellinger 2002). In microvascular lesions in AD comprise cortical and subcortical microinfarcts, subcortical lacunes and white matter lesions or leukoencephalopathy.

These observations support the idea that in AD, the structural integrity of the BBB is compromised and may induce transient leakage (Scheibel 1987; Scheibel et al., 1987). An absence of specific endothelial cell markers CD31 and CD34 support this idea (Kalaria 1999; 2000). Compromised morphology of the tight junctions of the endothelial cells further supports the concept of a BBB breakdown in AD (Claudio 1996). The number of tight junctions per standard vessel length is remarkably decreased in AD, however, the length of the junctions itself did not alter (Stewart et al., 1992). These vascular anomalies and morphological changes in the cerebral vessels suggest a leaky BBB in AD.

Existing Theories Regarding Origin of ABP

Two main theories are supported by several investigators on the origin of ABP causing cerebral microangiopathy. These include circulating blood levels of ABP and the vessel wall itself or the brain parenchyma (for details see Burgermeister et al., 2000; Zlokovic 2002).

The blood-borne ABP theory is supported by the data showing an increased level of ABP in AD patients (Kuo et al., 1996). Furthermore, experimentally infused ABP can be traced back in the cerebral vascular walls (Mackic et al., 1998). In addition, several transport mechanisms for ABP through the BBB, such as receptor mediated transcytosis or leakage caused by ABP toxicity has been demonstrated (Pluta et al., 1996; Zlokovic et al., 1996; Janscó et al., 1998; Straziella et al., 2000; Zlokovic et al., 2000).

According to the vessel wall hypothesis, the perivascular cells can also locally produce the accumulating ABP (Kalaria et al., 1996). Presence of mRNA of the amyloid precursor protein (APP) in endothelial cells, smooth muscle cells and pericytes isolated from brains of AD patients supports this idea (Natte et al., 1999). This observations suggests that APP present in vascular domain can produce ABP deposition. Demonstration of ABP immunoreactive material of endogenous origin in the smooth muscle cells of aged dogs in cell culture are in line with the vascular wall concept (Wisniewski et al., 2000).

The ABP deposition in smooth muscle cells of the vascular walls may be due to internalization and assembly of ABP via receptor mediated transcytosis (Urmoneit et al., 1997). Production of ABP through smooth muscle cells from APP can only induce cerebral amyloid angiopathy (CAA) by deposition of ABP in larger leptomeningeal or cortical vessels, but it is unlikely that this process can contribute to microangiopathy. It appears that even pericytes can take up APP and process to ABP (Perlmutter 1994). However, experimental evidences are still lacking to support this idea (Goldgaber et al., 1989; Natte et al., 1999).

Thus, there are reasons to believe that the main source of ABP in the cerebral capillary basal lamina is due to ABP-trafficking via the BBB, either from plasma to the brain, or conversely from the brain parenchyma to the cerebral circulation. The deposition of ABP is also influenced by ABP transport across the BBB in either direction together with the "sink" action of CSF and blood. The production, metabolism and aggregation of ABP are the main leading factors responsible for AD.

In addition, the toxic nature of ABP to the endothelium, smooth muscle cells and the pericytes (Kalaria 1997; Price et al., 1997; Janscó et al., 1998) can contribute to the pathological breakdown of the BBB and influence microvascular structural integrity commonly seen in AD. It would be interesting to see whether expression of various stress proteins, e.g., heat shock protein (HSP) occurs in the brains or spinal cord of AD patients. This will give new insight in progression and pathogenesis of AD in relation to stress reaction.

To combat the devastating disaster of the society that affects millions of people World-wide new therapeutic strategies to manipulate the ABP transport at the BBB to decrease systemic influx and enhance the CNS efflux may be one way to minimize the pathogenesis of AD in the near future.

Heat Stress and Neurodegeneration

Heat stress and associated heat stroke in which body temperature rises above 40° C are life-threatening illnesses. Severe CNS dysfunction, e.g., delirium, convulsion, coma and death of more than 50 % of the victims can be seen within short duration in spite of lowering of the body temperature and therapeutic intervention (see Bouchama and Knochel 2002). Postmortem studies show profound brain damage, microhaemorrhages, vascular pathology, BBB disruption, nerve cell damage and cell death. The survivors often exhibit severe cognitive deficits, dementia and other abnormal mental functions (see Sharma and Hoopes 2003; Sharma 2004).

There are reasons to believe that the pathological mechanisms behind brain damage caused by heat stress induced hyperthermia is quite comparable to that seen in several neurodegenerative diseases. Thus, experimental models of heat stress induced brain damage could be used to study the pathophysiological principles of brain dysfunction in neurodegenerative diseases.

Blood-Brain Barrier in Heat Stress

Our laboratory was the first to demonstrate breakdown of the BBB during experimental or environmental heat stress in rats without developing heat stroke (Sharma and Dey 1978; Sharma 1982; Sharma and Dey 1984). This indicates that environmental heat exposure during summer months in many parts of the World could influence neuronal function and/or neurodegeneration due to BBB disruption (Sharma and Dey 1978; Sharma 1982; Sharma and Dey 1984). However, the role of external (environmental) or internal (fever, hyperpyrexia) factors leading to heat stress on the development of neurodegenerative diseases are not known and require further investigation.

Therapeutic hyperthermia using WBH is commonly employed as an adjunct to cytotoxic therapy for cancer treatment (see Katschinski et al., 1999; Sharma and Hoopes 2003 for review). However, DNA damage, inhibition of DNA repair, increased drug permeability and decreased resistance to DNA damaging agents are common during a combination of WBH and cytotoxic therapy for cancer treatment (Robins et al.,1995; 1997; see Sharma and Hoopes 2003 for details). Interestingly, effects of WBH on BBB functions during cancer therapy are still not well known (see Sminia et al., 1994). Since WBH appears to be a promising therapy for cancer patients, further studies in animal models are needed to examine BBB and brain dysfunction in details.

Experimental Studies on Heat Stress and Brain Dysfunction

A rat model to simulate WBH without having heat stroke is developed in our laboratory (Sharma 1982; Sharma and Dey 1986). In this model, rats were exposed to heat stress in a biological oxygen demand (BOD) incubator at 38 ° C for 1 h, 2 h and 4 h (Sharma 1982; Sharma and Dey 1986b; 1987b). The relative humidity (45-47 %) and wind velocity (20 to 26 cm/sec) was fairly kept constant (Sharma 1982; Sharma and Dey 1986b; 1987b).

Heat exposed young rats showed hyperthermia (>3.5 ° C; <42 ° C), behavioural symptoms and massive haemorrhagic petachae in the stomach wall after 4 h and not before (Table 9). Adult animals when exposed to 4 h heat stress did not show much symptoms indicating that stress reaction in WBH is dependent on the duration and age of the animals (see Sharma and Hoopes 2003).

Table 9. Stress symptoms in heat stressed rats

Parameters examined	Control n = 8	Heat stress at 38° C in BOD chamber		
		1 h n = 6	2 h n = 8	4 h n = 12
A. Stress symptoms				
Rectal T° C	37.42±0.23	38.41±0.32*	39.24±0.21**	41.48±0.23***
Salivation	nil	++	+++	+++
Prostration	nil	Nil	Nil	+++
Gastric haemorrhage	nil	4±3	8±3	(microhaemorrhages)

nil = absent, ++ = mild, +++ = moderate, ++++ = severe; * = P < 0.05, ** = P <0.01, *** = P <0.001 Student's unpaired t-test

Modified after Sharma 1982: Sharma and Dey 1986;1987.

BBB Permeability and Cerebral Blood Flow

Young rats subjected to 4 h heat stress showed marked increase in the BBB to Evans blue albumin and radioiodine tracer that varied slightly in individual animals (Figs. 4 and 5). Extravasation of Evans blue is apparent in 8 brain regions, viz., cingulate cortex, occipital cortex, parietal cortex, cerebellum, temporal cortex, frontal cortex, hypothalamus and thalamus (Figs. 5 and 6). In heat stressed rats, the blood-CSF barrier also appears to be disrupted. This is evident from a mild to moderate blue staining of the ventricular walls. The lateral ventricles exhibited mild staining whereas the fourth ventricle showed deep blue staining. The dorsal surface of the hippocampus and caudate nucleus took mild to moderate blue staining as well. The structures around the third ventricles were stained moderately blue (Fig. 6).

This increase in the BBB permeability was not evident in animals subjected to 1 h or 2 h heat exposure. The adult animals showed only mild increase in the BBB permeability after 4 h heat stress. These observations indicate the duration and age of animals is important factors in BBB dysfunction in heat stress.

In heat stressed animals, the regional cerebral blood flow (CBF) decreased in most of the brain regions after 4 h in young animals. However, the magnitude of CBF reduction did not correlate with the intensity of BBB breakdown (Fig. 7).

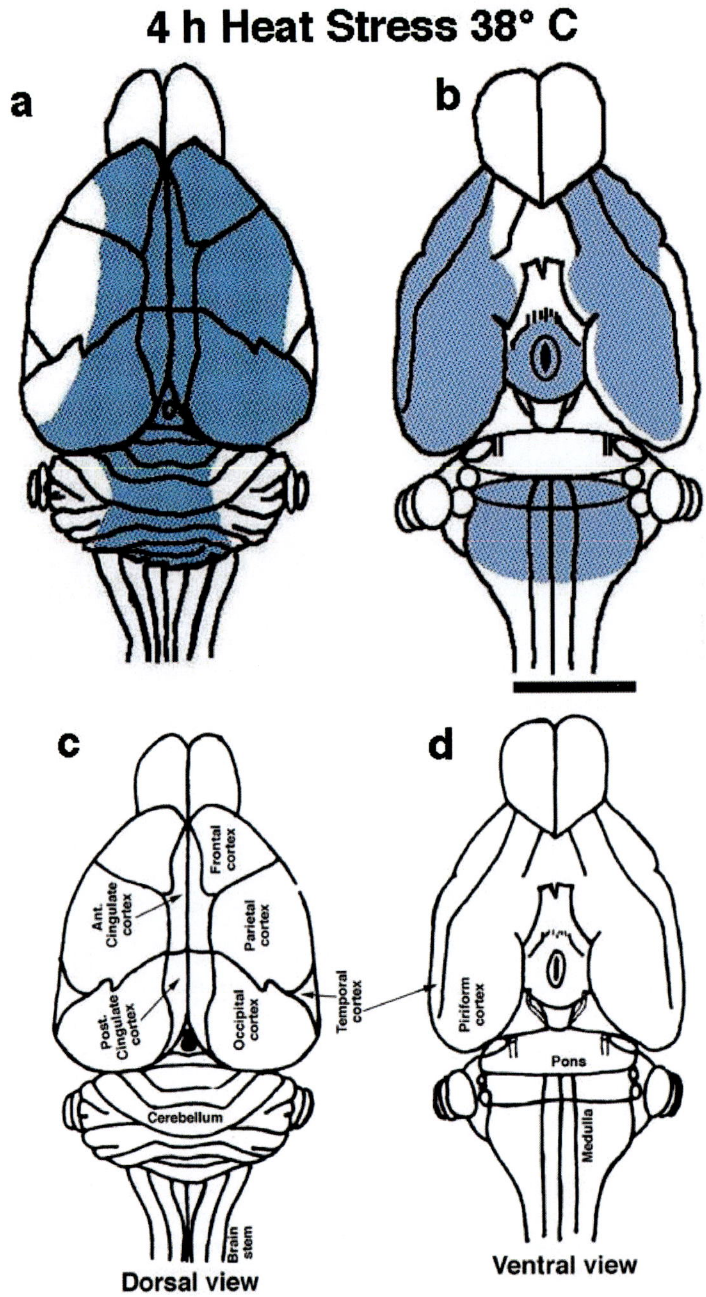

Fig. 4 Diagrammatic representation of Evans blue albumin (EBA) extravasation on the dorsal and ventral surfaces of the rat brain after 4 h heat stress (HS). Bar = 5 mm (After Sharma 2004). Different regions of the cerebral cortex are divided using hypothetical solid black lines. Bar = 4 mm (After Sharma 2004a).

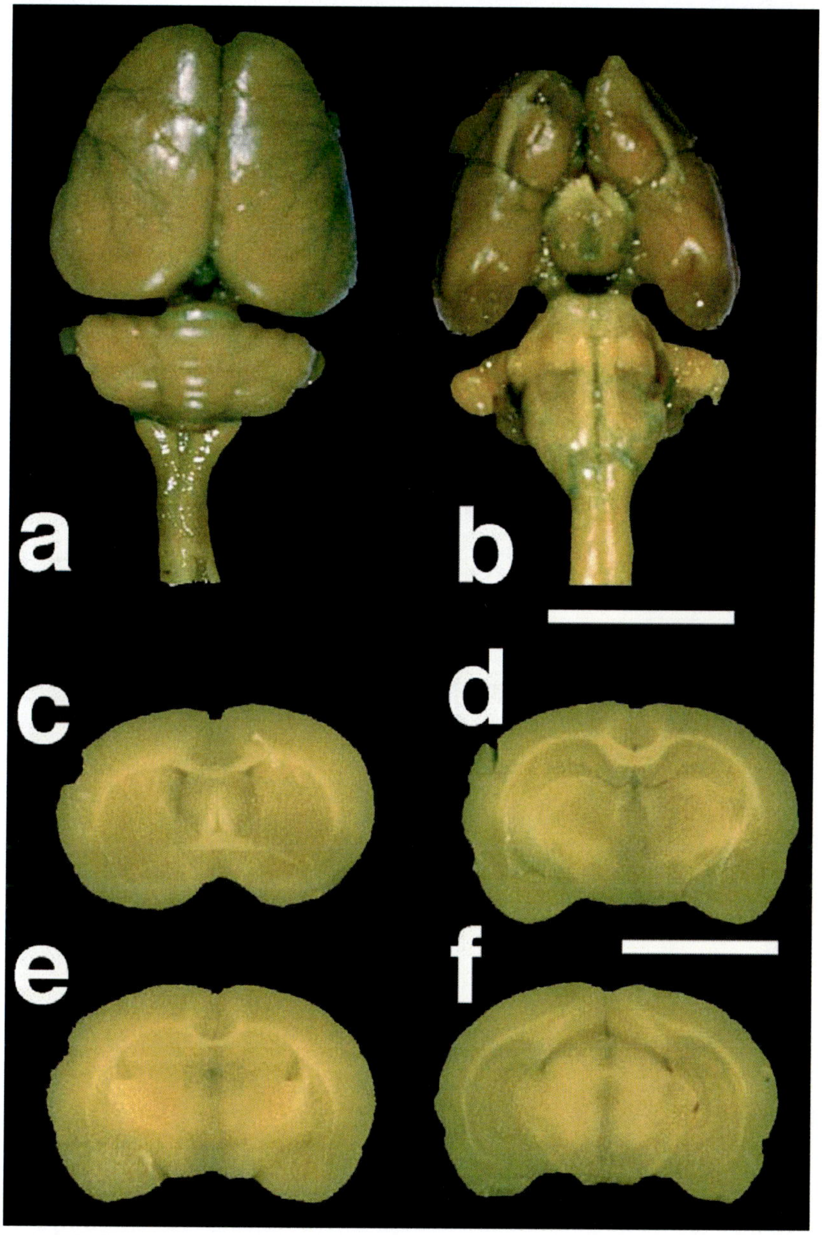

Fig. 5. One representative example of Evans blue albumin (EBA) extravasation on the dorsal and ventral surfaces as well as in the deeper parts of the rat brain following heat stress. Mild to moderate Evans blue staining of somatosensory cortex, piriform cortex, cerebellum, hypothalamus, pons and brain stem are evident (a,b). Coronal sections of rat brain from 4 different levels (c-f) showing EBA extravasation in deep brain structures, e.g., caudate putamen (c), hippocampus (d-e), thalamus (d-f), and hypothalamus (d-f). (Co-ordinates for coronal sections from Bregma: c = + 0.10 to +0.45; d -3.25 to -3.90; e = -4.20 to -4.60; f = -5.25 to - 6.65). Bar = 5 mm (Modified from Sharma 2004).

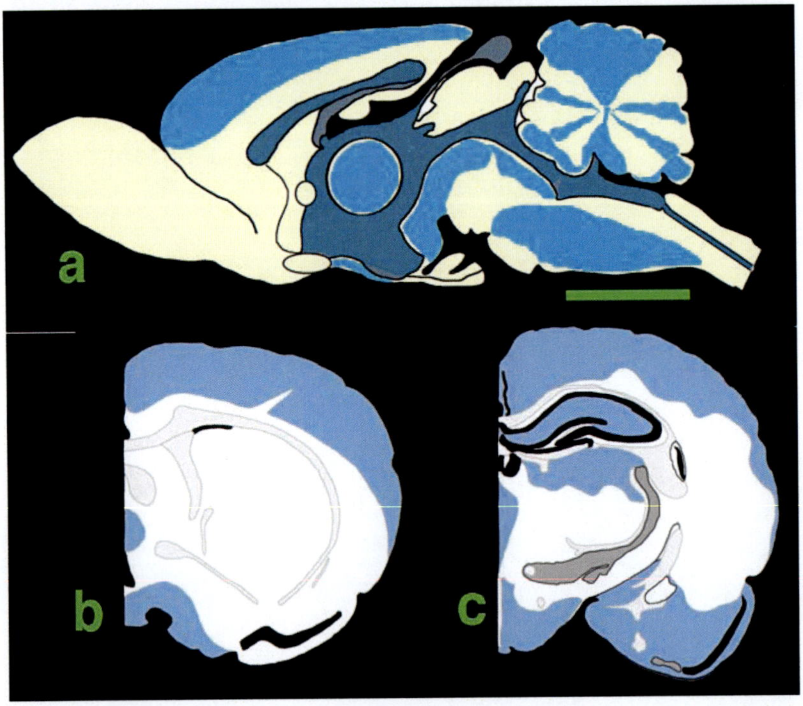

Fig. 6. Diagrammatic representation of mid-sagittal section of the rat brain showing extravasation of Evans blue albumin (EBA) following heat stress (HS, a). Staining of cerebroventricular walls of the lateral ventricles, 4th ventricle and median eminence is apparent. Bar = 5 mm. Cross sections of the brain passing through caudate-putamen (+0.45 from bregma, b) and hippocampal (-3.25 from bregma, c) levels showed leakage of EBA in the primary somato-sensory cortex, piriform cortex , hippocampus, hypothalamus and amygdala. Bar = 5 mm (Modified from Sharma 2004).

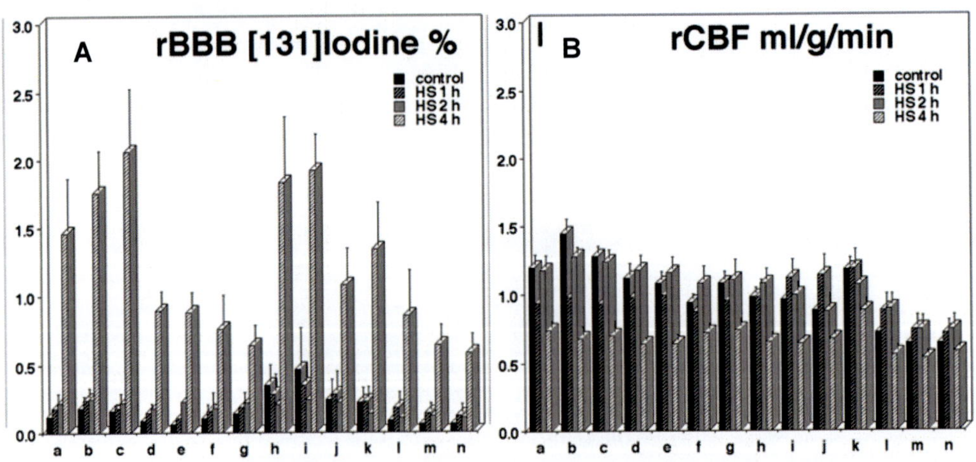

Fig. 7. Regional blood-brain barrier (rBBB, A) permeability and regional cerebral blood flow (rCBF, B) following heat stress. The rBBB permeability showed significant increase to [131]Iodine in all brain regions after 4 h heat stress. A significant decrease in the rCBF at this time is observed in identical regions. Alterations in the rBBB or rCBF during short periods of heat stress are not significant from the control group. a = frontal cortex, b = parietal cortex, c = occipital cortex, d = temporal cortex, e = cingulate cortex, f = hippocampus, g = caudate nucleus, h = thalamus, i = hypothalamus, j = sup. colliculus, k = inf. colliculus, l = cerebellum, m = pons, n = medulla. Values are mean±SD of 10 to 12 rats. Modified after Sharma 2004.

Brain Edema

Extravasation of endogenous serum proteins is associated with vasogenic edema formation (see Sharma et al., 1998). It appears that volume swelling of brain in closed cranial compartment is responsible for instant death of heat stroke victims due to compression of the vital centers. Thus, in heat stressed rats, brain edema was examined using measurement of the brain water content. The brain water content increased significantly in rats subjected to 4 h heat stress (Fig. 8). No increase in brain water is observed in animals subjected to 1 h or 2 h heat exposure. In adult animals, or rats exposed to chronic heat stress, the magnitude and severity of edema formation are much less evident (Fig. 8). These observations suggest that edema formation following BBB breakdown is important factor, in heat stress induced pathophysiology of brain damage.

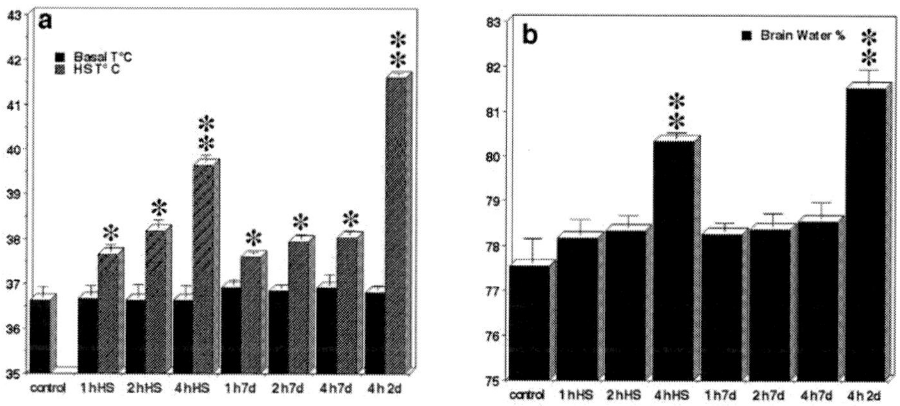

Fig. 8. Changes rectal temperature (a) and brain edema formation (b) in acute and chronic heat exposed rats. Significant increase in rectal temperature and brain water content is apparent following 4 h heat stress. No increase in body temperature or brain water content is seen in following 1 to 4 h heat exposure in heat adapted rats. Rats were adapted to heat by exposing them 1 h at 38° C for 7 days. However, when the adapted rats were subjected to an additional 4 h heat exposure on the 2nd day, profound hyperthermia and edema formation can be seen. Values are Mean±SD of 6 to 8 rats. Data modified after Sharma et al., 1986; 1992e.

Heat Stress Activates Spontaneous Electroencephalogram

Changes in the spontaneous electroencephalogram (EEG) or sensory evoked potentials occur following rise in brain temperature caused by exercise in hot environment (González-Alonso et al., 1999; Nielsen et al., 2001; Dubois et al., 1980; 1981; Febbraio et al., 1994). However, alterations in EEG activity at the time of the BBB breakdown in heat stress are still not well explored.

We recorded EEG in rats following heat stress using bipolar screw electrodes placed over the right and left cingulate and the parietal cortices (Fig. 9). The EEG in conscious rats consists an amplitude of 50 to 60 μV and a frequency of 6-7 Hz (Fig. 9). Exposure of rats to 1 h heat stress resulted in slight reduction in the EEG voltage (40 to 50 µV) with a mild increase in frequency (8-9 Hz). A significant reduction in EEG voltage is seen after 2 h heat exposure that was most marked in the cingulate cortex (20-30 µV; 8-9 Hz) (Fig. 9). At the end of 4 h heat exposure, the EEG amplitude reduced considerably (10-12 µV) in both the cingulate and parietal cortices with a slight increase in frequency (10-12 Hz) (Fig. 9). At this time, extravasation of Evans blue albumin is apparent in these areas of the cerebral cortex. This indicates that activation of EEG in heat stress occurs at the time of the BBB breakdown. Desynchronisation of neuronal activity in heat stress due to breakdown of the BBB permeability is likely to activate the cortical EEG.

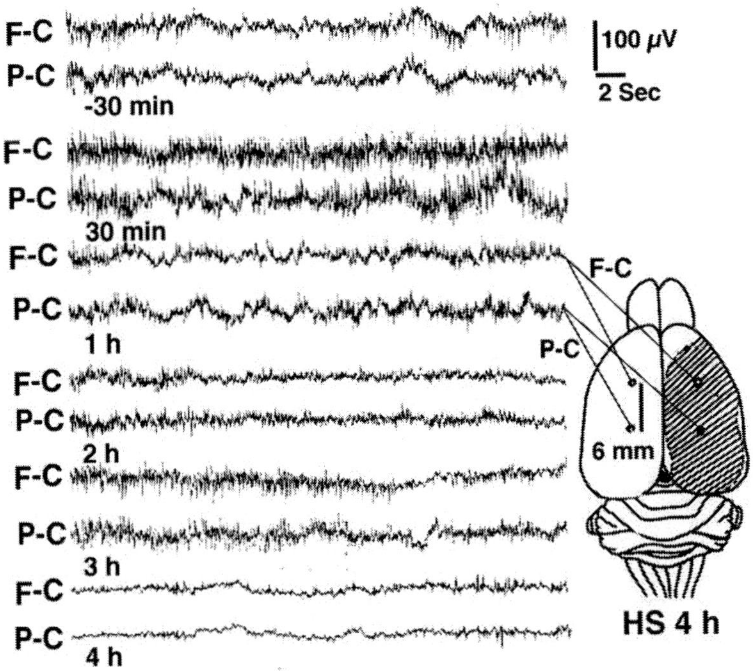

Fig. 9. Representative example of EEG tracings from bipolar electrodes placed on the frontal cortex (F-C) and parietal cortex (P-C) in acute heat stress. The EEG activity represents high voltage and slow activity (HVSA) before heat exposure (- 30 min). Flattening of EEG appeared at the end of 4 h heat exposure. At this time, BBB disruption to Evans blue dye is apparent (Modified after Sharma 2004).

Heat Stress Induces Selective Brain Damage

Heat stressed rats that exhibited BBB breakdown showed profound neuronal, glial and myelin damage (Figs. 10-12). These cell changes are commonly seen in the regions showing edematous expansion and BBB leakage e.g., cerebral cortex, brain stem, cerebellum, thalamus and hypothalamus (Figs. 10 and 11). Hippocampus showed a selective nerve cell damage in the CA-4 subfield (Fig. 10). Adult animals showed mild cell injury compared to young rats following heat exposure (Sharma 2004a).

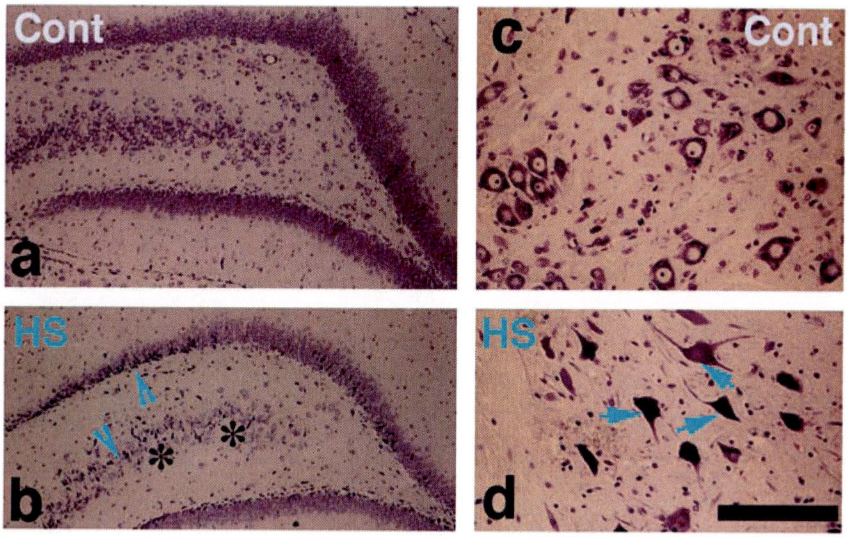

Fig. 10. Representative example of neuronal changes in 4 h heat stress (HS) in hippocampus (a,b) and in brain stem (c,d). Neuronal damage and degeneration (arrow heads) in dentate gyrus and CA-4 region (*) of the hippocampus (b) as well as several damaged and distorted nerve cells in the brain stem (d) are apparent (arrows) compared to respective controls (a, c). Nissl stain on 3 μm thick paraffin sections. Bars: A. a-b 50 μm; c-d 25 μm (Modified after Sharma 2004).

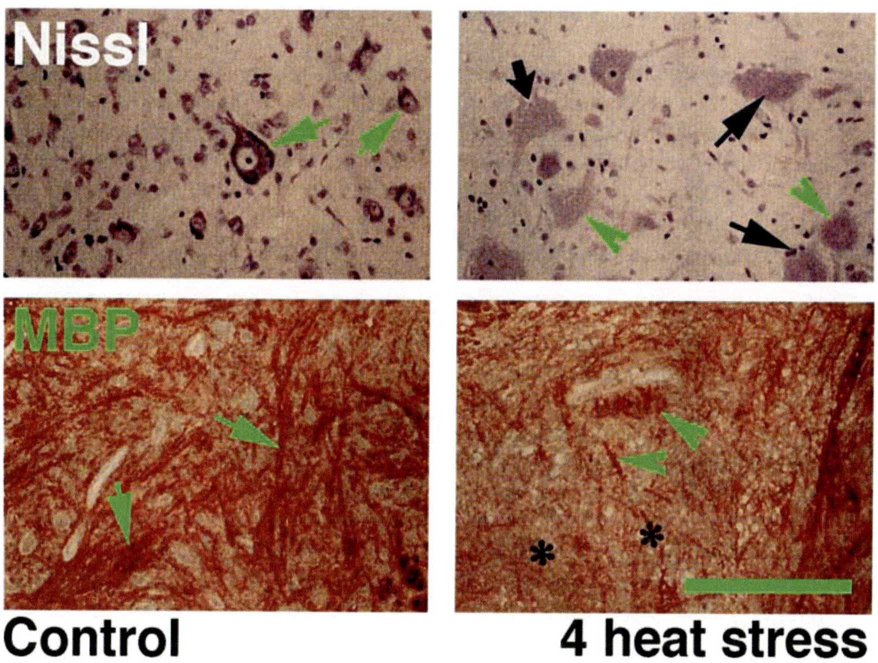

Fig. 11. Representative example of neuronal changes and myelin damage in 4 h heat stress (HS) compared to control. Degeneration of Nissl substance, vacuolation and edema around neurons (arrow heads) are apparent in the brain stem reticular formation (b) compared to control (arrows, a). Immunostaining of myelin basic protein (MBP) shows degeneration and loss of several myelinated fibers (arrow heads) in the thalamus of the heat stressed rats (d) compared to control (arrows, c). Bars: 50 μm; (Modified after Sharma et al., 1998c).

Profound axonal injuries in several parts of the brain are seen in young rats following heat exposure as evident with degradation of myelin basic protein (MBP) is immunohistochemistry (Sharma et al., 1992b; 1998a) (Fig. 11). This effect is much less apparent in adult animals (Fig. 11).

Glial cell activation seen with glial fibrillary acidic protein (GFAP) immunoreactivity is common in many parts of the brain exhibiting BBB breakdown (Sharma et al., 1992c). However, the magnitude of glial cell reaction in some brain regions does not coincide with the severity of BBB dysfunction or nerve cell damage (Fig. 12). This suggests that selective difference in the vulnerability of neurones, endothelial cells and glial cells exist in heat stress.

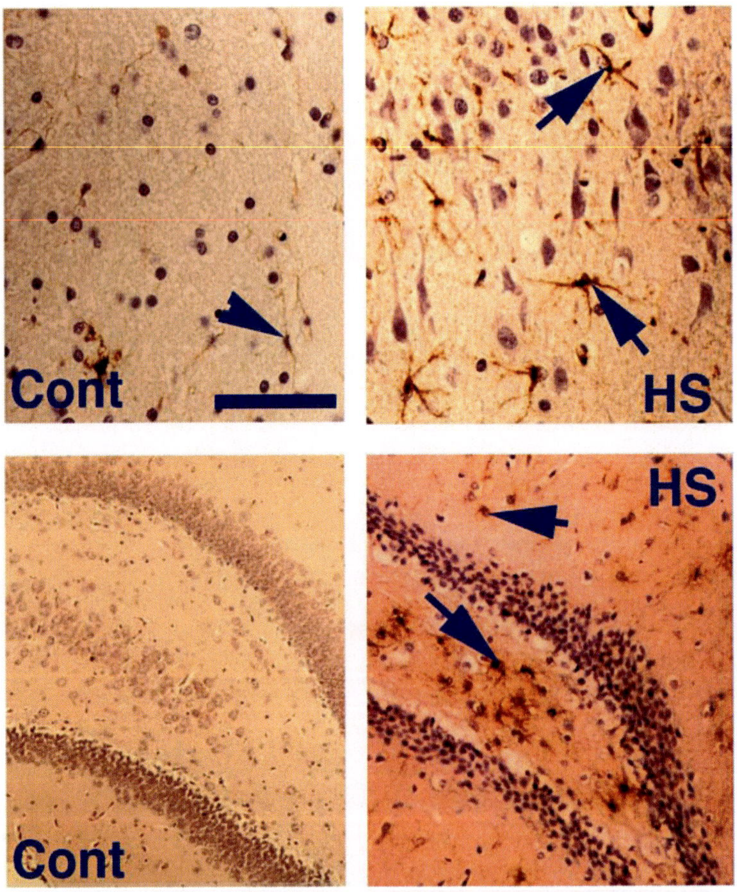

Fig. 12. Representative examples of astrocytic activation examined using glial fibrillary acidic protein (GFAP) immunoreactivity in heat stress. In heat stressed rats, star shaped astrocytes showing intense GFAP immunoreaction can be seen in the cortex (b) and hippocampus (d) compared to control (a,c). The GFAP immunostaining is prominent in the regions associated with BBB disruption and edema formation. Bar = 40 μm.

Ultratstructural Damage of Neuropil in Heat Stress

Ultratstructural studies demonstrated marked cell injury in several parts of the brain in young rats subjected to 4 h heat exposure. In the cerebral cortex, hippocampus, cerebellum, thalamus, hypothalamus, and brain stem many nerve cells with degenerated nuclei are present that often contain eccentric nucleolus (Fig. 13). Dark neurones containing vacuolated cytoplasm and degenerated nucleus with irregular foldings of the nuclear membrane are common findings in heat stress (Fig. 13). However, damage of one nerve cell appears to be very selective since the adjacent neuron may completely be normal in appearance in several brain regions.

In many regions damage to both pre- and post-synaptic membranes are quite common indicating gross dysfunction of neurochemical transmission in heat stress (Fig. 13). In some of brain regions damage to post-synaptic dendrites is also evident. Axonal damage, demyelination and vesiculation are most pronounced in the brain stem reticular formation, pons, medulla and the spinal cord (Fig. 13). Several unmyelinated axons are also swollen. These observations are in line with the idea that breakdown of the BBB is an important factor in brain damage.

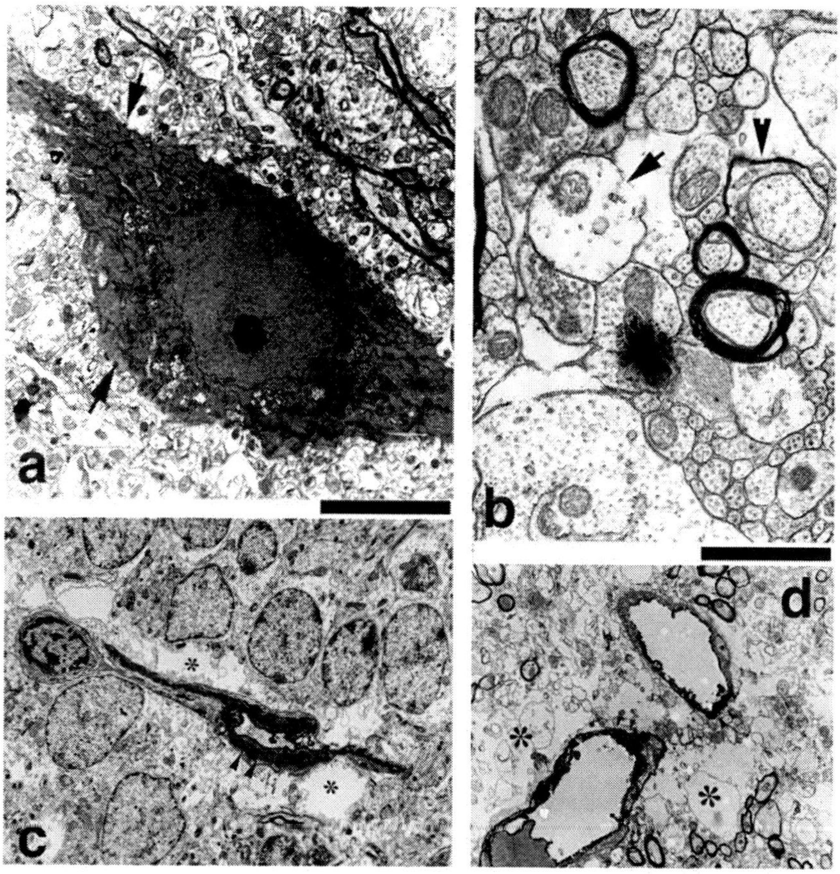

Fig. 13. Representative example of ultrastructural changes in the rat brain following 4 h heat stress (HS). One nerve cell with dark and electron dense cytoplasm (arrows) is seen in the cerebral cortex (a) along with other degenerative changes in the neuropil (b-d). High power electron micrograph from the parietal cerebral cortex cellular layer III shows damaged synapses (arrows), vesiculation of myelin and membrane damage (b). A completely collapsed microvessel (arrow heads) and distorted granule cells in the cerebellum are apparent (c). Perivascular edema (*), membrane damage and leakage of lanthanum across the microvessels (d) are apparent. Bars : a = 0.6 µm; b = 0.4 µm nm; c,d = 1 µm (Modified after Sharma et al., 1998; Sharma 2004).

Ultrastructural Changes in the Cerebral Endothelium

The microvascular pathology in heat stress is prominent in several brain regions. Several microvessels exhibit exudation of lanthanum across the cerebral endothelium in a very specific and selective manner (Figs. 13 and 14). Thus, in one microvessel often one endothelial cell is leaky to lanthanum, whereas the adjacent endothelial cells appear normal (see Fig. 14). In some brain regions, only one out of several microvessels may display lanthanum extravasation within the neuropil. This suggests that heat stress may influence selective activation of endothelial cell transporters, permeability factors, neurochemical receptors or ions channels in the brain.

In most vascular profiles, lanthanum is stopped at the luminal side of the tight junctions (Figs. 13 and 14) indicating that heat stress does not influence junctional widening. Thus, the increased endothelial cell membrane permeability rather than junctional widening plays important roles in lanthanum extravasation in heat stress. This mode of membrane permeability can be influenced by drugs modifying neurochemical receptors and /or signal transduction.

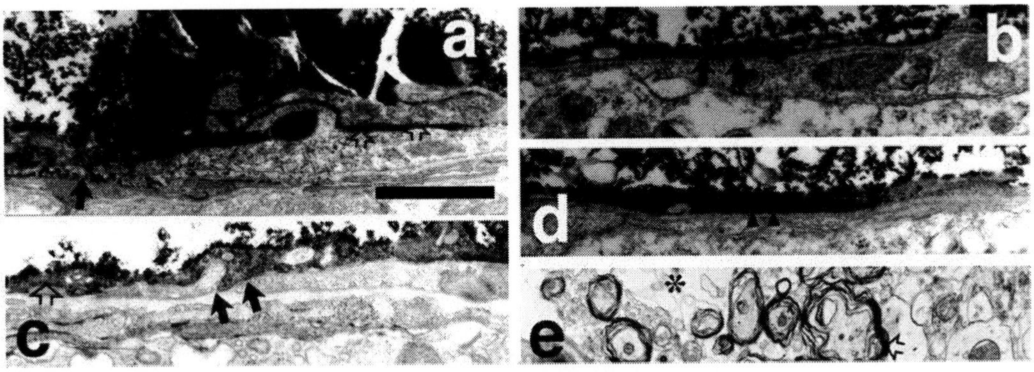

Fig. 14. Ultratstructural studies on the cerebral endothelial cells in heat stress showing distribution of the electron dense tracer, Lanthanum across the BBB. Lanthanum diffusely infiltrated within the cell membranes containing tight junction complex and enters into the endothelial cell cytoplasm (a). The tight junctions are not widened as lanthanum within the intercellular cleft is stopped at the junction (blank arrows, a). In other cases, the endothelial cell membrane became permeable to lanthanum (arrows, b,c). One endothelial cell showed lanthanum permeability in a certain segment of the endothelium (d arrow heads). Damage to neuropil (*) and myelin vesiculation are prominent in the adjacent area (e) exhibiting BBB disruption to lanthanum. Bars: A = 0.3 μm. Modified after Sharma et al., 1998a; Sharma 1999.

HSP Expression in Heat Stress

Several stressful stimuli, including hyperthermia induce HSP response that may serve as marker of cell injury or may have some role in repair and protective mechanisms (see Sharma and Hoopes 2003). There are reasons to believe that breakdown of the BBB may influence HSP expression in hyperthermia or other neurodegenerative diseases. Upregulation of HSP and another glial cell protein, vimentin in microvasculature following hyperthermic stress in rats are in line with this idea (Bechtold and Brown 2003).

We have taken a series of investigations to understand the role of BBB breakdown in relation to HSP expression in several models of CNS injuries including hyperthermia. The salient new findings in hyperthermia induced BBB disruption and HSP expression is discussed below.

HSP Immunohistochemistry

Immunohistochemistry was applied to study the HSP expression in the brain and spinal cord using antibodies directed against HSP-72 kD (Amersham, England; for details see Sharma et al., 1995). In brief, after routine fixation procedures (see Sharma et al., 1995), the desired tissue pieces from brain and spinal cord were dissected out and sectioned transversely (40 to 60 µm thick) on a Vibratome (Oxford Instruments, UK). These sections were transferred to the primary antibody solution (mouse anti-HSP antiserum 1:500) and normal swine serum (1:30 in phosphate buffer saline, PBS) and incubated free floating under agitation for 36 h at room temperature (Sharma et al., 1995). Immuno-complexes were developed using peroxidase-antiperoxidase (PAP) technique (Sharma et al., 1998). For electron microscopy, the sections were washed in 0.15 M sodium cacodylate buffer and post-fixed for 20 min in 2 % OsO_4 in cacodylate buffer, dehydrated in a graded series of ethanol and embedded in epon between acetate foils and polymerised at 60° C for 48 h (Sharma et al., 1995). For light microscopy, few sections in each block were not osmicated. In these sections, the immunoreaction against a light background was examined.

For ultrastructural investigation of labelled neurons, osmicated sections were used. The desired part of the tissue sections containing labelled neurones was trimmed out and the ultrathin sections were cut using a diamond knife (LKB, Ultramicrotome, Sweden). The ultrathin sections are collected on one hole grid and examined under a transmission electron microscope either unstained or counter stained with uranyl acetate and lead citrate (Sharma et al., 1995).

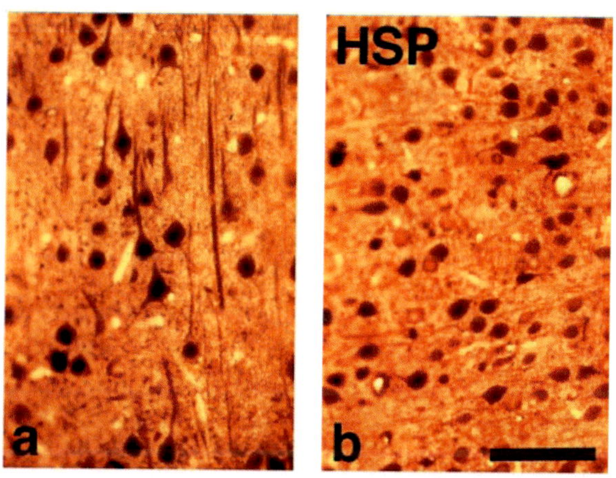

Fig. 15. Upregulation of heat shock proteins (HSP 72 kD) in heat stress in the cerebral cortex. Several nerve cells (arrows) exhibited pronounced HSP expression (a). The immunoreaction product is seen in both cytoplasm and karyoplasm (b). HSP expression in small cells (may be astrocytes) as well dendrites are celery visible (b). Bar: 40 µm (Modified after Sharma and Westman 2004).

Hyperthermia Induced HSP Expression

Subjection of young rats to 4 h heat exposure induced marked HSP expression in nerve cell nucleus as well as in the neuronal cytoplasm in several regions of the brain and spinal cord (Figs. 15 and 16; Table 10). Interestingly, the expression of HSP is most pronounced in the regions showing breakdown of the BBB. This indicates that disruption of the BBB plays an important role in HSP overexpression.

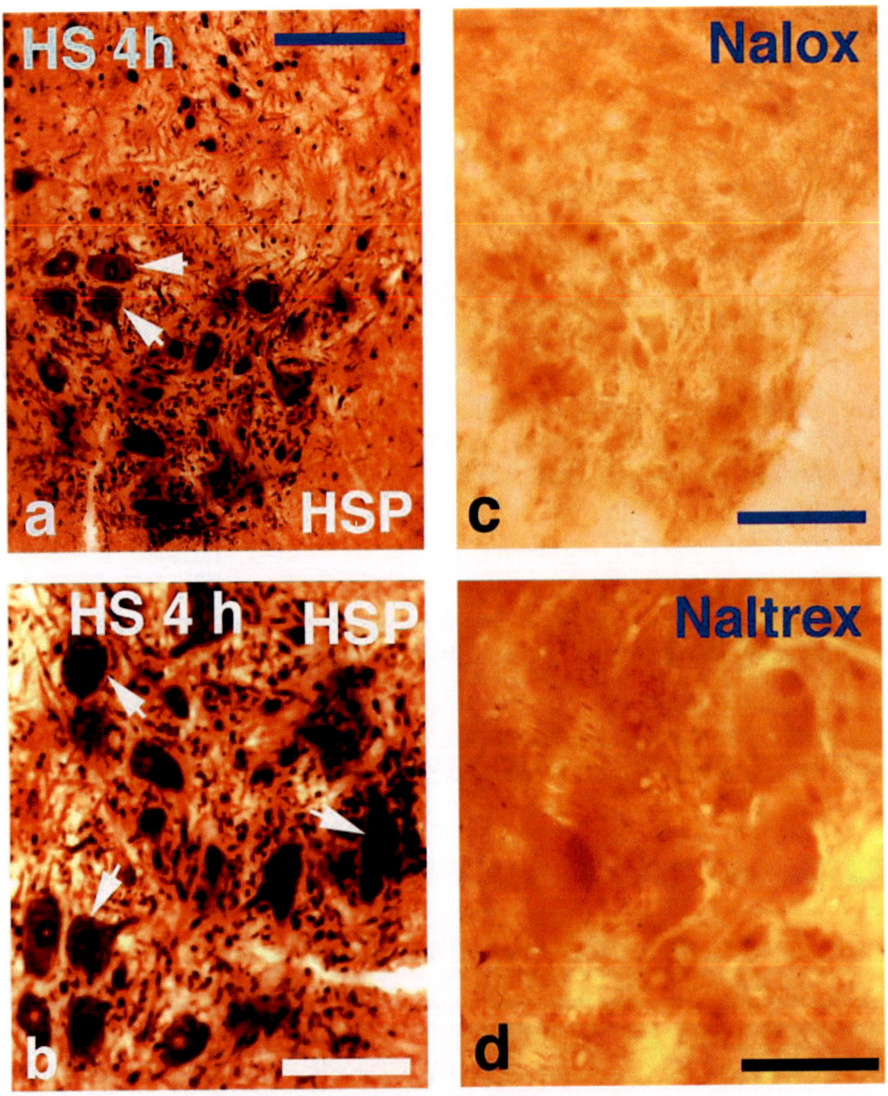

Fig. 16. HSP expression in spinal cord following heat stress (a,c) and its modification with drugs. Several HSP positive nerve cells (arrows) and dendrites in the ventral horn of the spinal cord (T8) are visible. Pretreatment with naloxone (Nalox, c) or naltrexone (Naltrex, d) prevented the upregulation of hyperthermia induced HSP expression in the spinal cord. Bar: A: a-d = 50 µm (Modified after Sharma and Westman 2004).

Table 10. Upregulation of HSP 72 (kDa) in the CNS of heat stress.

CNS regions	Control n = 5	heat stress conscious n = 6
Cerebral cortex		
cingulate anterior	+++	
cingulate posterior		+++
frontal	-/+?	+
parietal	-	+++
occipital	-	+++
temporal	-/+	+++
pyriform	++	
Cerebellum		
vermis	-	+++
cortex	-/+	+++
Hippocampus		
CA1	-	+
CA2	-	++
CA3	-/+?	++
CA4	-	+++
dentate gyrus	-	++
hilus	-	++
caudate nucleus		++
amygdala	-	+++
Colliculus		
colliculi superior	-	++
colliculi inferior	-	+++
Thalamus		
massa intermedia	-	+++
dorsal thalamic nuclei	-/+	++
ventral thalamic nuclei	-	+++
lateral thalamic nuclei	-	+++
Hypothalamus		
preoptic anterior	-	++
posterior hypothalamic nuclei	-	+++
brain stem	-/+	+++
reticular formation	-	+++
medulla	-	+++
Pons	-	+++
Spinal cord		
dorsal horn	-	++
ventral horn	-	+++
lateral horn	-	+++
white matter	-	+
central canal	-	++

- = negative, + = mild, ++ = moderate,+++ = profound immunostaining, ? = found in few cases only.

Modified after Westman and Sharma 1998; Sharma 2004

At the ultratstructural level, dark HSP reaction product in dendrites, endothelial cells as well as in the cytoplasm of nerve cell bodies are clearly evident (Fig. 17). The reaction product is largely attached to the surface of organelles including cytoskeleton and the endoplasmic reticulum (Fig. 17). Marked upregulation of HSP reaction product in the endothelial cells of cerebral and spinal capillaries at the ultratstructural level clearly indicates that compromise of the BBB in heat stress is somehow influences HSP expression.

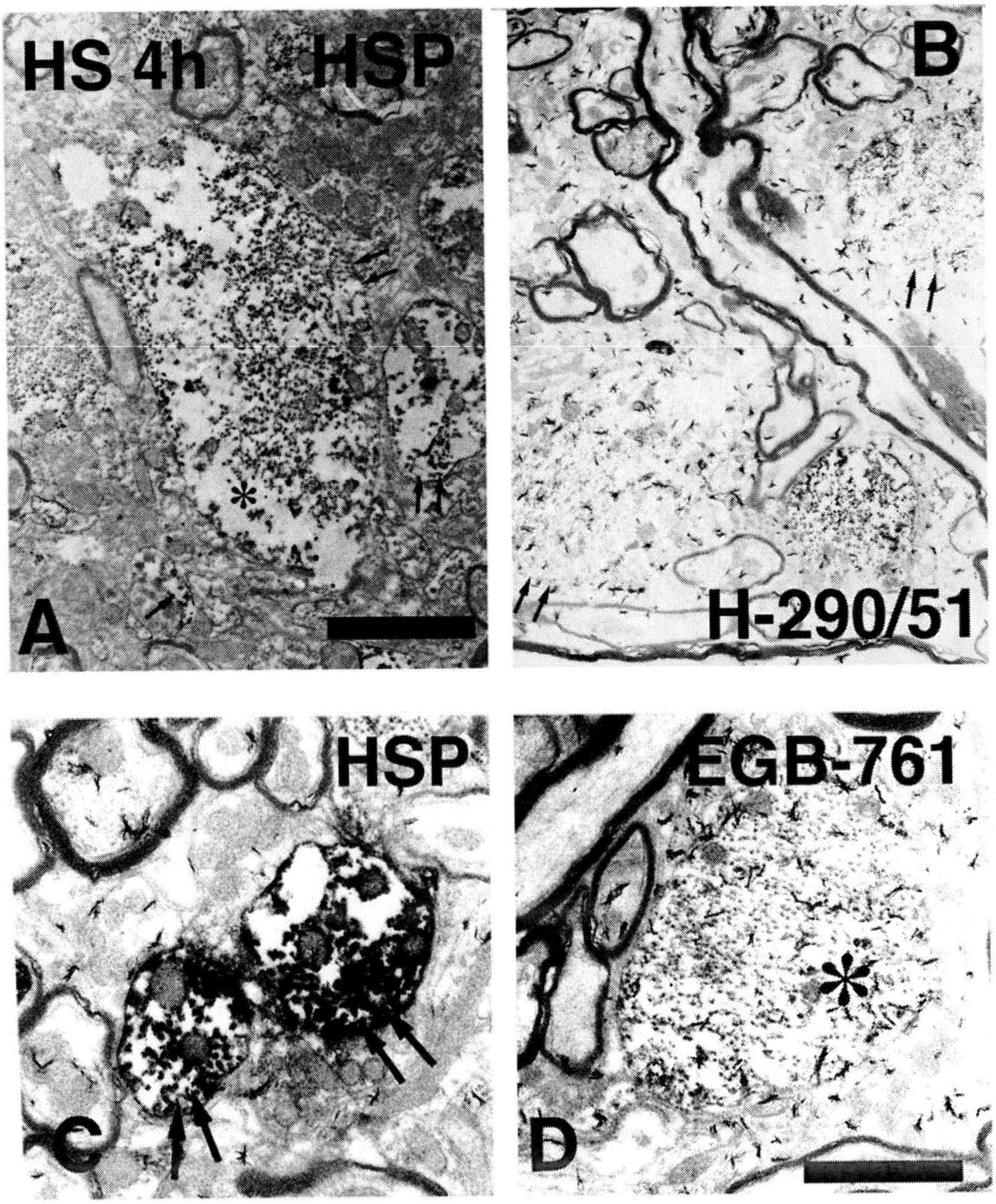

Fig. 17. Ultratstructural localisation of HSP immunoreactivity in heat stress (HS) and its modification with drugs. HSP immunoreactivity (seen as black immunoreaction products) is confined within the dendrites and attached to the cell cytoplasm (arrows, A, C). Pretreatment with H-290/51 (B) or EGB-761 (D) markedly attenuated the magnitude and intensity of HSP immunoreaction (Arrows, *, B,D). Bar: A-D= 0.5 μm. Data modified after Alm et al., 2000; Sharma 1999; Sharma and Westman 2004.

Factors Influencing HSP Expression

Several factors, e.g., extravasation of serum proteins and spread of edema fluids in the brain microenvironment or cellular injury signals following heat stress appear to play important roles in HSP induction (Sharma 1982; Sharma et al., 1992a). This hypothesis is examined using pharmacological manipulation of microvascular permeability disturbances, edema formation and cell injury.

Opioids and HSP Expression

To understand the role of opioids in hyperthermia induced HSP expression, separate groups of young animals were pretreated with multiple opioid receptor blocker drugs, e.g., naloxone (1 mg, 5 mg and 10 mg /kg, i.p.) or naltrexone (1 mg, 5 mg and 10 mg/kg, i.p.) (Martin 1983; Sharma et al., 1997a). Pretreatment with high dose of naloxone or naltrexone (10 mg/kg, i.p.) significantly attenuated HSP expression in the brain that was most pronounced in the spinal cord, cerebral cortex, hippocampus and in the hypothalamus (Fig. 16). The effects of naloxone are far more superior that naltrexone on inhibition of HSP expression in heat stress (Figs. 16). However, equimolar dose of naloxone and naltrexone is required to clarify the dose-related effectiveness of the opioid antagonists on HSP expression.

The ability of these opioids antagonists in attenuating stress response, BBB permeability, edema formation and cell injury appears to be important factors in inhibiting HSP expression. The HSP expression in normal animals are not influenced by these drugs indicates that a direct inhibitory effect of naloxone or naltrexone is unlikely.

Oxidative Stress and HSP Expression

The influence of oxidative stress on HSP expression in heat stress is examined using potent antioxidant compounds H-290/51 (Svensson et al., 1993; Sharma et al., 1997b) and EGB-761 and BN-52021 (Sharma et al., 2000).

Pretreatment with H-290/51, a chain breaking antioxidant significantly reduced the HSP expression of HSP following heat exposure (Fig. 18). HSP expression in nerve cells and dendrites at the ultrastructural level are also much less evident in H-290/51 pretreated group indicating that oxidative stress contributes to HSP induction.

Production of free radical and lipid peroxidation can directly damage the endothelial cell membrane causing disruption of the BBB. Pretreatment with H-290/51 significantly attenuated BBB permeability and cell injury (Sharma et al., 2001). This suggests that oxidative stress induced cellular damage and BBB disruption is important factors in attenuating HSP expression in heat stress (Hedlund et al., 1999; see Mautes and Noble 2000; Matz et al., 2001a,b).

To further confirm the role of oxidative stress in HSP induction, we used two potent antioxidant substances EGB-761 and Ginkgolide B that are known free radical scavengers with some capacity to inhibit lipid peroxidation (DeFudis 1998). The EGB-761 is a standardised extract from Ginkgo biloba leaves that contains falvonoids (24 % of flavonol hetrosides and about 7 % proanthocyanidins) and 6 % terpene trilactones (Ginkgolides A, B, C and bilobalide) (DeFudis 1998; Sharma et al., 1999; 2000e). The flavonoids posses radical scavangering activity and the Ginkgolides are known to inhibit free radical formation and to block lipid peroxidation (Köse and Dogan 1995; DeFudis 1998).

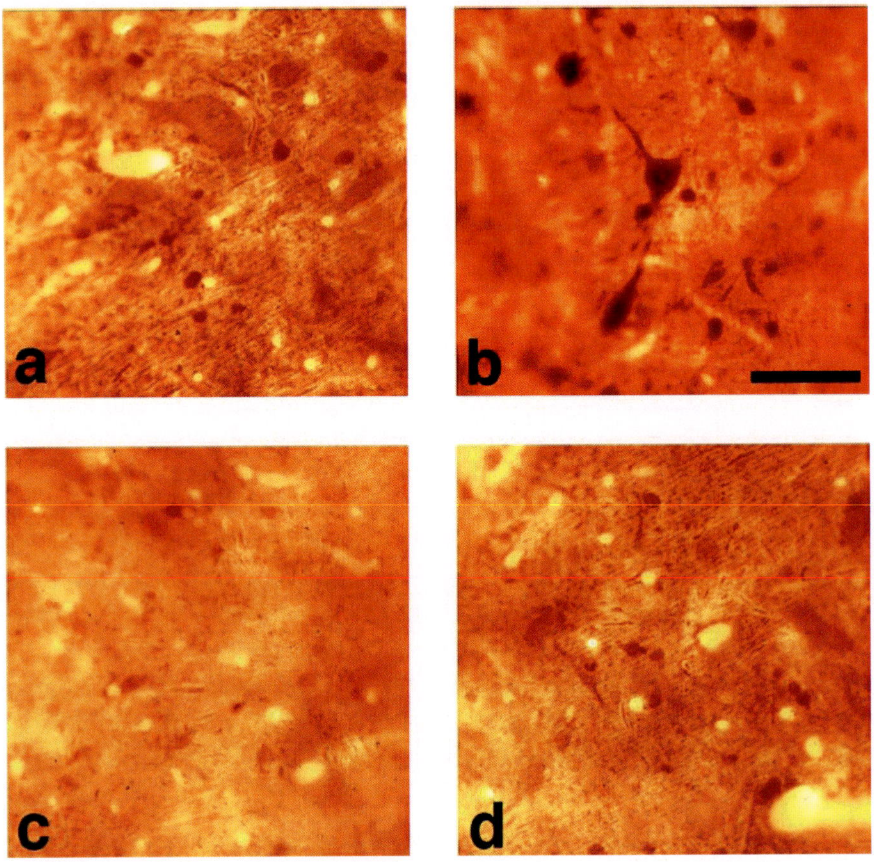

Fig. 18. HSP immunoreaction product in the brain and spinal cord of 4 h heat stressed rats and its modification with anaesthesia and drugs. The HSP upregulation is markedly attenuated in heat stressed animals pretreated with either EGB-761 (a), BN-52021 (b) or H-290/51 (c). Urethane anaesthetised animals (d) did not exhibit upregulation of HSP in heat stress. Bar: a,b = 60 µm; c,d = 30 µm. Data modified after Westman and Sharma 1998; Sharma 1999; Sharma and Westman 2004.

Pretreatment with EGB-761 or Ginkgolide B significantly attenuated the HSP expression in heat stress (Fig. 18). The effect of EGB-761 on HSP expression was far more superior than Ginkgolide B pretreatment (Fig. 18).

These observations support the idea that generation of free radicals and lipid peroxidation are important cellular or molecular signals for abnormal production of HSP. The capability of EGB-761 and BN-52021 to reduce hyperthermia induced BBB disruption, brain edema and cell injury suggest that these factors are important in HSP induction in heat stress. Obviously, free radical formation and lipid peroxidation contribute to BBB damage and cell injury.

Functional Significance of HSP Expression

Our observations are the first to demonstrate that the induction of HSP 72 kDa in neurons in heat stress is prevented by drugs capable to attenuate BBB disruption, edema formation and cell injury. This indicates that HSP response following heat stress or other neurodegenerative diseases is associated with breakdown of the BBB, local cellular stress and /or injury (Sharma et al., 1992a, Sharma et al., 1995; Sharma and Westman 1997).

These observations are in line with the hypothesis that induction of HSP is related to the magnitude and threshold of cell survival. Thus, when the HSP response is induced in the cell following thermal or other noxious insults to the CNS, further induction by the similar intensity of the stimuli is not possible because of desensitization of either the stress protein or the stress reaction itself (Welch 1992; Marcuccilli and Miller 1994; Sharma and Westman 2000). The threshold for cell damage is also enhanced by repeated thermal insult (Manzerra et al., 1993; Westman and Sharma 1998).

Drugs that thwart HSP expression in hyperthermia may be able to attenuate the cellular or molecular signal responsible for cellular stress needed to induce HSP expression. Obviously, disruption of the cellular microenvironment due to BBB breakdown and exposure of neuronal elements to edema fluid could be other important signals responsible for HSP induction.

This is further supported by the fact that drugs or compounds that attenuated the cellular stress, BBB dysfunction and/or cell injury considerably reduced the HSP induction (Chen et al., 1998; Shen et al., 1998; Stücker et al., 1998). It may be that edema by itself or a component of the edema fluid triggers the cellular stress response (Sharma et al., 1995). Induction of HSP response in various neural or non-neural cells by ACTH, catecholamines and cytokines is in line with this hypothesis (Blake et al., 1994; D'Souza et al., 1994; Udelsman et al., 1994; Marcuccilli and Miller 1994).

In conclusion, it appears that extravasation of serum components and spread of edema fluids are crucial factors in inducing HSP expression in the CNS. To further understand the molecular mechanisms of HSP expression it remains to be seen whether other members of HSP family, i.e., 27 kDa, 60 kDa, 90 kDa and 110 kDa are also expressed in hyperthermia under similar conditions.

CONCLUSION

Evidences presented in this review clearly suggest that the BBB disruption during stress is instrumental in causing selective neural injury leading to long-term consequences leading to abnormal brain function. Alterations in fluid microenvironment of the brain together with edema formation results in several cellular and molecular changes in the brain responsible for HSP induction, cell injury and/or cell death. Restoration of normal BBB function in hyperthermia or other CNS diseases by drugs could be one of the promising approaches to minimise neurodegenerative changes. Taken together, it appears that disruption of BBB is the gateway for brain dysfunction and on neurological disorders leading to neurodegeneration.

ACKNOWLEDGEMENTS

Research reported in this review was supported by Grants form Swedish Medical Research Council (Nr. 2710); AstraZeneca, Mölndal, Sweden; Alexander von Humboldt Foundation, Bonn, Germany; IPSEN-Medical, Paris, France; The University Grants Commission, New Delhi, India and The Indian Council of Medical Research, New Delhi, India. Technical assistance of Kärstin Flink, Kerstin Rystedt, Madeleine Thörnwall and Ulla

Johanssson and secretarial assistance of Aruna Sharma and Suraj Sharma is highly appreciated. Critically reading of the manuscript and constructive suggestions on section on Alzheimer's disease by Professor Berislav Zlokovic, University of Rochester Medical School, Rochester, USA and on other sections by Dr Rajendra D Badgaiyan, Harvard Medical School, Harvard University, Boston, USA are acknowledged with thanks.

REFERENCES

Abe H, Rusak B, Robertson HA (1991) Photic induction of Fos protein in the suprachiasmatic nucleus is inhibited by the NMDA receptor antagonist MK-801. *Neurosci Lett 127(1)*:9-12

Abercrombie ED, Jacobs BL (1987) Single-unit response of noradrenergic neurons in the locus coeruleus of freely moving cats. II. Adaptation to chronically presented stressful stimuli. J *Neurosci 7(9)*:2844-8

Ahlemeyer B, Krieglstein J (2003) Pharmacological studies supporting the therapeutic use of Ginkgo biloba extract for Alzheimer's disease. *Pharmacopsychiatry. 36* Suppl 1:S8-14.

Alzheimer A (1907) Uber eine eigenartig Erkrankung der Hirnrinde. Allg Z *Psychiatrie Psych Ger Med 64:* 146-148.

Anthony SG, Schipper HM, Tavares R, Hovanesian V, Cortez SC, Stopa EG, Johanson CE (2003) Stress protein expression in the Alzheimer-diseased choroid plexus. *J Alzheimers Dis. 5(3)*:171-7.

Banks WA, Kastin AJ, Barrera CM (1991) Delivering peptides to the central nervous system: dilemma and strategies. *Pharmacol Res 8*: 1345-1350.

Bechtold DA, Brown IR (2003) Induction of Hsp27 and Hsp32 stress proteins and vimentin in glial cells of the rat hippocampus following hyperthermia. *Neurochem Res*. 2003 Aug;28(8):1163-73.

Beere HM, Wolf BB, Cain K, Mosser DD, Mahboubi A, Kuwana T, Tailor P, Morimoto RI, Cohen GM, Green DR (2000) Heat-shock protein 70 inhibits apoptosis by preventing recruitment of procaspase-9 to the Apaf-1 apoptosome. *Nat Cell Biol 2(8)*:469-75

Blake MJ, Buckley AR, Buckley DJ, LaVoi KP, Bartlett T (1994) Neural and endocrine mechanisms of cocaine-induced 70-kDa heat shock protein expression in aorta and adrenal gland. *J Pharmacol Exp Ther 268(1)*:522-9

Blalock JE (1984) The immune system as a sensory organ. *J Immunol 132*: 1067-1070.

Blennow K, Wallin A, Fredman P, Karlssom I, Gottfries CG, Svennerholm L (1990) Blood-brain barrier disturbances in patients with Alzheimer's disease is related to vascular factors. *Acta neurol Scand 81*: 323-326.

Bouchama A, Knochel JP (2002) Heat stroke. *N Engl J Med 346(25)*:1978-88

Bradbury MWB (1979) *The Concept of a Blood-Brain Barrier*, Chicester, UK.

Bradbury MWB (1990) Physiology and pharmacology of the blood-brain barrier. *Handbook Exp Pharmacol 103:* 1-450, Springer, Heidelberg.

Bronstein JM, Farber DB, Wasterlain CG (1993) Regulation of type-II calmodulin kinase: functional implications. *Brain Res Rev 18(1)*:135-47.

Brown IR, Rush S, Ivy GO (1989) Induction of a heat shock gene at the site of tissue injury in the rat brain. *Neuron 2(6)*:1559-64

Buée L, Hof PR, Delacourte AD (1997) Brain microvascular changes in Alzheimer's disease and other dementias. *Ann NY Acad Sci 826*:7-24.

Burgermeister P, Calhoun ME, Winkler DT, Jucker M (2000) Mechanisms of cerebrovascular amyloid deposition. Lessons from mouse models. *Ann NY Acad Sci 903*:307-316.

Busciglio J, Yeh J, Yankner BA (1993) beta-amyloid neurotoxicity in human culture is not mediated by excitotoxins. *J Neurochem 61*: 1565-1568.

Carlsson C, Hagerdal M, Siesjö BK (1975) Increase in cerebral oxygen uptake and blood flow in immobilization stress. *Acta Physiol Scand 95(2):*206-8

Carlsson C, Hgerdal M, Kaasik AE, Siesjö BK (1976a) The effects of diazepam on cerebral blood flow and oxygen consumption in rats and its synergistic interaction with nitrous oxide. *Anesthesiology 45(3):*319-25

Carlsson C, Hagerdal M, Siesjö BK (1976b) Protective effect of hypothermia in cerebral oxygen deficiency caused by arterial hypoxia. *Anesthesiology 44(1):*27-35

Castano EM, Prelli F, Soto C, Beavis R, Matsubara E, Shoji M, Frangione B (1996) The length of amyloid-beta in hereditary cerebral hemorrhage with amyloidosis. Dutch type. Implications for the role of amyloid-b-1-42 in Alzheimer's disease. *J Bio Chem 271*: 32185-32191.

Charney DS, Deutch AY, Krystal JH, Southwick SM, Davis M (1993) Psychobiologic mechanisms of posttraumatic stress disorder. *Arch Gen Psychiatry 50*:295-305.

Chen JX, Chen WZ, Huang HL, Chen LX, Xie ZZ, Zhu BY (1998) Protective effects of Ginkgo biloba extract against lysophosphatidylcholine-induced vascular endothelial cell damage. *Acta Pharmacol Sinica 19*: 359-363.

Clarimon J, Bertranpetit J, Boada M, Tarraga L, Comas D. (2003) HSP70-2 (HSPA1B) is associated with noncognitive symptoms in late-onset Alzheimer's disease. *J Geriatr Psychiatry Neurol. 16(3):*146-50.

Ciocca DR, Oesterreich S, Chamness GC, McGuire WL, Fuqua SA (1993) Biological and clinical implications of heat shock protein 27,000 (Hsp27): a review. *J Natl Cancer Inst 85(19)*:1558-70

Claudio L (1996) Ultrastructural features of the blood-brain barrier in biopsy tissue from Alzheimer's disease patients. *Acta Neuropathol (Berl) 91*: 6-14.

Craig EA (1985) The heat shock response. CRC Crit Rev Biochem 18(3):239-80

Cullinan WE, Herman JP, Battaglia DF, Akil H, Watson SJ (1995) Pattern and time course of immediate early gene expression in rat brain following acute stress. *Neuroscience 64(2):*477-505

Corrodi H, Fuxe K, Lidbrink P, Olson L (1971) Minor tranquillizers, stress and central catecholamine neurons. *Brain Res 29(1):*1-16

Coussons-Read ME, Maslonek KA, Fecho K, Perez L, Lysle DT (1994) Evidence for the involvement of macrophage-derived nitric oxide in the modulation of immune status by a condition aversive stimulus. *J Neuroimmunol 50*: 51-58.

Crone C, Olesen SP (1982) Electrical resistance of brain microvascular endothelium. *Brain Res 241:* 49-55.

DeFudis, F. V. (1998) Gingko biloba extract. *From Chemistry to the Clinic*. Ullstein Medical Publishers, Weisbaden, pp. 1-395.

de la Torre JC (1999) Critical threshold cerebral hypoperfusion causes Alzheimer's disease. *Acta Neuropathol (Berl) 98*: 1-8.

de la Torre J C (2002) Alzheimer Disease as a vascular disorder. Nosological evidence. *Stroke 33:* 1152-1162.

D'Souza, S. D., Antel, J. P. and Freedman, M. S. (1994) Cytokine induction of heat shock protein expression in human oligodendrocytes: an interleukin-1-mediated mechanism. *J. Neuroimmunol. 50:* 17-24.

Dubois M, Sato S, Lees DE, Bull JM, Smith R, White BG, Moore H, Macnamara TE (1980) Electroencephalographic changes during whole body hyperthermia in humans. *Electroencephalogr Clin Neurophysiol 50(5-6):*486-95

Dubois M, Coppola R, Buchsbaum MS, Lees DE (1981) Somatosensory evoked potentials during whole body hyperthermia in humans. *Electroencephalogr Clin Neurophysiol 52(2):*157-62

Dunn AJ (1993) Role of cytokines in infection-induced stress. An NY Acad Sci 697: 189-202.

El Khoury J Hickman SE, Thomas CA, Cao L, Silverstein SC, Loke JD (1996) Scavenger receptor-mediated adhesion of microglia to b-amyloid fibrils. *Nature 382*: 716-719.

Engelhardt B, Laschinger M, Vajkoczy P (2003) Investigation of molecular mechanisms involved in T lymphocyte recruitment across the blood-spinal cord and brain barriers in health and disease. In: H S Sharma and J Westman (Eds) *The Blood-Spinal Cord and Brain Barriers in Health and Disease*, Elsevier Academic Press, San Diego, pp 117-158.

Farkas E, De Jong GI, Apró E, De Vos RAI, Jansen Steur ENH, Luiten PGM (2000) Similar ultrastructural breakdown of cerebrovascular capillaries in Alzheimer's disease, Parkinson's disease, and experimental hypertension. What is the functional link? *Ann NY Acad Sci 903*: 72-82.

Farkas E, Luiten PGM (2001) Cerebral microvascular pathology in aging and Alzheimer's disease. *Prog Neurobiol 64*: 575-611.

Febbraio MA, Snow RJ, Stathis CG, Hargreaves M, Carey MF (1994) Effect of heat stress on muscle energy metabolism during exercise. *J Appl Physiol 77(6):*2827-31

Frey KA (1998) Neurochemical imaging of Alzheimer's disease and other degenerative dementias. *Q J Nucl Med 42*: 166-178.

Frisoni GB, Calabresi L, Geroldi C, Bianchetti A, D'Acquarica AL, Govoni S, Sirtori CR, Trabucchi M, Franceschini G (1994) Apolipoprotein E e4 allele in Alzheimer's disease and vascular dementia. *dementia 5:* 240-242.

Garthwaite J (1991) Glutamate, nitric oxide and cell-cell signalling in the nervous system. *Trends Neurosci 14*:60-7.

Gatti S, Bartfai T (1993) Induction of tumor necrosis factor-a mRNA in the brain after peripheral endotoxin treatment: comparison with interleukin-1 family and interleukin-6. *Brain Res 624*: 291-294.

Gazzaley AH, Weiland NG, McEwen BS, Morrison JH (1996) Differential regulation of NMDAR1 mRNA and protein by estradiol in the rat hippocampus. *J Neurosci 16:* 6830-6838.

Goldgaber D, Harris HW, Hla T, Maciag T, Donnelly RJ, Jacobson JS, Vitek MP, Gajdusek DC (1989) Interleukin 1 regulates synthesis of amyloid beta-protein precursor mRNA in human endothelial cells. *Proc Natl Acad Sci USA 529*: 31-39.

Gonzalez MF, Shiraishi K, Hisanaga K, Sagar SM, Mandabach M, Sharp FR (1989) Heat shock proteins as markers of neural injury. *Brain Res Mol Brain Res 6(1):*93-100

Gonzalez-Alonso J, Teller C, Andersen SL, Jensen FB, Hyldig T, Nielsen B (1999) Influence of body temperature on the development of fatigue during prolonged exercise in the heat. *J Appl Physiol 86(3):*1032-9

Haas J, Storch-Hagenlocher B, Biessmann A, Wildermann B (2002) Inducible nitric oxide synthase and argininosuccinate synthetase: co-induction in brain tissue of patients with Alzheimer's dementia and following stimulation with b-amyloid 1-42 in vitro. *Neurosci Lett 322:* 121-125.

Hampel H, Muller-Spahn F, Berger C, Haberl A, Ackenheil M, Hock C (1995) Evidence of blood-cerebrospinal fluid barrier impairment in a subgroup of patients with dementia of the Alzheimer type and major depression: a possible indicator for immunoactivation. *Dementia 6*: 348-454.

Hashimura T, Kimura T, Miyakawa T (1991) Morphological changes of blood vessels in the brain with Alzheimer's disease. *Jpn J Psychiatry Neurol 45*: 661-665.

Hedlund S, Sharma H S, Sjöquist P-O, Westman J (1999) A new antioxidant compound h-290/51 attenuates heat shock protein (HSP 72 kD) response, breakdown of the blood-brain barrier permeability, edema and cell injury following acute heat exposure. an experimental study using light and electron microscopy in the rat. *J Therm Biol 24*: 409-414.

Helmbrecht K, Zeise E, Rensing L (2000) Chaperones in cell cycle regulation and mitogenic signal transduction: a review. *Cell Prolif 33(6)*:341-65

Herman JP, Cullinan WE (1997) Neurocircuitry of stress: central control of the hypothalamo-pituitary-adrenocortical axis. *Trends Neurosci 20*:78-84.

Hachinski V, Munoz D (1997) Cerebrovascular pathology in Alzheimer's disease: cause, effect and epiphenomenon. *Ann NY Acad Sci 826*: 1-6.

Hardy JA, Mann DM, Wester P, Winblad B (1986) An integrative hypothesis concerning the pathogenesis and progression of Alzheimer's disease. *Neurobiol Aging 7:* 489-502.

Hughes P, Dragunow M (1995) Induction of immediate-early genes and the control of neurotransmitter-regulated gene expression within the nervous system. *Pharmacol Rev 47(1)*:133-78.

Jaattela M, Wissing D, Kokholm K, Kallunki T, Egeblad M (1998) Hsp70 exerts its anti-apoptotic function downstream of caspase-3-like proteases. *EMBO J 17*(21):6124-34

Janscó G, Domoki F, Sántha P, Varga J, Fischer J, Orosz K, Penke B, Becskel A, Dux M, Tóth L (1998) b-amyloid (1-42) peptide impairs blood-brain barrier function after intracarotid infusion in rats. *Neurosci Lett 253:* 139-141.

Jellinger KA (2002) Alzheimer disease and cerebrovascular pathology: an update. *J Neural Transm.* 2002 May;109(5-6):813-36.

Jolly C, Morimoto RI (2000) Role of the heat shock response and molecular chaperones in oncogenesis and cell death. *J Natl Cancer Inst 92(19):*1564-72

Kalaria RN (1992) The blood-brain barrier and cerebral microcirculation in Alzheimer's disease. *Cerebrovasc Brain Metab Rev 4*: 226-260.

Kalaria RN (1996) Cerebral vessels in ageing and Alzheimer's disease. *Pharmacol Ther 72*: 193-214.

Kalaria RN (1997) Apolipoprotein E, arteriosclerosis, and Alzheimer's disease. *Lancet 349*: 1174-1175.

Kalaria RN (1999) The blood-brain barrier and cerebrovascular pathology in Alzheimer's disease. *Ann N Y Acad Sci 893*:113-125

Kalaria RN (2000) The role of cerebral ischemia in Alzheimer's disease. *Neurobiol Aging 21*: 321-330.

Kalaria RN, Harik SI (1989) Reduced glucose transporter at the blood-brain barrier and cerebral cortex in Alzheimer's disease. *J Neurochem 53*: 1083-1088.

Kalaria RN, Hedera PJ (1995) Differential degeneration of the cerebral microvasculature in Alzheimer's disease. *NeuroReport 6*: 477-480.

Kalaria RN, Pax AB (1995) Increased collagen content of cerebral microvessels in Alzheimer's disease. *Brain Res 707*: 349-352.

Kalaria RN, Pax AB, Premkumar DRD, Lieberburg I (1996) Production and increased detection of amyloid b-protein and amyloidogenic fragments in brain microvessels, meningeal vessels and choroid plexus in Alzheimer disease. *Mol Brain Res 35*: 58-68.

Katschinski DM, Wiedemann GJ, Longo W, d'Oleire FR, Spriggs D, Robins HI (1999) Whole body hyperthermia cytokine induction: a review, and unifying hypothesis for myeloprotection in the setting of cytotoxic therapy. *Cytokine Growth Factor Rev 10(2):*93-7

Kaufmann SH (1992) Heat shock proteins in health and disease. *Int J Clin Lab Res 21(3)*:221-6

Kawai M, Kalaria RN, Harik SI, Perry G (1993) The relationship of amyloid plaques to cerebral capillaries in Alzheimer's disease. *Am J Pathol 37*: 1435-1446.

Kathol RG, Jaeckle RS, Lopez JF, Meller WH (1989) Consistent reduction of ACTH responses to stimulation with CRH, vasopressin and hypoglycaemia in patients with major depression. *Br J Psychiatry 155*:468-78.

Kidd VJ, Lahti JM, Teitz T (2000) Proteolytic regulation of apoptosis. *Semin Cell Dev Biol 11(3)*:191-201

Kimura T, Hashimura T, Miyalawa T (1991) Observation of microvessels in the brain with Alzheimer's disease by scanning electron microscopy. *Jpn J Psychiatry Neurol 45*: 671-676.

Kluger MJ (1991) Fever: role of pyrogens and cryogens. *Physiol rev 71*: 93-127.

Kobari M, Meyer JS, Ishijo M, Kawamura J (2000) Distinguishing patients with senile dementia of Alzheimer type and normal elderly subjects utilizing xenon CT-CBF and multivariate analysis. Keio *J Med 49 (Suppl 1)*: A101-A104.

Korf J, Aghajanian GK, Roth RH (1979) Increased turnover of norepinephrine in the rat cerebral cortex during stress: role of the locus coeruleus. *Neuropharmacology 12(10)*:933-8

Köse K., Dogan P. (1995) Lipid peroxidation induced by hydrogen peroxide in human erythrocyte membranes. 1. Protective effect of Gingko Biloba extract (EGb 761). *J. Int. Med. Res. 23*: 1-8.

Kingsley RJ, Afif E, Cox BC, Kothari S, Kriechbaum K, Kuchinsky K, Neill AT, Puri AF, Kish VM (2003) Expression of heat shock and cold shock proteins in the gorgonian Leptogorgia virgulata. *J Exp Zool 296A(2):*98-107

Kuo YM, Emmerling MR, Vigo-Pelfry C, Kasunic TC, Kilpatrick JB, Murdoch GH, Ball MJ, Roher AE (1996) Water-soluble Ab (N-40, N-42) oligomers in normal and Alzheimer disease brains. *J Biol Chem 271*: 4077-4081.

LeBlanc AC (2003) Natural cellular inhibitors of caspases. Prog Neuropsychopharmacol *Biol Psychiatry 27(2)*:215-29

Li GC, Li L, Liu RY, Rehman M, Lee WM (1992) Heat shock protein hsp70 protects cells from thermal stress even after deletion of its ATP-binding domain. *Proc Natl Acad Sci U S A 89(6)*:2036-40

Lüth H-J, Holzer M, Gärtner U, Staufenbiel M, Arendt T (2001) Expression of endothelial and inducible NOS-isoforms is increased in Alzheimer's disease, in APP23 transgenic mice and after experimental brain lesion in rat: evidence for an induction by amyloid pathology. *Brain Res 913*: 57-67.

Lüth H-J, Holzer M, Gertz HJ, Arendt T (2000) aberrant expression of nNOS in pyramidal neurons in Alzheimer's disease is highly colocalized with p21 ras and p16INK4a. *Brain Res 852*: 45-55.

London JA, Biegel D, Pachter JS (1996) Neurocytopathic effects of b-amyloid-stimulated monocytes: a potential mechanism for central nervous system damage in Alzheimer disease. *Proc Natl Acad Sci USA 93*: 4147-4152

Luine V, Vilegas M, Martinez C, McEwen BS (1994) Repeated stress causes reversible impairments of spatial memory performance. *Brain Res 639*: 167-170.

Landfield PW, Eldridge JC (1991) The glucocorticoid hypothesis of brain aging and neurodegeneration: recent modifications. *Acta Endocrinol (Copenh) 125* Suppl 1:54-64.

Lindvall O, Kokaia Z, Bengzon J, Elmer E, Kokaia M (1994) Neurotrophins and brain insults. *Trends Neurosci 17*: 490-496.

Lindquist S (1986) The heat-shock response. *Annu Rev Biochem 55*:1151-91

Lindquist S, Craig EA (1988) The heat-shock proteins. *Annu Rev Genet 22*:631-77

Lindquist S, Craig EA (1988) The heat-shock proteins. *Annu Rev Genet 22*:631-77

Loberg EM, Torvik A (1991) Uptake of plasma proteins into damaged neurons. An experimental study on cryogenic lesions in rats. *Acta Neuropathol (Berl) 81(5)*:479-85

Lysle DT, Cunnick JE, Fowler H, Rabin BS (1988) Pavlovian conditioning of shock-induced suppression of lymphocyte reactivity: Acquisition, extinction and preexposure effects. *Life Sci 42*: 2185-2194.

Mackic JB, Stins M, McComb JC, Calero M, Ghiso J, Kim KS, Yan SD, Stern D, Schmidt AM, Frangione B, Zlokovic BV (1998a) Human blood-brain barrier receptors for Alzheimer's amyloid b1-40. Asymmetrical binding, endocytosis and transcytosis at the apical side of brain microvascular endothelial cell minolayer. *J Clin Invest 102*: 734-743.

Magarinos AM, McEwen BS, Flugge G, Fuchs E (1996) Chronic psychological stress causes apical dendritic atrophy of hippocampal CA3 pyramidal neurons in subordinate tree shrews. *J Neurosci 16*: 3534-3540.

Maier SF, Fleshner M, Watkins LW (1998) Neural, endocrine, and immune mechanisms of stress induced immunomodulation. In: New frontiers in Stress Research. *Modulation of Brain Function.* Eds: A Levy, E Grauer, D Ben-Nathan, E R de Kloet, Harwood Academic Publishers, The Netherlands, pp. 175-185.

Maness LM, Banks JB, Podlisny MB, Selkoe DJ, Kastin AJ (1994) Passage of human amyloid B-proetin 1-40 across murine blood-brain barrier. *Life Sci 55*: 1643-1650.

Martel CL, Mackic JB, McComb JG, Ghiso J, Zlokovic BV (1996) Blood-brain barrier uptake of the 40 and 42 amino acid sequences of circulating Alzheimer's amyloid B in guinea pigs. *Neurosci Lett 206*: 157-160.

Martin, W. R (1983) Pharmacology of opioids. *Pharmacol. Rec., 35*: 283-323.

Masters CL, Simms G, Weinman NA, Multhaup G, McDonald BL, Beyreuther K (1985) Amyloid plaque core protein in Alzheimer's disease and down syndrome. *Proc Natl Acad Sci USA 82*: 4245-4249.

Mattila KM, Pirttila T, Blennow K, wallin A, Viitanen M, Frey H (1994) Altered blood-brain barrier function in Alzheimer's disease? *Acta Neurol Scand 89*: 192-198.

Mattson MP, Rydel RE (1996) Alzheimer's disease. Amyloid ox-tox transducers. *Nature 382*: 674-675.

Matz PG, Lewen A, Chan PH (2001a) Neuronal, but not microglial, accumulation of extravasated serum proteins after intracerebral hemolysate exposure is accompanied by cytochrome c release and DNA fragmentation. *J Cereb Blood Flow Metab 21(8):*921-8

Matz PG, Fujimura M, Lewen A, Morita-Fujimura Y, Chan PH (2001b) Increased cytochrome c-mediated DNA fragmentation and cell death in manganese-superoxide dismutase-deficient mice after exposure to subarachnoid hemolysate. *Stroke 32(2):*506-15

Manzerra P, Rush SJ, Brown IR (1993) Temporal and spatial distribution of heat shock mRNA and protein (hsp70) in the rabbit cerebellum in response to hyperthermia. *J Neurosci Res 36(4)*:480-90

Marcuccilli CJ, Miller RJ (1994) CNS stress response: too hot to handle? Trends Neurosci 17(4):135-8

Marcuccilli CJ, Mathur SK, Morimoto RI, Miller RJ (1996) Regulatory differences in the stress response of hippocampal neurons and glial cells after heat shock. *J Neurosci 16(2):*478-85

Mautes AE, Noble LJ (2000) Co-induction of HSP70 and heme oxygenase-1 in macrophages and glia after spinal cord contusion in the rat. *Brain Res 883(2):*233-7

Mautes AE, Bergeron M, Sharp FR, Panter SS, Weinzierl M, Guenther K, Noble LJ (2000) Sustained induction of heme oxygenase-1 in the traumatized spinal cord. *Exp Neurol 166(2):*254-65

McEwen BS (1999) Stress and hippocampal plasticity. *Annu Rev Neurosci 22*:105-122.

McEwen BS, Stellar E (1993) Stress and the individual. Mechanisms leading to disease. *Arch Intern Med 153*:2093-101.

Meda L, Cassatella MA, Sendrei GI, Otvos Jr L, Baron P, Villalba M, ferrari D, Rossi F (1995) activation of microglial cells by b-amyloid protein and interferon-g. *Nature 374*: 647-650.

Miyakawa T, Uehara Y, Desaki J, Kimura T, Kuramoto R (1988) Morphological changes of microvessels in the brain with Alzheimer's disease. *Jpn J Psychiatry Neurol 42*: 819-824.

Mielke R, Heiss WD (1998) Positron emisson tomography for diagnosis of Alzheimer's disease and vascular dementia. *J neural Transm Suppl 53*: 237-250.

Minowada G, Welch WJ (1995) Clinical implications of the stress response. *J Clin Invest 95(1)*:3-12

Morita-Fujimura Y, Fujimura M, Kawase M, Chan PH (1999) Early decrease in apurinic/apyrimidinic endonuclease is followed by DNA fragmentation after cold injury-induced brain trauma in mice. *Neuroscience 93(4):*1465-73

Mosser DD, Caron AW, Bourget L, Meriin AB, Sherman MY, Morimoto RI, Massie B (2000) The chaperone function of hsp70 is required for protection against stress-induced apoptosis. *Mol Cell Biol 20(19):*7146-59

Munoz DG, Erkinjuntti T, Gaytan-Garcia S, Hachinski V. (1997) Serum protein leakage in Alzheimer's disease revisited.*Ann N Y Acad Sci. 826*:173-89.

Natte R, de Boer WI, Maat-Schieman ML, Baelde HJ, Vinters HV, Roos RA, van Duinen SG (1999) Amyloid beta precursor protein-mRNA is expressed throughout cerebral vessel walls. *Brain Res 821*: 179-183.

Nibuya M, Morinobu S, Duman RS (1995) Regulation of BDNF and trkB in rat brain by chronic electroconvulsive seizures and antidepressant drug treatments. *J Neurosci 15*: 7539-7547.

Nielsen B, Hyldig T, Bidstrup F, Gonzalez-Alonso J, Christoffersen GR (2001) Brain activity and fatigue during prolonged exercise in the heat. *Pflugers Arch 442(1):*41-8

Nowak TS Jr, Bond U, Schlesinger MJ (1990) Heat shock RNA levels in brain and other tissues after hyperthermia and transient ischemia. *J Neurochem 54(2)*:451-8

Nylandsted J, Rohde M, Brand K, Bastholm L, Elling F, Jaattela M (2000) Selective depletion of heat shock protein 70 (Hsp70) activates a tumor-specific death program that is independent of caspases and bypasses Bcl-2. *Proc Natl Acad Sci U S A 297(14):*7871-6

Ohata M, Fredericks WR, Sundaram U, Rapoport SI (1981) Effects of immobilization stress on regional cerebral blood flow in the conscious rat. *J Cereb Blood Flow Metab 1(2):*187-94

Olesen SP (1989) An electrophysiological study of microvascular permeability and its modulation by chemical mediators. *Acta Physiol Scand 136 (Suppl) 579*: 1-28.

Otake K, Kin K, Nakamura Y (2002) Fos expression in afferents to the rat midline thalamus following immobilization stress. *Neurosci Res 43(3):*269-82

Pappolla MA, Sos M, Omar RA, Sambamurti K (1996) The heat shock/oxidative stress connection. Relevance to Alzheimer disease. *Mol Chem Neuropathol.* 1996 28(1-3):21-34.

Patel MN, McNamara JO (1995) Selective enhancement of axonal branching of cultured dentate gyrus neurons by neurotrophic factors. *Neuroscience 69:* 763-770.

Perlmutter LS (1994) Microvascular pathology and vascular basement membrane components in Alzheimer's disease. *Mol Neurobiol 9*: 33-40.

Perlmutter LS, Myers MA, Barron E (1994) Vascular basement membrane components and the lesions of Alzheimer's disease. *Microsc Res Tech 28*: 204-215

Perry G, Smith MA, McCann CE, Siedlak SL, Jones PK, Friedland RP (1998) Cerebrovascular muscle atrophy is a feature of Alzheimer's disease. *Brain Res 791*: 63-66.

Pluta R, Barcikowska M, Januszewski S, Misicka A, Lipkowski AW (1996) Evidence of blood-brain barrier permeability/leakage for circulating human Alzheimer's beta-amyloid-(1-42)-peptide. *NeuroReport 7*: 1261-1265.

Prelli F, Castano E, Gleener GG, Frangione B (1988) Differences between vascular and plaque core amyloid in Alzheimer's disease. *J Neurochem 51*: 648-651.

Popov VI, Bocharova LS, Bragin AG (1992) Repeated changes of dendritic morphology in the hippocampus of ground squirrels in the course of hibernation. *Neuroscience 48*: 45-51.

Price JM, Sutton ET, Hellermann A, Thomas T (1997) beta-Amyloid induces cerebrovascular endothelial dysfunction in the rat brain. *Neurol res 19:* 534-538.

Prior R, Durso D, Frank R, Prikulis I, Cleven S, Ihl R, Pavlakovic G (1996) Selective binding of soluble Ab1-40 and Ab1-42 to a subset of senile plaques. *Am J Pathol 148*: 1749-1756.

Ranger AM, Malynn BA, Korsmeyer SJ (2001) Mouse models of cell death. *Nat Genet 28(2)*:113-8

Rapoport SI (1976) *Blood-Brain Barrier in Physiology and Medicine*, Raven Press, New York.

Robins HI, Kutz M, Wiedemann GJ, Katschinski DM, Paul D, Grosen E, Tiggelaar CL, Spriggs D, Gillis W, d'Oleire F (1995) Cytokine induction by 41.8 degrees C whole body hyperthermia. *Cancer Lett 97*(2):195-201

Robins HI, Rushing D, Kutz M, Tutsch KD, Tiggelaar CL, Paul D, Spriggs D, Kraemer C, Gillis W, Feierabend C, Arzoomanian RZ, Longo W, Alberti D, d'Oleire F, Qu RP, Wilding G, Stewart JA (1997) Phase I clinical trial of melphalan and 41.8 degrees C whole-body hyperthermia in cancer patients. *J Clin Oncol 15(1)*:158-64

Roses AD (1998) Alzheimer's disease: a model of gene mutations and susceptibility polymorphisms for complex psychiatric diseases. *Am J Med Genet 81*: 49-57

Rosenberg RN (2000) The molecular and genetic basis of AD: the end of the begining. *Neurobiology 54*: 2045-2054.

Saas P, Boucraut J, Quiquerez AL, Schnuriger V, Perrin G, Desplat-Jego S, Bernard D, Walker PR, Dietrich PY (1999) CD95 (Fas/Apo-1) as a receptor governing astrocyte apoptotic or inflammatory responses: a key role in brain inflammation? *J Immunol 162(4)*:2326-33

Sapolsky RM (1992) *Stress, the aging brain, and the mechanisms of neuronal death.* Cambridge, Mass, MIT Press.

Sapolsky RM (1996b) Why stress is bad for your brain. *Science 273*: 749-750.

Selkoe DJ (1998) The cell biology of b-amyloid precursor protein and presenilin in Alzheimer's disease. trends *Cell Biol 8*: 447-453.

Selye H (1976) *Stress in Health and Disease,* Butterworths, London

Scheibel AB, Duong TH, Tomiyasu U (1987) Denervation microangigraphy in senile dementia. Alzheimer type. *Alz Dis Assoc Dis 1*: 19-37.

Scheibel AB (1987) Alterations of the cerebral capillary bed in the senile dementia of Alzheimer. *Ital J Neurol Sci 8*: 457-463.

Scheibel AB, Duong TH, Jacobs R (1989) Alzheimer's disease as a capillary dementia. *Ann Med 21:* 103-107.

Seubert P, Vigo-Pelfrey S, Esch F, Lee M, Dovey H, Davis D, Sinha S, Schlossmacher M, Whaley JSwindlehurst C, McCormack R, Wolfert P, Selkoe D, Liedeberg I, Schenk D (1992) Isolation and quantification of soluble Alzheimer's b-peptide from biological fluids. *Nature 359:* 325-328.

Sharma H S (1982) *Blood-Brain Barrier in Stress*, Ph D Thesis, Banaras Hindu University, p. 1-85, Varanasi, India.

Sharma H S (1999) Pathophysiology of blood brain barrier, brain edema and cell injury following hyperthermia: New role of heat shock protein, nitric oxide and carbon monoxide. an experimental study in the rat using light and electron microscopy, *Acta Universitatis Upsaliensis 830:* 1-94 .

Sharma H S (2000a) Bradykinin2 receptor antagonist HOE-140 attenuates blood-spinal cord barrier permeability following trauma to the rat spinal cord. *Acta Neurochir (Wien) Suppl. 76*: 159-163.

Sharma H S (2000b) Degeneration and Regeneration in the CNS. New Roles of Heat Shock Proteins, Nitric oxide and Carbon Monoxide. *AminoAcids: 19*: 335-337.

Sharma H S (2004) Blood-brain and spinal cord barriers in stress. In: *The Blood-Spinal Cord and Brain Barriers in Health and Disease*, H S Sharma and J Westman (Eds), Elsevier Academic Press, San Diego, pp. 231-298.

Sharma H S (2004a) Influence of serotonin on the blood-brain and blood-spinal cord barriers. In: H S Sharma and J Westman (Eds) *The Blood-Spinal Cord and Brain Barriers in Health and Disease*, Elsevier Academic Press, San Diego, pp 117-158.

Sharma H S (2003) Neurotrophic factors attenuate microvascular permeability disturbances and axonal injury following trauma to the rat spinal cord. *Acta Neurochir (Wien), Suppl. 86*: 383-388.

Sharma H S, Alm P (2004) Role of nitric oxide on the blood-brain and the spinal cord barriers. In: *The Blood-Spinal Cord and Brain Barriers in Health and Disease*, Eds. H S Sharma and J Westman, Elsevier Academic Press, San Diego, pp. 191-230.

Sharma HS, Cervós-Navarro J (1990) Brain oedema and cellular changes induced by acute heat stress in young rats. *Acta Neurochir Suppl (Wien) 51*:383-6

Sharma H S, Dey P K (1978) Influence of heat and immobilization stressors on the permeability of blood-brain and blood-CSF barriers. *Indian Journal of Physiology and Pharmacology, 22, Supplement II,* p. 59-60.

Sharma H S, Dey P K (1981) Impairment of blood-brain barrier by immobilization stress: Role of serotonin. *Indian Journal of Physiology and Pharmacology 25*: 111-122.

Sharma H S, Dey P K (1984) Role of 5-HT on increased permeability of blood-brain barrier under heat stress. *Indian Journal of Physiology and Pharmacology 28*: 259-267.

Sharma H S, Dey P K (1986b) Influence of long-term immobilization stress on regional blood-brain barrier permeability, cerebral blood flow and 5-HT level in conscious normotensive young rats. *Journal of the Neurological Sciences 72*:61-76.

Sharma H S, Dey P K (1986a) Probable involvement of 5-hydroxytryptamine in increased permeability of blood-brain barrier under heat stress. *Neuropharmacology 25*:161-167.

Sharma H S, Dey P K (1987) Influence of long-term acute heat exposure on regional blood-brain barrier permeability, cerebral blood flow and 5-HT level in conscious normotensive young rats. *Brain Research 424*:153-162.

Sharma H S, Dey P K (1988) EEG changes following increased blood-brain barrier permeability under long-term immobilization stress in young rats. *Neuroscience Research 5*:224-239.

Sharma H S, Hoopes P J (2003) Hyperthermia induced pathophysiology of the central nervous system. *Int J Hypertherm 19*: 325-354.

Sharma H S, Westman J (2004) The heat shock proteins and hemeoxygenase response in central nervous system injuries. In: *The Blood-Spinal Cord and Brain Barriers in Health and Disease*, H S Sharma and J Westman (Eds), Elsevier Academic Press, San Diego, pp. 329-360.

Sharma H S, Westman J (2000) Pathophysiology of hyperthermic brain injury. Current concepts, molecular mechanisms and pharmacological strategies. *Research in Legal*

Medicine Vol. 21 Hyperthermia, Burning and Carbon Monoxide (Ed. M. Oehmichen) Lübeck Medical University Publications, Schmidt-Römhild Verlag, Lübeck, Germany , pp. 79-120.

Sharma HS, Westman J (1997) Prostaglandins modulate constitutive isoform of heat shock protein (72 kD) response following trauma to the rat spinal cord. *Acta Neurochir Suppl (Wien) 70*:134-7

Sharma H S, Cervós-Navarro J, Dey P K (1991a) Increased blood-brain barrier permeability following acute short-term forced-swimming exercise in conscious normotensive young rats. *Neuroscience Research 10*: 211-221.

Sharma H S, Westman J, Cervós-Navarro J, Gosztonyi G (1992a) Acute systemic heat exposure increases heat shock protein (HSP-70 kD) immunoreactivity in the brain and spinal cord of young rats. *Clin Neuropathol 11*: 174-175.

Sharma H S, Kretzschmar R, Cervós-Navarro J, Ermisch A, Rühle H-J, Dey P K (1992b) Age-related pathophysiology of the blood-brain barrier in heat stress. *Prog Brain Res* 189-196.

Sharma H S, Westman J, Nyberg F, Cervós-Navarro J, Dey P K (1992c) Role of serotonin in heat adaptation: An experimental study in the conscious young rat. *Endocrine Regulations 26*: 133-142.

Sharma H S, Cervós-Navarro J, Gosztonyi G, Dey P K (1992d) Role of serotonin in traumatic brain injury. An experimental study in the rat. In: *The Role of Neurotransmitters in Brain Injury,* M Globus and W D Dietrich (Eds), Plenum Press, New York, pp. 147-152.

Sharma H S, Nyberg F, Cervós-Navarro J, Dey P K (1992e) Histamine modulates heat stress induced changes in blood-brain barrier permeability, cerebral blood flow, brain oedema and serotonin levels: An experimental study in conscious young rats. *Neuroscience 50*: 445-454.

Sharma H S, Zimmer C, Westman J, Cervós-Navarro J (1992f) Acute systemic heat stress increases glial fibrillary acidic protein immunoreactivity in brain. An experimental study in the conscious normotensive young rats. *Neuroscience 48*: 889-901.

Sharma H S, Westman J, Nyberg F, Zimmer C, Cervós-Navarro J, Dey P K (1994a) Selective vulnerability of rat hippocampus in heat stress. In: Temperature Regulation [Ed. A S Milton], *Advances in Pharmacological Sciences*, Birkhauser, pp. 267-272, Basel.

Sharma H S, Westman J, Nyberg F, Cervós-Navarro J, Dey P K (1994b) Role of serotonin and prostaglandins in brain edema induced by heat stress. An experimental study in the rat. *Acta Neurochirurgica (Suppl). 60*: 65-70.

Sharma H S, Olsson Y, Westman J (1995) A serotonin synthesis inhibitor, p-chlorophenylalanine reduces heat shock protein response following trauma to the rat spinal cord. An immunohistochemical and ultrastructural study in the rat. *Neurosci Res 21*: 241-249

Sharma H S, Nyberg F, Gordh T, Alm P, Westman J (1997a) Topical application of insulin like growth factor-1 reduces edema and upregulation of neuronal nitric oxide synthase following trauma to the rat spinal cord. *Acta Neurochir, Suppl 70*, 130-133

Sharma H S, Westman J, Cervós-Navarro J, Dey P K, Nyberg F (1997b) Opioid receptor antagonists attenuate heat stress-induced reduction in cerebral blood flow, increased blood-brain barrier permeability, vasogenic brain edema and cell changes in the rat. *Ann NY Acad Sci 813*: 559-571.

Sharma H S, Westman J, Cervós-Navarro J, Nyberg F (1997c) Role of neurochemicals in brain edema and cell changes following hyperthermic brain injury in the rat. *Acta Neurochir, Suppl 70,* 269-274

Sharma H S, Westman J, Nyberg F (1998a) Pathophysiology of Brain Edema and Cell Changes following Hyperthermic Brain Injury, In: Brain Functions in Hot Environment, Eds: Sharma H S, Westman *J, Progress in Brain Research, 115*: 351-412

Sharma H S, Alm P, Westman (1998b) Nitric oxide and carbon monoxide in the pathophysiology of brain functions in heat stress, In: Brain Functions in Hot Environment, Eds: Sharma H S, Westman *J, Progress in Brain Research, 115*: 297-333.

Sharma H S, Westman J, Cervós-Navarro J, Dey P K, F. Nyberg F (1998c) Blood-brain barrier in stress: a gateway to various brain diseases. In: *New Frontiers of Stress Research: Modulation of Brain Function,* Eds. A Levy, E Grauer, D Ben-Nathan, E R de Kloet, Harwood Academic Publishers Inc, Amsterdam, pp. 259-276.

Sharma H S, Nyberg F, Gordh T, Alm P, Westman, J (1998d) Neurotrophic factors attenuate neuronal nitric oxide synthase upregulation, microvascular permeability disturbances, edema formation and cell injury in the spinal cord following trauma. In: *Spinal Cord Monitoring. Basic Principles, Regeneration, Pathophysiology and Clinical Aspects,* Eds: Stålberg E, Sharma H S, Olsson Y, Springer Wien New York , pp. 118-148.

Sharma H S, Nyberg F, Westman J, Alm P, Gordh T, Lindholm D (1998e) Brain derived neurotrophic factor and insulin like growth factor-1 attenuate upregulation of nitric oxide synthase and cell injury following trauma to the spinal cord. *Amino Acids 14:* 121-130.

Sharma H S, Drieu K, Alm P, Westman J (2000a) Role of nitric oxide in blood-brain barrier permeability, brain edema and cell damage following hyperthermic brain injury. An experimental study using EGB-761 and Gingkolide B pretreatment in the rat. *Acta Neurochir (Wien) Suppl. 76*: 81-86.

Sharma H S, Nyberg F, Gordh T, Alm P, Westman J (2000b) Neurotrophic factors influence upregulation of constitutive isoform of heme oxygenase and cellular stress response in the spinal cord following trauma. An experimental study using immunohistochemistry in the rat. *AminoAcids 19*: 351-361.

Sharma H S, Westman J, Gordh T, Alm P (2000c) Topical application of brain derived neurotrophic factor influences upregulation of constitutive isoform of heme oxygenase in the spinal cord following trauma. An experimental study using immunohistochemistry in the rat. *Acta Neurochir (Wien) Suppl. 76*: 365-369.

Shen JG, Wang J, Zhao BL, Hou JW, Gao TL, Xin WJ (1998) Effects of EGb 761 on nitric oxide and oxygen free radicals, myocardial damage and arrhythmia in ischemia-reperfusion injury in vivo. *Biochim Biophys Acta 1406*: 228-236.

Shi Y (2002) Mechanisms of caspase activation and inhibition during apoptosis. *Mol Cell 9(3):*459-70

Shibata M, Yamada S, Kumar SR, Calero M, bading J, Frangione B, Holtzman DM, Miller CA, Strickland DK, Ghiso J, Zlokovic BV (2000) Clearance of Alzheimer's amyloid-b1-40 peptide from brain by LDL receptor-related protein-1 at the blood-brain barrier. *J Clin Invest 106:* 1489-1499.

Shoji M, Golde TE, Ghiso J, Cheung TT, estus S, Shaffer LM, Cai XD, McKay DM, Tintner R, Frangione B (1992) Production of the Alzheimer amyloid-b protein by normal proteolytic processing. *Science 258*: 126-129.

Shoji M, Kawarabayashi T, Sato M, Sasaki A, matsubara E, Ikzuka T, Harigaya Y, Hirai S (1996) Systemic overexpression of a C-termianl fragment of human amyloid beta-protein precursor causes accumulation of Alzheimer beta-amyloid fibrils in pancreas of transgenic mice. *Gerontology 42* Suppl 1: 48-56.

Sminia P, van der Zee J, Wondergem J, Haveman J (1994) Effect of hyperthermia on the central nervous system: a review. *Int J Hyperthermia 10*(1):1-30

Smith MA, Cizza G (1996) Stress-induced changes in brain-derived neurotrophic factor are attenuated in aged Fischer 344/N rats. *Neurobiol Aging 17*: 859-864.

Smith MA, Brady LS, Glowa J, Gold PW, Herkenham M (1991) Effects of stress and adrenalectomy on tyrosine hydroxylase mRNA levels in the locus coeruleus by in situ hybridization. *Brain Res 544(1):*26-32

Smith MA, Makino S, Kvetnansky R, Post RM (1995a) Stress and glucocorticoid affect the expression of brain-derived neurotrophic factor and neurotrophin-3 mRNA levels in the hippocampus. *J Neurosci 15*: 1768-1777.

Smith MA, Makino S, Kim S-Y, Kvetnansky R (1995b) Stress increases brain-derived neurotrophic factor mRNA in the hypothalamus and pituitary. *Endocrinology 136*: 3743-3750.

Snoeckx LH, Cornelussen RN, Van Nieuwenhoven FA, Reneman RS, Van Der Vusse GJ (2001) Heat shock proteins and cardiovascular pathophysiology. *Physiol Rev 81(4):*1461-97

States BA, Honkaniemi J, Weinstein PR, Sharp FR (1996) DNA fragmentation and HSP70 protein induction in hippocampus and cortex occurs in separate neurons following permanent middle cerebral artery occlusions. *J Cereb Blood Flow Metab 16(6):*1165-75

Stennicke HR, Ryan CA, Salvesen GS (2002) Reprieval from execution: the molecular basis of caspase inhibition. *Trends Biochem Sci 27(2)*:94-101

Stewart PA, Hayakawa K, Akers MA, Vinters HV (1992) A morphometric study of the blood-brain barrier in Alzheimer's disease. *Lab Invest 67*: 734-742.

Straziella N, Ghersi-Egea JF, Ghiso J, Dehouck MP, Frangione B, Patlak C, Fenstermacher J, Gorevic P (2000) In vitro evidence that beta-amyloid peptide 1-40 diffuses across the blood-brain barrier and affects its permeability. *J Neuropathol Exp Neurol 59*: 29-38.

Strittmatter WJ (2001) Apolipoprotein E and Alzheimer's disease: signal transduction mechanisms. *Biochem Soc Symp 67*:101-109.

Stücker O., Pons C., Duverger, J.-P., Drieu K. (1998) *Antioxidant effects of Ginkgolide B. Consequences on vascular regulation in rat cremastre muscle.* Proc. 25th Eur. Conf. Microcirc., Paris, France, pp. 319-323

Seubert P, Vigo-Pelfrey S, Esch F, Lee M, Dovey H, Davis D, Sinha S, Schlossmacher M, Whaley JSwindlehurst C, McCormack R, Wolfert P, Selkoe D, Liedeberg I, Schenk D (1992) Isolation and quantification of soluble Alzheimer's b-peptide from biological fluids. *Nature* 359: 325-328.

Sugawara T, Fujimura M, Morita-Fujimura Y, Kawase M, Chan PH (1999) Mitochondrial release of cytochrome c corresponds to the selective vulnerability of hippocampal CA1 neurons in rats after transient global cerebral ischemia. *J Neurosci 19(22)*:RC39

Suzuki N, Iwatsubo T, Odaka A, Ishibashi Y, Kitada C, Ihara Y (1994) High tissue content of soluble beta 1-40 is linked to cerebral amyloid angiopathy. *Am J Pathol 145*: 452-460.

Tabaton M, Nunzi MG, Xue R, Usiak M, Autilio-Gambetti L, Gambetti P (1994) Soluble amyloid b-protein is a marker of Alzheimer amyloid in brain but not in cerebrospinal fluid. *Biochem Biophys Res Commun 200:* 1598-1603.

Teller JK, Russo C, DeBusk LM, Angelini G, Zaccheo D, Dagna-Bricarelli F, Scartezzini P, Bertolini S, Mann DM, Tabaton M, Gambetti P (1996) Presence of soluble amyloid beta-peptide precedes amyloid plaque formation in Down's syndrome. *Nat Med 2*: 93-95.

Tissiéres A, Mitchell HK, Tracy UM (1974) Protein synthesis in salivary glands of Drosophila melanogaster: relation to chromosome puffs. *J Mol Biol 84(3):*389-98

Udelsman, R., Blake, M. J., Stagg, C. A. and Holbrook, N. J. (1994) Endocrine control of stress-induced heat shock protein 70 expression in vivo. *Surgery, 115* : 611-616.

Urmoneit B, Prikulis I, Wihl G, D'Urso D, Frank R, Heeren J, Beisiegel U, Prior R (1997) Cerebrovascular smooth muscle cells internalize Alzheimer amyloid beta protein via a lipoprotein pathway: implications for cerebral amyloid angiopathy. *Lab Invest 77*: 157-166.

Uno H, Tarara R, Else JG, Suleman MA, Sapolsky RM (1989) Hippocampal damage associated with prolonged and fatal stress in primates. *J Neurosci 9*: 1705-1711.

Van de Craen M, Declercq W, Van den brande I, Fiers W, Vandenabeele P (1999) The proteolytic procaspase activation network: an in vitro analysis. *Cell Death Differ 6(11):*1117-24

Vargas-Roig LM, Gago FE, Tello O, Aznar JC, Ciocca DR (1998) Heat shock protein expression and drug resistance in breast cancer patients treated with induction chemotherapy. *Int J Cancer 79(5):*468-75

Vigo-Pelfrey C, Lee D, Keim P, Lieberburg I, Schenk DB (1993) Characterization of b-amyloid peptide from human cerebrospinal fluid. *J neurochem 61*: 1965-1968.

Vinters HV (1987) Cerebral amyloid angiopathy. A critical review. Stroke 18: 311-324.

Wallace MN, Geddes JG, Farqhar DA, Masson MR (1997) Nitric oxide synthase in reactive astrocytes adjacent to beta-amyloid plaques. *Exp Neurol 144*: 266-272.

Watkins LR, Maier SF, Goehler LE (1995) Cytokine-to-brain communication: a review and analysis os alternative mechanisms. *Life Sci 57*: 1011-1026.

Welch WJ (1992) Mammalian stress response: cell physiology, structure/function of stress proteins, and implications for medicine and disease. *Physiol Rev 72(4):*1063-81

Westman J, Sharma HS (1998) Heat shock protein response in the central nervous system following hyperthermia. *Prog Brain Res 115*:207-39

Whitesell L, Sutphin PD, Pulcini EJ, Martinez JD, Cook PH (1998) The physical association of multiple molecular chaperone proteins with mutant p53 is altered by geldanamycin, an hsp90-binding agent. *Mol Cell Biol 18(3):*1517-24

Wisniewski HM, Kozlowski PB (1982) Evidence for blood-brain barrier changes in senile dementia of the Alzheimer type (SDAT*). Ann NY Acad Sci 396*: 119-131.

Wisniewski T, Ghiso J, Frangione B (1997) Biology of A-b amyloid in Alzheimer's disease. *Neurobiol Dis 4:* 313-328.

Wisniewski HM, Wegiel J, Vorbrodt AW, Mazur-Kolecka B, Frackowiak J (2000) Role of perovascular cells and myocytes in vascular amyloidosis. *Ann NY Acad Sci 903:* 6-18.

Xia MQ, Qin SX, Wu LJ, Mackay CR, Hyman BT (1998) Immunohistochemical study of the beta-chemikine receptors CCR3 and CCR5 and their ligands in normal and Alzheimer's disease brains. *Am J Pathol 153*: 31-37.

Yamashita K, Miyakawa T, Katsuragi S (1991) Vascular changes in the brains with Alzheimer's disease. *Jpn J Psychiatry Neurol 45*: 79-84.

Yan SD, Chen X, Fu J, Chen M, Zhu H, Roher A, Slattery T, Zhao L, Nagashima M, Morser J, Migheli A et al. (1996) RAGE and amyloid-b peptide neurotoxicity in Alzheimer's disease. *Nature 382*: 685-691.

Younkin SG (1998) The role of A beta 42 in Alzheimer's disease. *J Physiol (Paris) 92:* 3293-3299.

Yoo BC, Seidl R, Cairns N, Lubec G (1999) Heat-shock protein 70 levels in brain of patients with Down syndrome and Alzheimer's disease. *J Neural Transm Suppl. 57*:315-22.

Volloch VZ, Sherman MY (1999) Oncogenic potential of Hsp72. *Oncogene 18(24)*:3648-51

Zlokovic BV (1997) Can blood-brain barrier play a role in the development of cerebral amyloidosos and Alzheimer's disease pathology? *Neurobiol Dis 4:* 23-26.

Zlokovic BV (2002) Vascular disorder in Alzheimer's disease: role in pathogenesis of dementia and therapeutic targets.*Drug Deliv Rev 54(12):*1553-1559.

Zlokovic BV, Martel CL, Matsubara E, McComb JG, Zheng G, McCluskey RT, Frangione B, Ghiso J (1996) Glycoprotein 330/megalin: probable role in receptor-mediated transport of apolipoprotein J alone and in a complex with Alzheimer disease amyloif-b at the blood-brain and blood-cerebrospinal fluid barriers. *Proc Natl Acad Sci USA 93*: 4229-4234.

Zlokovic BV, Yamada S, Holtzman D, Ghiso J, Frangione B (2000) Clearance of amyloid-b peptide from brain: transport or metabolism? *Nat Med 6:* 718-719.

Zylicz M, King FW, Wawrzynow A (2001) Hsp70 interactions with the p53 tumour suppressor protein. *EMBO J 20(17)*:4634-8

In: Depression and Dementia
Editor: Suptendra Nath Sarbadhikari, p. 153-181
ISBN 1-59454-114-0

Chapter 6

MULTI-PRONGED APPROACH FOR STUDYING LATERALIZATION IN DEPRESSION

Subodh Kumar* and Manas K. Mandal**

* Department of Clinical Psychology, Institute of Mental Health, Amritsar-143 001. India.

** Corresponding author, Director, Defence Institute of Psychological Research, DRDO, Timarpur, Delhi-110 054. India.

ABSTRACT

The concept of distinct functional specialization of the two sides of the human brain has increasingly been found helpful in understanding the brain-behaviour relationship in general, and specifically in psychiatric illness. Left hemisphere superiority in cognitive functions and right hemisphere advantage, although not very clear, for affect processing have generally been accepted (Borod, 1992). Empirical support for right hemisphere superiority in emotional processing has been drawn from studies conducted on both normal and clinical subjects. Brain-damaged patients were taken in most of the clinical studies. Relatively few of them were conducted on patients with affective disorders. Considering the phenomenon of cerebral lateralization somewhat recognized for emotional processing, it appears surprising (Mandal, Asthana, Pandey, & Sarbadhikari, 1996).

Although the research techniques that utilize the differential specialization of the cerebral hemispheres in processing emotional cues have to be methodologically improved for providing more conclusive results, some observations may be useful in resolving some of the neuropsychiatric issues. To see whether patients with affective illness, such as depressives, show any right hemisphere dysfunction would be revealing. In this review, studies that relate to lateralization of brain functions in depressive illness were selected. The chapter is divided into three sections. The first section deals with the lateralization of affect. The second section accounts the lateralization studies in depression using different methods: brain-damage, behavioural, electrophysiological, and functional neuroimaging. Finally, we present a critical evaluation of the existing literature and provide suggestions for future research. Some of the research in this area has been reviewed earlier by Coffey (1987) and Mandal, Asthana, Pandey, & Sarbadhikari (1996). Since functional neuroimaging techniques have been used relatively recently in lateralization research, we examined such studies, and also recent observations through other methods.

Lateralization and Emotion

Researchers studying the involvement of the hemispheric side in emotional processing have interpreted the findings in different ways. There are two major speculations: (a) the right hemisphere hypothesis suggests the superiority of right hemisphere for all kinds/dimensions of emotions (Strauss & Moscovitch, 1981; Suberi & McKeever, 1977) and (b) the valence hypothesis which proposes the advantage of right hemisphere for negative emotions (such as sadness, fear, or anger) and a left hemisphere or bilateral superiority for positive emotions such as happiness (see Borod, 1992). Both clinical (Borod, Martin, Alpert, Brozgold, & Welkowitz, 1993; Mandal, Borod, Asthana, Mohanty, Mohanty, & Koff, 1999) as well as experimental (Davidson, 1984; Reuter-Lorenz & Davidson, 1981; a review by Moretti, Charlton, & Taylor, 1996) studies have provided evidence for the distinct hemispheric involvement as a function of emotion type.

Lateralization studies on emotional perception were mostly conducted on normal and brain-damaged subjects. Two sensory modalities - visual with split-field technique, and auditory with dichotic-listening technique - were generally used in these studies. In the visual split-field technique, emotional stimuli are exposed techistoscopically in a specific visual field for a very brief period (below 150 msec) implicating the contralateral hemispheric side. Studies based on this technique suggested that emotions are perceived generally in a better way in the left visual field (a right hemisphere function). When subjects were asked to memorize facial expressions of emotions, left visual field advantage was found (Suberi & McKeever, 1977). Similar results were obtained when facial emotions were identified with reaction time as a dependent measure (Buchtel, Campari, De Risio, & Rota, 1978; Strauss & Moscovitch, 1981). With chimeric faces (such as a combination of an emotional hemiface with a neutral hemiface of the same poser) also, researchers found that emotional hemifaces are more accurately processed in the right hemisphere (Campbell, 1978; Heller & Levy, 1981). But visual-field superiority may be a function of stimulus type. Right hemisphere superiority for facial stimuli and left hemisphere advantage for lexical stimuli have been reported in normal subjects (Dutta & Mandal, 2002). In auditory dichotic-listening technique, although the two ears are stimulated simultaneously with different stimuli, emotional stimuli (such as emotional tone) are presented to a specific hemisphere (Wexler, 1980). In such conditions, inhibited ipsilateral cortical projections allow the contralateral projections to process the stimuli (Bryden, 1982; Kimura, 1961). Using this technique also, right hemisphere superiority for judgement of emotional tone of speech (Bryden, Ley, & Sugarman, 1982; Safer & Leventhal, 1977; Saxby & Bryden, 1984), nonverbal vocalizations, and musical processes (Borod, 1992) was observed.

Involvement of the right hemisphere in emotional processing was also supported by the findings of studies conducted on focal brain-damaged patients. Right-hemisphere-damaged (RHD) patients have been found deficient in remembering emotional material (Wechsler, 1973), comprehending emotional tone of the voice (Heilman, Bowers, Speedie, & Coslett, 1984), apprcciating humorous stimuli (Bihrlc, Brownell, Powelson, & Gardner, 1986), and perceiving or judging emotional faces (Borod, Koff, Perlman Lorch, & Nicholas, 1986; Bowers, Bauer, Coslett, & Heilman, 1985; Kucharska-Pietura & David, 2003). Further, studies also showed that RHD patients were less accurate on measures of frequency (Blonder, Bower, & Heilman, 1991; Borod, Koff, Perlman Lorch, Nicholas, & Welkowitz, 1988) and accuracy (Borod et al., 1986; Buck & Duffy, 1980) of facial expressions of emotions. Right hemispheric superiority has not only been observed across affective valence but also across expressive channels (such as, facial, prosodic, lexical) of emotions (Borod, 1992; Borod et al., 1998).

Empirical evidence also supports the valence hypothesis in brain-damaged patients. RHD patients were found significantly more inaccurate in the perception of negative emotions but not in the perception of positive emotions, compared to left-hemisphere-damaged (LHD) patients and normal controls (Adolphs, Jansari, & Tranel, 2001; Borod et al., 1986; Mandal, Tandon, & Asthana, 1991). In addition, Borod and colleagues (Borod & Koff, 1990; Borod et al., 1986; Borod et al., 1988; Borod, Koff, & White, 1983) showed a right hemisphere (RH) involvement for the expression of negative emotions and a left hemisphere (LH)/bilateral involvement for expression of positive emotions. Borod (1992, p. 341) had two speculations in favour of this finding. (1) Negative emotions are associated with a survival mechanism which requires a gestalt and synthetic processing (a function of the RH), (2) Positive emotions are more linguistic/communicative than emotional, and thus LH becomes more dominant.

Relative task difficulty for brain-damaged patients seems to account the hemispheric involvement in emotional processing. When asked to match photographs of top-bottom facial parts of emotional expressions, the LHD patients were found inferior to RHD patients (Asthana, Mandal, Tandon, & Asthana,1991). In this study, it is possible that the hemifacial judgement of emotional expressions needed greater processing load, and this difficulty was coupled with relative supremacy of the intact hemisphere. It is suggested that the performance of left hemisphere decreases more in comparison to right hemisphere when task difficulty with facial processing increases (Benton, 1986).

Notably, findings of some studies suggest that RHD and LHD patients did not differ significantly in their ability to express facial emotions (Weddell, Miller, & Trevarthen, 1990) or match hemifacial photographs of emotional expressions (Mandal, Asthana, Tandon, & Asthana, 1992). Rather, in these studies, patients with anterior region damage were more impaired than the patients with posterior region damage and normal controls. It has been found that anterior lesion sites are important for the expression of emotions and posterior lesion sites for the perception (Borod, 1992). A review by Borod (1993) indicated that "the valence hypothesis of right hemisphere superiority for processing negative emotions is more systematic among normal subjects but not among brain-damaged patients" (p. 458). The fact that lesion side, site, and size in the brain differ across studies (Mandal, Asthana, Pandey, & Sarbadhikari, 1996) may be responsible for this observation.

Lateralization in Depression

Although a number of studies have been devoted to investigate cerebral laterality in schizophrenia (see Glass, 1987; Gur & Chin, 1999; Sommer et al., 2001), researchers have comparatively less attempted the lateralization of brain functions in depression. The available literature on this issue may be classified into four broad categories: lesion studies, behavioural studies, electrophysiological studies, and functional neuroimaging studies.

Lesion Studies

In general, patients with LHD have showed more depressive symptoms in comparison to patients with RHD (Black, 1975; Burton & Labar, 1999; Gainotti, 1972; Gasparrini, Satz, Heilman, & Coolidge, 1978; House et al., 1989; Mandal, Mohanty, Pandey, & Mohanty, 1996; Sackeim et al., 1982; Spalletta, Guida, & Caltagirone, 2003; Starkstein et al., 1988). Additionally, studies conducted on patients with unilateral epileptogenic focus reported significantly more sadness and depression in the patients with left-sided lesions during the interictal period than the patients with right-sided lesions (Altshuler, Devinsky, Post, & Theodore, 1990; Mendez et al., 1994; Perrini, 1986; Perrini & Mendius, 1984; Victoroff et al., 1994). Contrarily, right hemisphere epileptic foci are also found associated with depression (Abrams & Taylor, 1979; Flor-Henry, 1969; Kohler et al., 1999).

PET findings suggest the interictal hypometabolism in epileptic lesions (Engel, 1984; Victoroff et al., 1994). Studies favoring an association between decreased left-sided activation and depression, however, did not provide simultaneous evaluation of cerebral functions, and thus left possibility that the observed mood changes may be result of changes elsewhere in the brain (Davidson & Henriques, 2000). Further, there is strong evidence that RHD patients show significant impairment in recognizing facial expressions of sadness and other emotions as well (Borod, 1992; Borod et al., 1998; Mandal et al., 1999; Mandal, Tandon, & Asthana, 1991), and discriminating sad faces shown on the left side (Adolphs, Jansari, & Tranel, 2001).

In some studies, researchers have used sodium amytal to selectively inactivate a hemisphere. These studies indicate that inactivation of the left hemisphere produces dysphoric mood or crying, and inactivation of the right hemisphere is linked with elated mood or laughter in some subjects (Alema & Rosadini, 1964; Christianson et al., 1993; Lee et al., 1990; Terzian, 1964). Though such findings may be considered in support of the right hemisphere involvement in sadness and depression (Flor-Henry, 1979), the occurrence of dysphoric responses when the anesthetized left hemisphere resumes functioning (Terzian, 1964) suggests the role of diminished activation of the left hemisphere also (Davidson & Henriques, 2000).

Behavioural Studies

Behavioural studies on lateralization pattern in depression were mostly conducted using dichotic-listening and visual half-field techniques. The ear advantage found in dichotic-listening studies was associated with hemisphere-specific processing ability in depressive patients (Kimura, 1961; Wexler & Halwes, 1985). Left ear advantage (a RH function) was found for musical tones or click stimuli in normal right-handed subjects (Bryden, 1982; Springer & Deutsch, 1990). Depressed subjects generally did not show left ear advantage for such nonverbal dichotic tasks (Bruder et al., 1981; Johnson & Crockett, 1982; Yozawitz et al., 1979). On the other hand, depressives failed to show right ear advantage (a LH function) for verbal dichotic tasks (Johnson & Crockett, 1982; Moscovitch, Strauss, & Olds, 1981), which normals generally do (Bryden, 1982). But recent findings support the increased LH advantage for fused words (Bruder et al., 1999; Pine et al., 2000).

In studies using visual half-field method, depressed patients were found significantly impaired in recognizing facial emotions presented to the right hemisphere (Bruder et al.,

2002; Kucharska-Pietura & David, 2003; Mikhailova et al., 1996). With reaction time as a dependent measure, patients with unipolar depression without anxiety showed marked slowness of reactivity to the left visual field (RH) stimuli, while anxious depressives showed opposite trend (Liotti, Sava, Rizzolatti, & Caffarra, 1991). Depressed patients also selected positive words more quickly presented to the left than right visual-field in comparison to remitted and nondepressed controls (Enloe et al., 2001). But when patients were asked to *express* facial emotions, valence hypothesis was supported (Yecker et al., 1999). They produced positive emotions with greater right-hemiface intensity and negative emotions with greater intensity on left-hemiface. Intensity of facial expressions, further, has been found related to facial asymmetry in normals (Mandal, Asthana, & Pandey, 1995).

Some studies employing lateral eye movement (Myslobdsky & Horesh, 1978; Silverstein & Meltzer, 1983) have extended support for the right hemisphere involvement in depression. Some authors (Hatta, 1984; Raine, 1991) did not find this method a sensitive and valid index of functional cerebral asymmetry. However, left and right lateral eye movements were linked with emotional arousal and cognitive processes respectively (Wilbur & Roberts-Wilbur, 1985). Also, lateral eye movement is found strongly correlated with dichotic listening (Lefevre, Starck, Lambert, & Genesee, 1977) and EEG asymmetries (Neubauer, Schulter, & Pfurtscheller, 1988). In a study using line-bisection task, right hemisphere dysfunction was not found in the patients with major depression (Ramos-Brieva, Olivan, Palomares, & Vela, 1984).

Further, some researchers have reported bilateral hemispheric dysfunction in depression using neuropsychological tests (Fromm-Auch, 1983; Silverstein & Meltzer, 1983; Taylor & Abrams, 1983; cited in Coffey, 1987). The inconsistencies in findings are generally attributed to the clinical states of the patients studied or to the stimuli/tasks eliciting hemispheric specificity. Studies conducted by Bruder and associates suggest the impact of subtypes and course of the depressive illness on perceptual asymmetry. They observed that patients with bipolar depression did not show RH advantage for visual hemifield (Bruder et al., 1992; Bruder et al., 1989) and dichotic listening (Bruder et al., 1981) tasks compared to unipolar depressives and normal controls. In addition, patients with atypical depression showed pathological increase in right hemisphere bias for perceiving emotional chimeric faces compared to patients with typical depression and controls (Bruder et al., 2002). In an another study done on atypical depressives, those with early onset of illness reported less left hemispheric advantage on a dichotic listening task than those with late onset (Stewart, Bruder, McGrath, & Quitkin, 2003). Fused nonsense syllabi and dichotic words are not found to be processed by the same (i. e., left) hemisphere (Wexler & Halwes, 1985).

Electrophysiological Studies

EEG abnormalities have been noted in both hemispheres of the depressed patients. Studies indicating right-sided EEG abnormalities in depression provide findings such as greater alpha desynchrony in right frontal region (Tucker, Stenslie, Roth, & Shearer, 1981), less activation in the right precentral region in depression (Monakhov et al., 1979; Perris, 1974), a significant increase of alpha band in the right hemisphere (Bauer & Hesselbrock, 2002; Tucker, 1983), lower alpha burst occurrence variability in the right hemisphere (Cazard, 1989), increased activation of right frontal region (Schaffer, Davidson, & Saron,

1983), decreased (Henriques & Davidson, 1990, 1997) and increased (Pozzi et al., 1995) activation in right posterior region, and so forth. A significant right-sided polymodality in the distribution of EEG amplitudes was also found in depressed patients (Von Knorring, 1983).

Findings of the relatively greater right hemisphere EEG activation in depression were not interpreted similarly. Tucker (1981) suggested that greater right hemisphere EEG activation is a result of inhibiting positive affect processes of the right hemisphere. In contrast, Davidson (1984) believed that the finding is congruent with the role of right hemisphere in processing negative emotions.

Regarding EEG changes in the left hemisphere, depression appears to be linked with both decreased and increased activation. Reduced left-sided anterior activation (e.g., Allen et al., 1991; Gotlib, Ranganath, & Rosenfeld, 1998; Henriques & Davidson, 1990, 1991; cited in Davidson & Henriques, 2000) is reported. On the other hand, greater left-sided activation of alpha, beta, and theta bands was found in elderly depressed patients (Roemer et al., 1992). Bilateral decrease of EEG activation is reported (Pollock & Schneider, 1989, 1990).

Though the literature on evoked potential in depression is larger than EEG (for reviews, see Henriques & Davidson, 1989; Zahn, 1986), relatively few studies have examined the issue of cerebral laterality in depression. Evoked potential studies during spatial and temporal discrimination tasks showed that control subjects with greater right hemisphere advantage for a complex tone task had greater right than left P3 amplitudes (Bruder et al., 1995; Tenke et al., 1993; cited in Davidson & Henriques, 2000). Patients with depression failed to show the normal greater right than left asymmetry and had lower P3 amplitudes than controls (Bruder et al., 1995). Greater N2 over the lateral sites of the right hemisphere to complex tone task (Bruder et al., 1998) and decrease of N2 component in right posterior region to the facial recognition-memory task (Deldin et al., 2000) have been found in depressed patients. In addition, bipolar depressives showed smaller N100 amplitudes for the test stimuli presented to the right than left hemisphere in comparison to patients with unipolar depression (Bruder et al., 1992).

On the other hand, Bruder et al. (1991) found that patients with typical depression showed longer P3 latency for an audiospatial task, not for temporal task, when the stimuli presented to the left hemisphere than to the right hemisphere. This asymmetry was not observed in atypical depressives and normal controls. Left hemisphere asymmetry in depression was also found using Bereitschaftspotential paradigm (Haag et al., 1994) during right fist clench task.

Functional Neuroimaging Studies

Studies of blood flow and glucose metabolism have the advantage over electrophysiological studies for providing better spatial resolution, but with a loss of temporal resolution and an increase in cost. Both metabolism and blood flow studies use a radioactive tracer to examine cerebral activation. The underlying assumption is that increased neuronal activation is associated with increase in blood flow (Davidson & Henriques, 2000). Most of these studies have been marked by regional brain dysfunctions, with left-, right-sided or bilateral changes. Prefrontal cortex (PFC) has been more frequently studied in depression than other brain regions, namely, anterior cingulated cortex (ACC), hippocampus, and amygdala. Studies of depression have typically reported decreased left frontal activation

(Bench et al., 1992, 1993; Delvenne et al., 1990; Holthoff et al., 1999; Passero, Nardini, & Battistini, 1995; Yazici et al., 1992). Decreased activation in right prefrontal (Kimbrell et al., 2002) and right parietal cortex (Galynker et al., 1998) has also been reported. Recovery after the treatment has been found to be associated with increased activation in the left frontal region (Bench et al., 1995; Kennedy et al., 2001; Passero, Nardini, & Battistini, 1995). In addition, Left-sided activation in pregenual region of the cingulate gyrus is found (Drevets et al. 1997). Bilateral decreases in frontal activation have also been reported in metabolism (Biver et al., 1994; Brody et al., 2001; Francois et al., 1995) and blood flow studies (Chabrol et al., 1986; Schroeder et al., 1989) of depression.

Decreased activation in ACC has been reported in depression with fMRI (Beauregard et al. 1998), and PET (Bench et al. 1992; Drevets et al. 1997; George et al. 1997; Smith et al., 1999) studies. Also in SPECT studies, decreased regional cerebral blood flow in the left (Curran et al. 1993; Mayberg et al. 1994) or right (Ito et al. 1996) ACC has been found in medicated depressed unipolar patients compared with controls. Interestingly, Mayberg and colleagues (1997) found that unipolar depressed patients who responded to treatment after six weeks showed higher pretreatment glucose metabolism in rostral region of the ACC compared with both nonresponders and nonpsychiatric controls.

"A comparable number of investigators have found that depressed subjects are characterized by global decreases in blood flow (Bonne & Krausz, 1997; Gustafson, Risberg, & Silfverskiold, 1981; Mathew et al., 1980; Mayberg et al., 1994; Rush et al., 1982; Sackeim et al., 1990; Warren et al., 1984). Global decreases in blood flow are also typical of elderly depressed subjects (Hoyer, Oesterreich, & Wagner, 1984; Lesser et al., 1994; Philpot et al., 1993)" (Davidson & Henriques, 2000, p. 283).

Further, studies have shown that depression is frequently associated with increased levels of cortisol in hippocampus (Carroll et al, 1976; Vakili et al. 2000). Although the hypercortisolemia may make hippocampal cells more vulnerable to insults caused by hypoxia, hypoglycemia, or excitatory neurotransmitters (Vakili et al. 2000), the precise nature of the association between sustained elevations of cortisol and hippocampal damage is not completely known (Sheline, 2000). For amygdala, a positive correlation between amygdalar activation and severity of depression (Drevets et al. 1992) was found. Abercrombie et al. (1998) observed that greater right amygdala activation may predict the expression of more negative affect in depressed patients, but is unrelated to changes in positive affect. In a study using affect discrimination task, Yurgelun-Todd et al. (2000) found higher left amygdalar activation in depressed bipolar patients than controls in response to fearful faces. Consistent with this, Sheline et al (2001) found that depressed patients showed left amygdala hyperarousal to masked emotional faces, indicating processing outside of conscious awareness. Right amygdala activation did not differ from control subjects in their study. Increased left amygdala activation for fearful faces is also reported in normal adults (Thomas et al., 2001); so the findings from such studies need careful examination.

In a comprehensive review, Davidson and colleagues (2002) have discussed the effects of regional brain dysfunctions, evidenced by structural and functional neuroimaging studies, on the psychological characteristics of depressive illness, and identified much work remaining in this area. "Abnormalities in prefrontal cortex function would be expected to compromise goal-instantiation in patients with depression. Left-sided hypoactivation would result in deficits in pre-goal attainment forms of positive affect, whereas right-sided hyperactivation would result in excessive behavioural inhibition and anticipatory anxiety. Hypoactivation in regions of the prefrontal cortex with which the amygdala is interconnected may result in a decrease in the regulatory influence on the amygdala and a prolonged time course of amygdala activation in response to challenge. This might be expressed phenomenologically as perseveration of negative affect and rumination" (Davidson et al. 2002, p. 562).

The ACC monitors the conflicting situations in the brain (Carter et al., 1999). In depressed patients, in which ACC activation is pathologically decreased, the incongruence between their mood state and environmental expectations would not be properly managed and thus, the usual ACC call to other brain regions, such as PFC, for further processing would not be issued (Davidson et al., 2002). The hippocampus is supposed to play an important role in making the emotional behaviour context-appropriate. The persistence of sadness in depressive patients in situations that would normally require happiness could partly be as a result of hippocampal dysfunction. Finally, amygdalar hyperactivation in some patients may be linked more with the fear-like and anxiety-related features of the symptoms than with the sad mood and anhedonia. (Davidson et al., 2002). Also, its excessive activation may produce hypervigilance toward threat-related cues, further increasing some symptoms of depression (Davidson et al., 2002).

It should be clear that all the affect-related brain structures are interconnected in regionally specific ways and exhibit bi-directional feedback (Davidson et al., 2002). The dysfunction may also be in the functional and/or anatomical connectivity between different brain regions. "New neuroimaging studies suggest that patterns of functional connectivity may differ between depressed patients and controls. Interhemispheric, cortical limbic and thalamocortical connectivity have all been found to be different in depressed patients compared to controls. Just which specific features of depression are associated with each of these different patterns of functional connectivity must by disentangled in the future research" (Davidson et al., 1999, p. 232). There is evidence that the different depressive symptoms may be associated with the patterns of lateralized regional cerebral blood flow (Bench et al., 1993).

An important task for neuroimaging studies appears to unravel the relationship between pathological morphometric and functional changes in a specific brain region, and also find out the clinical correlates of these dysfunctional changes, keeping in view the heterogeneity of depressive symptoms. In depressives, decreased left-sided activation in the pregenual region of the anterior cingulate gyrus appears partly to be result of the reduced volume of gray matter as indicated by MRI-derived morphometric measures (Drevets et al., 1997). The finding that remission of symptoms by successful treatment is not accompanied by normal activation in this area (Drevets et al., 1997) supports this notion. This may not provide, however, any direct measure of the causal relationship (Davidson et al., 2002). Likewise, persistence of increased left amygdalar activity during the remitted phase of depression (Drevets et al., 1992) indicates that amygdalar dysfunction in at least some subtypes of depression may be trait-like feature. Cerebral blood flow and glucose metabolic data demonstrate that "major depression is associated with reversible, mood state-dependent, neurophysiological abnormalities in some structures and irreversible, trait-like abnormalities in some structures. In some of the regions in which trait-like abnormalities appear, abnormal metabolic activity appears at least partly related to the anatomical abnormalities in MRI studies of depression" (Drevets, 1998, p. 341). As longitudinal studies measuring of brain structure and function in at-risk individuals have not been conducted, it is difficult to specify which dysfunction may be primary or trait-like (Davidson et al., 2002). Careful attention to investigating functional brain changes in depressive spectrum disorders, familial pure depressive disorder, and depressive disorder with history of environmental triggers (stress or trauma) is suggested for future research.

Critical Evaluation of the Existing Literature and Recommendations for Future Research

Summing up, most of the lesion studies have found depressive features in LHD patients. Leventhal & Tomarken (1986, p. 586) found that LH damage results in depression, pessimism, and crying, and RH damage results in joviality, indifference, and laughing. Such findings, however, have been interpreted differently. Some researchers consider LH as a center of depression because its damage results in sadness (Robinson et al., 1985). Others believe that the damage of LH disinhibits the dysphoric tendencies of the RH (Sackeim et al., 1982). Further, RHD patients were found significantly impaired in *perceiving* sadness and other emotions regardless of valence and expressive channels, facial, prosodic, and lexical (Borod, 1992; Borod et al., 1998). Conceptual and methodological limitations of recently developed neuropsychological tests to asses emotional processing in brain-damaged patients have been discussed by Borod, Tabert, Santschi, & Strauss (2000).

Dichotic listening studies generally support the right hemisphere involvement for nonverbal stimuli and left hemisphere involvement for verbal stimuli. In visual hemifield studies, *perception* of facial emotions presented to the right hemisphere was impaired, whereas patients *expressed* facial emotions in accordance with the valence hypothesis. Bilateral hemispheric involvement is also indicated by some neuropsychological studies. We found that verbal stimuli have rarely been taken in the visual hemifield experiments on depressive patients. Importantly, generalized performance reduction (especially in cognitive and motor aspects) in depressed patients was not taken into account in most of the studies. In a study, major depressives were found significantly deficient in both visuospatial and affective tasks in comparison to general medical patients (Asthana, Mandal, Khurana, & Haque-Nizamie, 1998). Bruder and colleagues (Bruder, 1983b; Bruder et al., 1981; Bruder et al., 1989; Bruderet al., 1992; Bruder et al., 2002) showed that the degree and pattern of perceptual asymmetry may depend on the clinical state of the patients and subtypes of the illness.

In electrophysiological studies, asymmetries have been found in the regions of both hemispheres of the depressed patients. Davidson (1988) reviewed the conceptual and methodological issues central to EEG studies of cerebral asymmetry. He differentiated hemispheric specialization from activation. "Specialization refers to the preparadeness of a hemisphere to process information of a specific type (e.g., verbal or spatial) or in a particular manner. Activation refers to the degree to which a particular hemisphere is working or engaged. Dissociations between these two aspects of cerebral asymmetry are common. The hemisphere specialized to process a particular stimulus is not necessarily the one most activated" (Davidson, 1988, p. 87). Secondly, he addressed the importance of rostral-caudal differences for the understanding of both cerebral specialization and activation. "The functional significance of cerebral asymmetry differs in the anterior and posterior cortical regions. Asymmetries in the frontal region are more closely associated with affective processing, while asymmetries in posterior regions are more related to the nature of the cognitive requirements of a task. Activation asymmetries in these different regions are not highly correlated and are sometimes even inversely correlated. Therefore, it makes little sense to talk of a whole hemisphere being activated or specialized for a particular function" (Davidson, 1988, p. 87).

In functional neuroimaging studies, regional cerebral changes have been noted indicating left, right, or bilateral involvement in depression. "A particularly important methodological issue in the assessment of lateralized changes in neuroimaging studies is how putatively asymmetrical changes are measured. In most neuroimaging studies, if a focus of activation exceeds an arbitrary statistical threshold in one hemisphere but not in the other, a lateralized effect is reported. A formal test of the Hemisphere X Condition or Hemisphere X Group interaction must, however, be performed. This interaction test formally assesses whether the change in one hemisphere is significantly different from the change in the opposite hemisphere. Without such a test of the interaction term, it is simply not possible to know whether a reported lateralized effect is indeed truly asymmetrical. For example, if a focus exceeds threshold in one hemisphere and falls just below threshold in the other hemisphere, a lateralized effect would be claimed yet a formal test of the interaction would show that the interaction was clearly not significant. In addition, it is possible there to be a significant interaction without any of the main effects being significant. Thus, we must exercise considerable caution in interpreting putatively lateralized changes that have been reported in the recent neuroimaging studies of depression" (Davidson & Henriques, 2000, p. 279).

Theorists differ in their opinion on hemispheric involvement in depressive illness. Some believe that the right hemisphere modulates all emotions. Others believe that the right hemisphere mediates negative emotions and the left hemisphere mediates positive emotions. Still others hold the view that positive emotions generate bilateral involvement. Bilateral involvement has also been reported in depression by some researchers. The main reason behind such differences of opinion may be attributed to the differences in research strategies and different viewpoints for interpreting the findings.

A considerable number of studies, importantly, have evinced that depression is not associated with left or right cerebral dysfunction. Some lesion studies (Angeleri et al., 1997; House et al., 1990; Indaco et al., 1992; Oyebode, Kennedy, & Davison, 1986; Paolucci et al., 1999) found no significant association between the laterality of cerebral damage and development of depressive symptoms. RHD and LHD patients also exhibited no significant difference on facial emotional tasks (Mandal, Asthana, Tandon, & Asthana, 1992; Weddell, Miller, & Trevarthen, 1990). Further, a group of patients with left- and right-sided lesions showed similar auditory P300 amplitudes or its distribution in the brain (Korpelainen et al., 2000). In a SPECT study, Maes et al (1993) found no difference in the right-left distribution of cerebral blood flow between unipolar depressives and normal controls.

Two potential reasons for the inconsistent findings from lateralization studies in depression may be considered: participant variable and stimulus variable. Diagnostic subtype, stage of the illness, clinical state or symptom severity, age and sex of the subjects may produce different results. Even in carefully diagnosed patients, considerable heterogeneity may exist in the symptoms of depression. Examining relations between specific symptom clusters (related to mood, negative cognition, or psychomotor retardation) and patterns of lateralization may particularly be helpful. Bench et al (1993), in an important study, found that the symptom clusters were associated with patterns of regional cerebral blood flow in major depressive patients. The impact of subtypes of depression (such as unipolar, bipolar, typical, atypical, endogenous, reactive) on results of functional laterality was evidenced by dichotic listening (for review, see Bruder, 1983b), visual hemifield (Bruder et al., 1989; Bruder et al., 1992), event-related potential (Bruder et al., 1991; Bruder et al., 1992), and electrodermal (Myslobodosky & Horesh, 1978) studies. The stage of the illness (such as acute, chronic, remitted) may also have an effect on lateral indices in dichotic listening studies (e.g., Bruder et al., 1981; Moscovitch et al., 1981). Findings of Wexler & Heninger (1979) supports the hypothesis that in acute illness stage the interhemispheric inhibition which generally mediates laterality collapses. Miller et al (2002) have recently found the influence of variability in clinical course on the patients' frontal EEG asymmetry. Remission of depression is found to be associated with nomalization of the observed left frontal hypoactivation (Baxter et al., 1989; Bench et al., 1995; Martinot et al., 1990; Passero, Nardini, & Battistini, 1995) and asymmetry on dichotic listening tasks (Bruder, 1983b).

Greater severity of depressive symptoms was found associated with less dichotic listening laterality (Bruder, 1983a, 1983b). In neuroimaging studies also, activation in the left prefrontal regions was found negatively correlated with severity of depression (Andreason et al., 1992; Baxter et al., 1989; Bench et al., 1993; Drevets et al., 1992; Kato et al., 1995; cited in Davidson & Henriques, 2000). Further, when facial expressions were rated with the Emotion Facial Action Coding System (EMFACS; Friesen, 1986), Berenbaum (1992) found a link between severity of depressive symptoms and the likelihood of expressing emotions. In this study, those depressives who did not show anger/contempt or disgust had significantly lower Beck Depression Inventory (Beck et al., 1961) scores than those who did. In contrast, depressives who showed happy expressions did not differ in severity from those who did not. This finding indicates that the intent to express anger/contempt/disgust may reflect a different underlying mechanism than the disposition to express happiness. However not investigated, this underlying mechanism may also have to do with supposedly the different lateralization patterns for expressing anger and happiness in the same depressive patients.

Cerebral laterality with dichotic listening technique has been found affected by the age of illness onset (Pine et al., 2000; Stewa, Bruder, McGrath, & Quitkin, 2003). Larsen (1984) reported that in normal children the magnitude of right ear advantage for correct responses decreased with increasing age on a dichotic listening task. This developmental change was more evident in right handers. As neuroimaging data suggest, older depressives showed more bilateral or global frontal hypoactivation than the younger patients (e.g., Hoyer, Oesterreich, & Wagner, 1984; Kumar et al., 1993; cited in Davidson & Henriques, 2000). In sleep EEG measures, interhemispheric coherence was found lowest in adolescent girls, not in children, with major depression (Armitage et al., 2000). Duda & Brown (1984) found a right hemisphere advantage for processing facial emotions in normal females than males, and further, they were more accurate in recognizing sad than happy expressions. Gender differences using dichotic listening method may be found as a result of confounding factors rather than the cerebral lateralization (Welsh & Elliott, 2001).

Functional laterality is also indicated through side- bias of the subjects. By side- bias, we mean the bias reflected in the differential use of paired organs (such as hand, foot, eye, or ear) as a function of preference, performance, or attentional/intentional factors (Mandal et al., 2000). Though inconsistent, findings in general showed an association between left/atypical handedness and some types of developmental disorders and psychopathology (see the review by Coren & Halpern, 1991). In addition, alcoholic subjects are found to have reduced right side- bias for all four measures, handedness, footedness, eyedness, and earedness (Mandal, Bhushan, Kumar, & Gupta, 2000), unlike heroin addicts and normal controls. Although some early studies have reported increased incidence of left handedness in schizoaffective and bipolar patients compared to normal controls (Lishman & McMeekan, 1976), and in bipolar I patients compared to bipolar II patients (Sackein & Decina, 1983; cited in Coffey, 1987), the proposition is perhaps not tested utilizing side- bias measures of all forms, hand, foot, eye and ear, on depressive patients.

Individual differences in the degree of cerebral lateralization has been noted in psychiatric patients, including depressives (Wexler & Heninger, 1979). In electrophysiological studies, consistent differences in baseline measures of activation asymmetry has been found in anterior cerebral regions (Davidson, 1992). Further, the role of attentional bias has been pointed out in dichotic listening studies (Bryden, Munhall, & Allard, 1983; Mondor & Bryden, 1991). A substantial decrease in right ear advantage was observed when the time period between onset of the actual trial of dichotic listening was made longer (Mondor & Bryden, 1991). "Individuals vary not only in their underlying perceptual asymmetries for auditory input, but also in the manner in which such asymmetries interact with other higher order cognitive functions" (Cowell & Hugdahl, 2000, p. 95).

The second potential source of variation is the stimulus or task. Dichotic-listening studies have mostly used verbal stimuli, and a few studies nonsense syllable task. The efficacy of such task had been emotional voice (Bryden, 1988). Different hemispheric involvement in depression was found for verbal and nonverbal dichotic listening tasks. Taking event-related potential, Bruder et al., (1991) reported longer P3 latency in an audiospatial, not temporal, task for the left hemisphere, than the right hemisphere, in typical depressive patients. Perceptual asymmetry in depressive patients is also understood convincingly through techistoscopic studies, very few however. Mandal & Palchoudhury (1985) observed that in a free-viewing condition depressive symptoms do not significantly impair the ability to identify facial emotions. The patients were, unlike normals, rather more accurate in recognizing sadness than happiness; and preferred more sad faces for interaction than normals (Mandal & Palchoudhury, 1986).

The issue of hemispheric control of emotional expression may be related to the degree to which emotions are posed or voluntarily expressed as compared to spontaneous expression. Brain lesion studies indicate the possibility of a dissociation between voluntary and involuntary control of emotional expressions (Gatz, 1970; Monrad-Krohn, 1924; Peele, 1961; cited in Sackeim & Gur, 1978). Recent studies have also argued in favour of a differential neurological involvement for posed and spontaneous facial expressions in terms of type of fibre projections (bilateral, ipsilateral or contralateral) and control of motor system (pyramidal extrapyramidal) (Asthana & Mandal, 1997; Borod et al., 1997). In a study on normal subjects, the intensity of facial expressions of both happy and sad emotions on the left side of the face (a RH function) was found stronger during the spontaneous than the posed expressions (Dopson, Beckwith, Tucker, & Bullard-Bates, 1984). Here, experimental induction of spontaneous affect was based on 'memory' of emotional experiences, and thus, the role of memorial cognitive processes in emotion elicitation could not be controlled. Although spontaneous facial expressions are difficult either to sample or to control for variables other than emotions (Mandal, Harizuka, Bhushan, & Mishra, 2001), investigating lateral asymmetry with posed and spontaneous emotional expressions on the same group of depressive subjects may be more informative. Further, it is important to include more than one emotion or dimension of emotion (such as positive/negative, aroused/ nonaroused, or approach/avoidance) in lateralization studies to ascertain whether the observed effects are indeed specific to sadness or are more general characteristics of emotion per se.

There is evidence that emotional experience and expression may be dissociated in brain-damaged patients (Gainotti, 1983; Ross, 1984) and schizophrenics (Berenbaum & Oltmanns, 1992; Kring, Kerr, Smith, & Neale, 1993; Kring & Neale, 1996; Sison, Alpert, Fudge, & Stern, 1996). Also, neurological evidence indicates that the systems controlling facial expressions and subjective experience may act independently (Ross & Mesulam, 1979; cited in Berenbaum & Oltmanns, 1992). Anterior and posterior lesion sites were found implicated for expression and perception of emotions respectively (Borod, 1992). The study of lateral indices of different aspects of emotion processing - perception, experience, and expression - in depressive patients may also provide interesting results. This speculation gets emphasis from two sources of evidence. First, people with depression have been found to have flat affect (e.g., Andreasen, 1979; Pogue-Geile & Harrow, 1984), as in schizophrenia. Secondly, depressive patients are reported to be less facially expressive to positive emotions such as happiness (Berenbaum, 1992; Berenbaum & Oltmanns, 1992; Ellgring, 1989) than normal controls. Depressives however exhibited more anger than normals (Berenbaum, 1992; Riley, Treiber, & Woods, 1989).

Borod et al. (1986) obtained lateral indices of affect perception and expression on brain-damaged patients. The RH hypothesis was supported for both perception and expression of emotion. The valence hypothesis was partly supported by the perception factor; that is, RHD patients were significantly more impaired than LHD patients or normal controls in perceiving negative emotions. In lateralization studies, little attempt has been made to explore the interdependence or independence of different aspects of affect processing - affect perception, experience, and expression. Independent research on affect perception with split-field/dichotic-listening technique and affect expression with hemifacial mobility were carried out, but very little research was undertaken on the same individuals for these measures. The inconsistencies in findings of studies on affect lateralization may be resolved if the research to examine all three aspects of affect processing (perception, experience, and expression of affect) is conducted on the same individual (Mandal, Asthana, Pandey, & Sarbadhikari, 1996; Mandal, Pandey, & Prasad, 1998). In such a case, the potential confounding of subject variables may be avoided to allow a better understanding of the lateralization of emotional processes.

In lateralization studies, relationship between normal emotional functions and affective illness, such as depression, is not clear (Mandal, Asthana, Pandey, & Sarbadhikari, 1996). Most of the studies on lateralization of emotional states were conducted on brain-damaged patients. Though, observations from such studies may not be directly applicable to patients without brain damage (Mandal, Asthana, Pandey, & Sarbadhikari, 1996). Further, impairment following a focal brain damage does not essentially provide information about that region (Sergent, 1988; cited in Mandal et al., 1996). Probably to avoid such problems, lateralization studies have also been conducted by inducing affect state in normal individuals. Lateralization of depression is tempted to be understood by inducing sadness in the subjects. One considerable issue in such procedure is the degree to which an experimentally induced negative affective state approximates negative affect in clinical depression, especially in terms of quality and severity of the affect (discussed by Scott & Ingram, 1998); although experimental control is one advantage in such procedure. Isolating specific features of sadness during controlling sensory, perceptual, and memorial processes associated with the specific form of emotion elicitation is the another methodological issue (Davidson & Henriques, 2000). Moreover, sadness is only a part of depression, and it is possible that other symptoms (such as loss of interest, negative cognition, psychomotor decrement) or cluster of symptoms (such as cognitive, motoric, or somatic) play a much larger role in reflecting lateralization pattern. It is difficult, therefore, to generalize the affective processes in depression on the basis of affect induction studies. Such studies perhaps have more advantage for understanding the mechanisms underlying affective functioning, than affective illness.

Etevenon (1983) proposed a three-step intracerebral interaction model: (a) intrahemispheric antero-posterior inhibition, (b) interhemispheric reciprocal inhibition, and (c) cross-hemispheric coupling (cited in Mandal et al, 1996). The cross-hemispheric coupling model was accepted by Tucker (1983) with a proposition that happy mood is a function of the positive coupling of left anterior/right posterior areas and negative coupling of left posterior/right anterior areas. In contrast, sad mood is a function of the reverse order of cross-hemispheric coupling. In addition to interhemispheric reciprocal situation (Leventhal & Tomarken, 1986) or cross-hemispheric coupling (Tucker, 1983), researchers have showed an intrahemispheric activation theory for depression. Shackman (2000) found that the left frontal region is the region that consistently distinguishes depressed from healthy individuals, on the basis of findings from both clinically (Henriques & Davidson, 1991) and subclinically (Davidson, Schaffer, & Saron, 1985; Schaffer, Davidson, & Saron, 1983) depressed subjects.

In a study, patients with anterior region brain-damage were found significantly inferior to the patients with posterior region brain-damage in the perceptual matching task with hemifacial affective stimuli, and interestingly, the difference between right and left hemisphere-damage patients was nonsignificant (Mandal, Asthana, Tandon, & Asthana, 1992). RHD and LHD patients also exhibited no significant difference in voluntarily expressing facial emotions, but those with anterior region damage showed more impairment than those with posterior region damage and normals (Weddell, Miller, & Trevarthen, 1990). Findings of hemiregional variations in facial expression of emotions in normal people (Asthana & Mandal, 1997) also underscore the involvement of several neuroanatomical regions, which may not be explained by their lateral side, in processing facial emotions. The view that depressive symptoms cluster into categories of mood, cognitive, motor, and somatic regulation also allows for identification of different brain regions which make up the disorder. Thus, there is convincing evidence for the importance of compartmentalizing the brain into regions, such as anterior-posterior, (for a review, see Davidson & Henriques, 2000), other than the left-right sides, to have a more comprehensive view of depression. Recently, Shenal, Harrison, & Demaree (2003) presented a model composed of three neuroanatomical divisions, left frontal, right frontal, and right posterior, and proposed that dysfunction in any of these quadrants may lead to depressive symptoms.

Russell (1995) argued that sadness is not such kind of emotion which is pancultural, and it does not provide "precise message" communicated through facial expressions. [The controversy regarding universality of emotions inferred from facial expressions, however, remains.] Affect lateralization research may potentially draw its attention to the examination of interaction pattern of neurocultural components of emotion. It has already been shown that left sided facial asymmetry (a RH function) is more akin to negative rather than positive emotions (Borod, Haywood, & Koff, 1997; Borod & Koff, 1990; Campbell, 1986). But there is dearth of evidence suggesting culture-specific pattern of hemifacial asymmetry. Taking normal subjects, Mandal, Harizuka, Bhushan, & Mishra (2001) observed culture-specificity with respect to hemifacial asymmetry and valence of emotion expressions: (1) Japanese showed a right hemifacial bias for negative emotions; Indians and North Americans showed left hemifacial bias for all emotions, and (2) negative emotion expressions were least distinctly identifiable in Japanese faces followed by Indian and North American faces. Keeping in view the identification of cross-cultural patterns of emotion recognition in normal (Elfenbein et al., 2002) and schizophrenic (Habel et al., 2000) subjects, the paradigm of standardized measures of emotion recognition may be extended in future to find out cross-cultural pattern of lateral indices in depressive illness.

As we discussed, there are a number of methodological confounds which make cerebral laterality of depression state-dependent. Further research is needed in this area to identify trait-like features of cortical indices. Researchers have yet to be sure that the performance on varied tasks measuring laterality is not affected by factors independent of actual hemispheric advantage (Leventhal & Tomarken, 1986; Stone, 1980). On the other hand, findings also indicate that several measures of cerebral laterality "may not all assess the same phenomenon" (Schneider, 1983, p. 287). The general claim of right hemisphere dysfunction in depression is not accepted without controversy. It is found that the relationship between affect processing and affective illness in terms of intra- and interhemispheric role is not straitforward (Mandal, Asthana, Pandey, & Sarbadhikari, 1996).

REFERENCES

Abercrombie, H. C., Schaefer, S. M., Larson, C. L., Oakes, T. R., Holden, J. E., et al. (1998). Metabolic rate in the right amygdala predicts negative affect in depressed patients. *NeuroReport*, 9, 3301-3307.

Abrams, R., & Taylor, M. A. (1979). Differential EEG patterns in affective disorder and schizophrenia. *Archives of General Psychiatry*, 36, 1355-1358.

Adolphs, R., Jansari, A., & Tranel, D. (2001). Hemispheric perception of emotional valence from facial expressions. *Neuropsychology,* 15, 516-524.

Alema, G., & Rosadini, G. (1964). Donnees cliniques et E.E.G. de l'introduction d'amytal sodium dans la circulation encephalique, concernant l'etat de conscience. *Acta Neurochirurgica,* 12, 241-257.

Allen, K. M., Blascovich, J., Tomaka, J., & Kelsey, R. M. (1991). Presence of human friends and pet dogs as moderators of autonomic responses to stress in women. *Journal of Personality and Social Psychology,* 61, 582-589.

Altshuler, L. L., Devinsky, O., Post, R. M., & Theodore, W. (1990). Depression, anxiety, and temporel lobe epilepsy. *Archives of Neurology*, 47, 284-288.

Andreasen, N. C. (1979). Affective flattening and the criteria for schizophrenia. *American Journal of Psychiatry*, 136, 944- 947.

Andreason, P. J., Altemus, M., Zametkin, A.j., King, A. C., Lucinio, J., & Cohen, R. M. (1992). Regional cerebral glucose metabolism in bulimia nervosa. *American Journal of Psychiatry*, 149, 1506-1516.

Angeleri, F., Angeleri, V. A., Foschi, N., Giaquinto, S., Nolfe, G., Saginario, A., & Signorino, M. (1997). Deprssion after stroke: an investigation through catamnesis. *Journal of Clinical Psychiatry*, 58, 261-265.

Armitage, R., Emslie, G. J., Hoffmann, R. F., Weinberg, W. A., Kowatch, R. A., Rintelmann, J., & Rush, A. J. (2000). Ultradian rhythms and temporal coherence in sleep EEG in depressed children and adolescents. *Biological Psychiatry,* 47, 338-350.

Asthana, H. S., & Mandal, M. K. (1997). Hemiregional variations in facial ___expression of emotions. *British Journal of Psychology*, 88, 519-525.

Asthana, H. S., Mandal, M. K., Khurana, H., & Haque-Nizamie, S. (1998). Visuospatial an daffect recognition deficit in depression. *Journal of Affective Disorder*, 48, 57-62.

Asthana, H. S., Mandal, M. K., Tandon, S. C., & Asthana, S. (1991). Matching top-bottom parts of facial ___expression of emotion by brain-damaged patients. *Behavioural Neurology*, 4, 255-263.

Bauer, L. O. & Hesselbrock, V. M. (2002). Lateral asymmetries in the frontal brain: effects of depression and a family history of alcoholism in female adolescents. Alcohol and Clinical Experimental Research, 26, 1662-1668.

Baxter, L. R., Schwartz, J. M., Phelps, M. E., Mazziotta, J. C., Guze, B. H., Selin, C. E., Gerner, R. H., & Sumida, R. M. (1989). Reduction of prefrontal cortex glucose metabolism common to three types of depression. *Archives of General Psychiatry*, 46, 243-250.

Beauregard, M., Leroux, J. M., Bergman, S., Arzoumanian, Y., Beaudoin, G., et al. (1998). The functional neuroanatomy of major depression: an fMRI study using an emotional activation paradigm. *NeuroReport*, 9, 3253-3258.

Beck, A.T., Ward, C.H., Mendelson, M., Mock, J.E., & Edward, J.K. (1961). An inventory for measuring depression. *Archives of General Psychiatry*, 4, 561-571.

Bench, C. J., Frackowiak, R. S., & Dolan, R J. (1995). Changes in regional cerebral blood flow on recovery from depression. *Psychological Medicine*, 25, 247-261.

Bench, C. J., Friston, K. J., Brown, R. G., Frackowiak, R. S., & Dolan, R. J. (1993). Regional cerebral blood flow in depression measured by positron emission tomography: The relationship with clinical dimensions. *Psychological Medicine*, 23, 579-590.

Bench, C. J., Friston, K. J., Brown, R. G., Scott, L. C., Frackowiak, R. S., & Dolan, R. J. (1992). The anatomy of melancholia- focal abnormalities of cerebral blood flow in major depression. *Psychological Medicine*, 22, 607-615.

Benton, A. (1986). Reaction times in brain disease: Some reflections. *Cortex,* 22, 129-140.

Berenbaum, H. (1992). Posed facial expressions of emotion in schizophrenia and depression. *Psychological Medicine*, 22, 929- 937.

Berenbaum, H., & Oltmanns, T. F. (1992). Emotional experience and ___expression in schizophrenia and depression. *Journal of Abnormal Psychology*, 101, 37- 44.

Bihrle, A. M., Brownell, H. H., Powelson, J. A., & Gardner, H.(1986). Comprehension of humorous and nonhumorous materials by left and right brain-damaged patients. *Brain and Cognition,* 5, 399-411.

Biver, R., Goldman, S., Delvenne, V., Luxen, A., De Maertelaer, V., Hubain, P., Mednlewicz, J. & Lotstra, F. (1994). Frontal and parietal metabolic disturbances in unipolar depression. *Biological Psychiatry*, 36, 381-388.

Black, F. W. (1975). Unilateral brain lesion and MMPI performance: A preliminary study. *Perceptual and Motor Skills*, 40, 87-90.

Blonder, L. X., Bower, D., & Heilman, K. M. (1991). The role of the right hemisphere in emotional communication. *Brain*, 114, 1115-1127.

Bonne, O., & Krausz, Y, (1997). Pathophysiological significance of cerebral perfusion abnormalities in major depression- Trait or state marker. *European Neuropsychopharmacology,* 7, 225-233.

Borod, J. C. (1992). Interhemispheric and intrahemispheric control of emotion: A focus on unilateral brain damage. *Journal of Consulting and Clinical Psychology*, 60, 339-348.

Borod, J. C. (1993). Cerebral mechanisms underlying facial, prosodic, and lexical emotional _expression: A review of neuropsychological studies and methodological issues.*Neuropsychologia,* 7, 445-463.

Borod, J. C., Cicero, B. A., Obler, L. K., Welkowitz, J., Erhan, H. M., Santschi, C., Grunwald, I. S., Agosti, R. M., & Whalen, J. R. (1998). Right hemisphere emotional perception: evidence across multiple channels. *Neuropsychology,* 12, 446-458.

Borod, J. C., Haywood, C. S., & Koff, E. (1997). Neuropsychological aspects of facial asymmetryduring emotional ___expression: A review of the normal and adult literature. *Neuropsychology Review*, 7, 41-59.

Borod, J. C., & Koff, E. (1990). Lateralization for facial emotional behaviour: A methodological perspective. *International Journal of Psychology*, 25, 157-177.

Borod, J. C., Koff, E., Perlman Lorch, M., & Nicholas, M. (1986). The ___expression and perception of facial emotion in brain-damaged patients. *Neuropsychologia,* 24, 169-180.

Borod, J. C., Koff, E., Perlman Lorch, M., & Nicholas, M., & Welkowitz, J. (1988). emotional and nonemotional facial behaviours in patients with brain-damage. *Journal of Neurology,Neurosurgery, and Psychiatry,* 51, 826-832.

Borod, J. C., Koff, E., & White, B. (1983). Facial asymmetry in posed and spontaneous expressions of emotion. *Brain and Cognition*, 2, 165-175.

Borod, J. C., Martin, C. C., Alpert, M., Brozgold, A., & Welkowitz, J. (1993). Perception of facial emotion in schizophrenic and right brain-damage patients. *Journal of Nervous and Mental Disease,* 18, 494-502.

Borod, J. C., Tabert, M. H., Santschi, C., & Strauss, E. H. (2000). Neuropsychological assessment of emotional processing in brain-damaged patients. In J. C. Borod (Ed.), *The neuropsychology of emotion* (pp. 80-105). New York: Oxford University Press.

Bowers, D., Bauer, R. M., Coslett, H. B., & Heilman, K. M. (1985). Processing of faces by patients with unilateral hemisphere lesions: Dissociation between judgements of facial affect and facial identity. *Brain and Cognition*, 4, 258-272.

Brody, A. L., Saxena, S., Stoessel, P., Gillies, L. A., Fairbanks, L. A., Alborzian, S., Phelps, M. E., Huang, S. C., Wu, H. M., Ho, M. L., Ho, M. K., Au, S. C., Maidment, K., & Baxter, L. R. Jr. (2001). Regional brain metabolic changes in patients with major deprerssion treated with either paroxetine or interpersonal therapy: preliminary findings. *Archive of General Psychiatry*, 58, 631-640.

Bruder, G. E. (1983a). Dichotic listening laterality in schizophrenia and affective disorders: The role of diagnostic subtype and clinical state. In P. Flor-Henry, & J. Gruzelier (Eds.), *Laterality and psychopathology* (pp. 411-426). Amsterdam: Elsevier.

Bruder, G. E. (1983b). Cerebral laterality and psychopathology: a review of dichotic listening studies. *Schizophrenia Bulletin*, 9, 134-151.

Bruder, G. E., Quitkin, F. M., Stewart, J. W., Martin, C., Voglamaier, M. M., & Harrison, W. M. (1989). Cerebral laterality in depression: Differences in perceptual asymmetry among diagnostic subtypes. *Journal of Abnormal Psychology*, 98, 177-186.

Bruder, G. E., Stewart, J. W., McGrath, P. J., Ma, G. L., Wexler, B. E., & Quitkin, F. M. (2002). Atypical depression: enhanced right hemispheric dominance for perceiving emotional chimeric faces. *Journal of Abnormal Psychology*, 111, 446-454.

Bruder, G. E., Stewart, J. W., Towey, J. P., Friedman, D., Tenke, C. E., Voglmaier, M. M., Leite, P., Cohen, P., & Quitkin, F. M. (1992). Abnormal cerebral laterality in bipolar depression: convergence of behavioural and brain event-related potential findings. *Biological psychiatry*, 32, 33-47.

Bruder, G. E., Sutton, S., Berger-Gross, P., Quitkin, F., & Davies, S. (1981). Lateralized auditory processing in depression: Dichotic click detection. *Psychiatry Research*, 4, 253-266.

Bruder, G. E., Tenke,C.E., Stewart, J. W., Towey, J. P., Leite, P., Voglmaier, M., & Quitkin, F. M (1995). Brain event-related potentials to complex tones in depressed patients: Relations to perceptual asymmetry and clinical features. *Psychophysiology,* 32, 373-381.

Bruder, G. E., Tenke, C. E., Towey, J. P., Leite, P., Fong, R., Srewart, J. E., McGrath, P. J., & Quitkin, F. M. (1998). Brain ERPs of depressed patients to complex tones in an oddball task: relation of reduced P3 asymmetry to physical anhedonia. *Psychophysiology*, 35, 54-63.

Bruder, G. E., Towey, J. P., Stewart, J. W., Friedman, D., Tenke, C., & Quitkin, F. M. (1991). Event-related potential in depression: Influence of task, stimulus hemifield, and clinical features on P3 latency. *Biological Psychiatry*, 30, 233-246.

Bruder, G. E., Wexler, B. E., Stewart, J. W., Price, L. H., & Quitkin, F. M. (1999). Perceptual asymmetry differences between major depresion with or without a comorbid anxiety disorder. *Journal of Abnormal Psychology*, 108, 233-239.

Bryden, M. P. (1982). *Laterality: Hemispheric specialization in the intact brain.* San Diego: Academic Press.

Bryden, M. P. (1988). Dichotic studies of the lateralization of affect in normal subjects. In K. Hugdahl (Ed.), *Handbook of dichotic listening* (pp. 1-44). Chichester, UK: Wiley.

Bryden, M. P., Ley, R. G., & Sugarman, J. H. (1982). A left ear advantage for identifying the emotional quality of tonal sequences. *Neuropsychologia,* 20, 83-87.

Bryden, M. P., Munhall, K., & Allard, F. (1983). Attentional biases and the right-ear effect in dichotic listening. *Brain and Cognition*, 18, 236-248.

Buchtel, H., Campari, F., De Risio. C., & Rota, R. (1978). Hemispheric differences in discriminative reaction time to facial expressions. *Italian Journal of Psychology*, 5, 159-169.

Buck, R., & Duffy, R. J. (1980). Nonverbal communication of affect in brain-damaged subjects. *Cortex*, 16, 351-362.

Burton, L. A. & Labar, D. (1999). Emotional status after right vs. left temporal lobectomy. *Seizure,* 8, 116-119.

Campbell, R. (1978). Asymmetries in interpreting and expressing a posed facial _expression. *Cortex,* 14, 327-342.

Campbell, R. (1986). Asymmetry of facial action: Some facts and fancy of normal face movement. In R. Bruyer (Ed.), *The neuropsychology of face perception and facial _expression* (pp. 247-267). Hillsdale, NJ: Erlbaum.

Carroll, B. J., Curtis, G. C., & Mendels, J. (1976). Cerebrospinal fluid and plasma free cortisol concentrations in depression. *Biological Medicine*, 6, 235-244.

Carter, C. S., Botvinick, M. M., & Cohen, J. D. (1999). The contribution of the anterior cingulated cortex to executive processes in cognition. *Review of Neuroscience*, 10, 49-57.

Cazard, P. (1989). Hemispheric asymmetry of alpha burst frequency of occurrence variations in depression. *International Journal of Neuroscience*, 47, 181-191.

Chabrol, H., Barrere, M., Guell, A., Bes, A., & Moron, P. (1986). Hypofrontality of cerebral blood flow in depressed adolescents [letter to the editor]. *American Journal of Psychiatry*, 143, 263-264.

Christianson, S. A., Saisa, J., Garvill, J., & Silfvinius, H. (1993). Hemispheric inactivation and mood-state changes. *Brain and Cognition,* 23, 127-144.

Coffey, C. E. (1987). Cerebral laterality and emotion: The neurology of depression. *Comprehensive Psychiatry*, 28, 197-219.

Coren, S., & Halpern, D. F. (1991). Left-handedness: A marker for decreased survival fitness. *Psychological Bulletin,* 109, 90-106. [Medline].

Cowell, P., & Hugdahl, K. (2000). Individual differences in neurobehavioural measures of laterality and interhemispheric function as measured by dichotic listening. *Developmental Neuropsychology*, 18, 95-112.

Curran, S. M., Murray, C. M., Van Beck, M., Dougall, N., O'Carroll, R. E., et al. (1993). A single photon emission computerized tomography study of regional brain function in elderly patients with major depression and with Alzheimer-type dementia. *British Journal of Psychiatry,* 163, 155-165.

Davidson, R. J. (1984). Affect, cognition and hemispheric specialization. In C. E. Izard, J. Kagan, & R. Zajonc (Eds.), *Emotions, cognition and behaviour* (pp. 320-365). Cambridge: Cambridge University Press.

Davidson, R. J. (1988). EEG measures of cerebral asymmetry: conceptual and methodological issues. *International Journal of Neuroscience*, 39, 71-89.

Davidson, R. J. (1992). Anterior cerebral asymmetry and the nature of emotion. *Brain and Cognition*, 20, 125-151.

Davidson, R. J., Abercrombie, H. C., Nitschke, J. B., & Putnam, K. M. (1999). Regional brain function, emotion and disorders of emotion. *Current Opinion in Neurobiology*, 9, 228-234.

Davidson, R. J., & Henriques, J. (2000). Regional brain function in sadness and depression. In J. C. Borod (Ed.), *The neuropsychology of emotion* (pp. 269-297). New York: Oxford University Press.

Davidson, R. J., Pizzagalli, D., Nitschke, J. B., & Putnam, K. (2002). Depression: perspectives from affective neuroscience. *Annual Review of Psychology,* 53, 545-574.

Davidson, R. J., Schaffer, C. E., & Saron, C. (1985). Effects of lateralized presentations of faces on self reports of emotion and EEG asymmetry in depressed and nondepressed subjects. *Psychophysiology,* 22, 353-364.

Deldin, P. J., Keller, J., Gergen, J. A., & Miller, G. A. (2000). Right-posterior face processing anomaly in depression. *Journal of Abnormal Psychology*, 109, 116-121.

Delvenne, V., Delecluse, F., Hubain, P. P., Schoutens, A., De Maertelaer, V., & Mendlewicz, J. (1990). Regional cerebral blood flow in patients with affective disorders. *British Journal of Psychiatry*, 157, 359-365).

Dopson, W.N., Beckwith, B. E., Tucker, D.M., & Bullard- Bates, P.C. (1984). Asymmetry of facial ___expression in spontaneous emotion. *Cortex*, 20, 243- 251.

Drevets, W. C. (1998). Functional neuroimaging studies of depression: the anatomy of Melancholia (abstract). *Annual Review of Medicine*, 49, 341-361.

Drevets, W. C., Price, J. L., Simpson, J. R. J., Todd, R. D., Reich, T., Vannier, M., & Raichle, M. (1997). Subgenual prefrontal cortex abnormalities in mood disorders. *Nature*, 386, 824-827.

Drevets, W. C., Videen, T. O., Price, J. L., Preskorn, S. H., Charnichael, T., & Raichle, M. E. (1992). A functional anatomical study of unipolar depression. *The Journal of Neuroscience*, 12, 3628-3641.

Duda, P. D., & Brown, J. (1984). Lateral asymmetry of positive and negative emotions. *Cortex*, 20, 253- 261.

Dutta, T., & Mandal, M. K. (2002). Visual-field superiority as a function of stimulus type and content. *International Journal of Neuroscience*, 112, 945-952.

Elfenbein, H. A., Mandal, M. K., Ambady, N., Harijuka, S., & Kumar, S. (2002). Cross cultural patterns in emotion recognition: Highlighting design and analytical techniques . *Emotion*, 2, 75- 84.

Ellgring, H. (1989). Nonverbal communication in depression. Cambridge: Cambridge University Press.

Engel, J. (1984). The use of positron emission tomographic scanning in epilepsy. *Annals of Neurology,* 15(suppl.), S180-S191.

Enloe, A. A. , Ilardi, S. S., Atchley, R. A., Cromwell, R. L., & Sewell, K. W. (2001). Word valence, attention, and hemispheric activity in depressed, remitted, and nondepressed controls. *Brain and Cognition*, 46, 129-133.

Etevenon, P. (1983). A model of intra- and inter-hemispheric relationships. In P. Flor-Henry & J. Gruzelier (Eds.), *Laterality and psychopathology* (pp. 291-300). Amsterdam: Elsevier.

Flor-Henry, P. (1969). Schizophrenic-like reactions and affective psychoses associated with temporal lobe epilepsy: Etiological factors. *American Journal of Psychiatry,* 126, 148-162.

Flor-Henry, P. (1979). Laterality, shifts of cerebral dominance, sinistrality, and psychosis. In J. Gruzelier, & P. Flor-Henry (Eds.), *Hemisphere asymmetries of function in psychopathology* (pp. 3-19). New York: Elsevier/North-Holland Biomedical Press.

Francois, A., Biver, F., Goldman, S., Luxen, A., Mendlewicz, J., & Lotstra, F. (1995). [Decrease in the frontal-superobasal metabolic ratio in unipolar depression] [in French]. *Acta Psychiatrica Belgica,* 95, 234-245.

Friesen, W. (1986). Recent developments in FACS- EMFACS. *Face value: Facial measurement newsletter*, 1, 1-2.

Fromm-Auch, D. (1983). Neuropsychological assessment of depressed patients before and after drug therapy. In P. Flor-Henry, & J. Gruzelier (Eds.), *Laterality and psychopathology* (pp. 82-102). Amsterdam: Elsevier.

Gainotti, G. (1972). Emotional behaviour and hemispheric side of the lesion. *Cortex*, 8, 41-55.

Gainotti, G. (1983). Laterality of affect: The emotional behaviour of right- and left- brain-damaged patients. In M. S. Myslobodsky (Ed.), *Hemisyndromes: Psychobiology, neurology, psychiatry.* San Diego: Academic Press.

Galynker, I. I., Cai, J., Ongseng, F., Finestone, H., Dutta, E., & Serseni, D. (1998). Hypofrontality and negative symptoms in major depressive disorder. *Journal of Nuclear Medicine*, 39, 608-612.

Gasparrini, W. G., Satz, P., Heilman, K. M., & Coolidge, F. L. (1978). Hemyspheric asymmetries of affective processing as determined by the Minnesota Multiphasic Personality Inventory. *Journal of Neurology, Neurosurgery, and Psychiatry*, 41, 470-473.

Gatz, A. J. (1970). *Manter's essentials of clinical neuroanatomy and neurophysiology*. Philadelphia: Davis.

George, M. S., Ketter, T. a., Parekh, P. I., Rosinsky, N., Ring, H. A., et al. (1997). Blunted left cingulated activation in mood disorder subjects during a response interference task (the Stroop). *Journal of Neuropsychiatry and Clinical Neuroscience*, 9, 55-63.

Glass, A. (1987). *Individual differences in hemispheric specialization*. New York: Plenum Press.

Gotlib, I. H., Ranganath, C., & Rosenfeld, J. P. (1998). Frontal EEG alpha asymmetry, depression, and cognitive functioning. *Cognition and Emotion*, 12, 449-478.

Gur, R. E., & Chin, S. (1999). Laterality in functional brain imaging studies of schizophrenia. *Schizophrenia Bulletin*, 25, 141-156.

Gustafson, L., Risberg, J., & Silfverskiold, P. (1981). Regional cerebral blood flow in organic dementia and affective disorders. *Advances in Biological Psychiatry*, 6, 109-116.

Haag, C., Kathmann, N., Hock, C., Gunther, W., Voderholzer, U., & Laakmann, G. (1994). Lateralization of the Bereitschafts-potential to the left hemisphere in patients with major depression. *Biological Psychiatry*, 36, 453-457.

Habel, U., Gur, R. C., Mandal, M. K., Salloum, J. B., Gur, R. E., Schneider, F. (2000). Emotional processing in schizophrenia across cultures : standardized measures of discrimination and experience. *Schizophrenia Research*, 42, 57-66.

Hatta, T. (1984). Lateral eye movements and hemispheric asymmetry: effects of question type, task type, and individual differences. *Cortex,* 20, 543-556.

Heilman, K. M., Bowers, D., Speedie, L., & Coslett, H. B. (1984). Comprehension of affective and nonaffective prosody. *Neurology,* 94, 917-921.

Heller, W., & Levy, J. (1981). Perception and ___expression of emotion in right handers and left handers. *Neuropsychologia,* 19, 263-272.

Henriques, J. B., & Davidson, R. J. (1989). Affective disorders. In G. Turpin (Ed.), *Handbook of clinical Psychophysiology* (pp. 357-392). London: Wiley.

Henriques, J. B., & Davidson, R. J. (1990). Regional brain electrical asymmetryies discriminate between previously depressed and healthy control subjects. *Journal of Abnormal Psychology*, 99, 22-31.

Henriques, J. B., & Davidson. R. J. (1991). Left frontal hypoactivation in depression. *Journal of Abnormal Psychology,* 100, 535-545.

Henriques, J. B., & Davidson. R. J. (1997). Brain electrical asymmetries during cognitive task performance in depressed and nondepressed subjects. *Biological Psychiatry*, 42, 1039-1050.

Holthoff, V. A., Beuthien-Baumann, B., Pietrzyk, U., Pinkert, J., Oehme, L., Franke, W. G., & Bach, O. (1999). Changes in regional cerebral perfusion in depression: SPECT monitoring of response to treatment [Article in German]. *DerNervenarzt*, 70, 620-626.

House, A., Dennis, M., Molyneux, A., Warlow, C., & Hawton, K. (1989). Emotionalism after stroke. *British Medical Journal*, 298, 991-994.

House, A., Dennis, M., Wariow, C., Hawton, K., & Molyneux, A. (1990). Mood disorders after stroke and their relation to lesion location. A CT scan study. *Brain*, 113, 1113-1129.

Hoyer, S., Oesterreich, K., & Wagner, O. (1984). Depression in old age and its relation to primary dementia: Variations in brain blood flow and oxidative metabolism. *Monographs of Neural Science,* 11, 187-192.

Indaco, A., Carrieri, P. B., Nappi, C., Gentile, S., & Striano, S. (1992). Interictal depression in epilepsy. *Epilepsy Research*, 12, 45-50.

Ito, H., Kawashima, R., Awata, S., Ono, S., Sato, K., Goto, R., Koyama, M., Sato, M., & Fukuda, H. (1996). Hypoperfusion in the limbic system and prefrontal cortex in depression: SPECT with anatomic standerdization technique. *Journal of Nuclear Medicine*, 37, 410-414.

Johnson, O., & Crockett, D. (1982). Changes in perceptual asymmetries with clinical improvement of depression and schizophrenia. *Journal of Abnormal Psychology*, 91, 45-54.

Kato, T., Shioiri, T., Murashita, H., Takahashi, Y., Inubushi, T., & Takahashi, S. (1995). Lateralized abnormality of high energy phosphate metabolism in the frontal lobes of patients with bipolar disorder detected by phase-encoded 31P-MRS. *Psychological Medicine*, 25, 557-566.

Kennedy, S. H., Evams, K. R., Kruger, S., Mayberg, H. S., Meyer, J. H., McCann, S., Arifuzzman, A. I., Houle, S., & Vaccarino, F. J. (2001). Changes in regional brain glucose metabolism measured with positron emission tomography after paroxetine treatment of major depression. *Americal Journal of Psychiatry*, 158, 899-905.

Kimbrell, T. A., Ketter, T. A., George, M. S., Little, J. T., Benson, B. E., Willis, M. W., Herscovitch, P., & Post, R. M. (2002). Regional cerebral glucose utilization in patients with a range of severities of unipolar depression. *Biological Psychiatry*, 51, 237-252.

Kimura, D. (1961). Cerebral dominance and the perception of verbal stimuli. *Canadian Journal of Psychology*, 15, 166-171.

Kohler, C., Norstrand, J. A., Baltuch, G., O' Connor, M. J., Gur, R. E., French, J. A., & Sperling, M. R. (1999). *Epilepsia*, 40, 336-340.

Korpelainen, J. T., Kauhanen, M. L., Tolonen, U., Brusin, E., Mononen, H., Hiltunen, P., Sotaniemi, K. A., Suominen, K., & Myllyla, V. V. (2000). Auditory P3000 event related potential in minor ischemic stroke. *Acta Neurologica Scandinavica*, 101, 202-208.

Kring, A. M., & Neale, J. M. (1996). Do schizophrenic patients show a disjunctive relationship among expressive, experiential and psychophysiological components of emotion ? *Journal of Abnormal Psychology*, 105, 249- 257.

Kring, A.M., Kerr, S., Smith, D.A., Neale, J.M. (1993). Flat affect in schizophrenia does not reflect discontinued subjective __expression of emotion. *Journal of Abnormal Psychology* , 102, 507- 517.

Kucharska-Pietura, K. & David, A. S. (2003). The perception of emotional chimeric faces in patients with depression, mania and unilateral brain damage. *Psychological Medicine*, 33, 739-745.

Kumar, A., Newberg, A., Alavi, A., Berlin, J., Smith, R., & Reivich, M. (1993). Regional cerebral glucose metabolism in late-life depression and alzheimer disease: A preliminary positron emission tomography study. *Proceedings of the National Academy do Sciences of the United States of America,* 90, 7019-7023.

Larsen, S. (1984). Developmental changes in the pattern of ear asymmetry as revealed by a dichotic listening task. *Cortex,* 20, 5-17.

Lee, G. P., Loring, D. W., Meader, K. J., & Brooks, B. B. (1990). Hemispheric specialization for emotion __expression: A reexamination of results from intracarotid administration of sodium amobarbital. *Brain and Cognition*, 12, 267-280.

Lefevre, E., Starck, R., Lambert, W. E., & Genesee, F. (1977). Lateral eye movements during verbal and nonverbal dichotic listening. *Perceptual and Motor Skills*, 44, 1115-1122.

Lesser, I. M., Mena, I., Boone, K. B., Miller, B. L., Mehringer, C. M., & Wohl, M. (1994). Reduction of cerebral blood flow in older depressed patients. *Archives of General Psychiatry*, 51, 677-686.

Leventhal, H., & Tomarken, A. J. (1986). Emotion: Today's problems. *Annual Review of Psychology*, 37, 565-610.

Liotti, M., Sava, D., Rizzolatti, G., & Caffarra, P. (1991). Differential hemispheric asymmetries in depression and anxiety: a reaction-time study. *Biological Psychiatry*, 29, 887-899.

Lishman, W. A., & McMeekan, E. R. L. (1976). Hand preference patterns in psychiatric patients. *British Journal of Psychiatry*, 129, 158-166.

Maes, M., Dierckx, R., Meltzer, H. Y., Ingels, M., Schotte, C., Vandewoude, M., Calabrese, J. & Cosyns, P. (1993). Regional cerebral blood flow in unipolar depression measured with Tc-99m-HMPAO single photon emission computed tomography: negative findings. *Psychiatry Research*, 50, 77-88.

Mandal, M. K., Asthana, H. S., & Pandey, R. (1995). Asymmetry in emotional face: its role in intensity of expression. *Journal of Psychology*, 129, 235-241.

Mandal, M. K., Asthana, H. S., Pandey, R., Sarbadhikari, S. (1996). Cerebral laterality in affect and affective illness: A review. *The Journal of Psychology*, 130, 447-459.

Mandal, M. K., Asthana, S. H., Tandon, S. C., & Asthana, S. (1992). Role of cerebral hemispheres and regions in processing hemifacial ___expression of emotion: Evidence from brain damage. *International Journal of Neuroscience*, 63, 187-195.

Mandal, M. K., Bhushan, B., Kumar, A., & Gupta, P. (2000). Side-bias in alcohol and heroin addicts. *Alcohol and Alcoholism*, 35, 381-383.

Mandal, M. K., Borod, J. C., Asthana, H. S., Mohanty, A., Mohanty, S., & Koff, E. (1999). Effects of lesion variables and emotion type on the perception of facial emotion. *Journal of Nervous and Mental Disease*, 187, 603-609.

Mandal,M. K., Harizuka, S., Bhushan, B., & Mishra, R. C. (2001). Cultural variation in hemifacial asymmetry of emotion expressions. *British Journal of Social Psychology*, 40, 385-398.

Mandal, M. K., Mohanty, A., Pandey, R., & Mohanty, S. (1996). Emotion-specific processing deficit in focal brain-damaged patients. *International Journal of Neuroscirnce*, 84, 87-95.

Mandal, M. K., & Palchoudhury, S. (1985). Responses to facial ___expression of emotion in depression. *Psychological Reports*, 56, 653-654.

Mandal, M. K., & Palchoudhury, S. (1986). Choice of facial affect and psychopathology. *Journal of Social Behaviour and Personality,* 1, 299-302.

Mandal, M. K., Pandey, R., Prasad, A. B. (1998). Facial expressions of emotions and schizophrenia: A review. *Schizophrenia Bulletin*, 24, 399- 412.

Mandal, M. K., Tandon, S. C., & Asthana, S. H. (1991). Right brain damage impairs recognition of negative emotions. *Cortex,* 27, 247-253.

Martinot, J. L., Hardy, P., Feline, A., Huret, J. D., Mazoyer, B., Attar-Levy, D., Pappata, S., & Syrota, A. (1990). Left prefrontal glucose hypometabolism in the depressed state: A confirmation. *American Journal of Psychiatry*, 147, 1313-1317.

Mathew, R. J., Meyer, J. S., Francis, D. J., Semchuk, K. M., Mortel, K., & Claghorn, J. L.(1980). Cerebral blood flow in depression. *American Journal of Psychiatry*, 137, 1449-1450.

Mayberg, H. S., Brennam, S. K., Mahurin, R. K., Jerabek, P. A., Brickman, J. S., et al (1997). Cingulate function in depression: a potential predictor of treatment response. *NeuroReport*, 8, 1057-1061.

Mayberg, H. S., Lewis, P. L., Regenold, W., & Wagner, H. N. (1994). Paralimbic hypoperfusion in unipolar depression. *Journal of Nuclear Medicine*, 35, 929-934.

Mendez, M. F., Taylor, J. L., Doss, R. C., & Salguero, P. (1994). Depression in secondary epilepsy: Relation to lesion laterality. *Journal of Neurology, Neurosurgery, and Psychiatry*, 57, 232-233

Mikhailova, E. S., Vladimirova, T. V., Iznak, A. F., Tsusulkovskaya, E. J., & Sushko, N. V. (1996). Abnormal recognition of facial expression of emotions in depressed patients with major depression disorder and schizotypal personality disorder. *Biological Psychiatry,* 40, 697-705.

Miller, A., Fox, N. A., Cohn, J. F., Forbes, E. E., Sherrill, J. T., & Kovacs, M. (2002). Regional patterns of brain activity in adults with a history of childhood-onset depression: gender differences and clinical variability. *American Journal of Psychiatry,* 159, 934-940.

Monakhov, K., Perris, C., Botskarev, V. R., Von Knorring, L., & Nikiforov, A. I. (1979). Functional interhemispheric differences in relation to various psychopathological components of the depressive syndrome. *Neuropsychobiology,* 5, 143-155

Mondor, T. A., & Bryden, M. P. (1991). The influence of attention on the dichotic REA. *Neuropsychologia,* 29, 1179-1190.

Monrad,-Krohn, G. H. (1924). On the dissociation of voluntary and emotional innervations in facial paresis of central origin. *Brain*, 47, 22-45.

Moretti, M., Charlton, S., & Taylor, S. (1996). The effects of hemispheric asymmetries and depression on the perception of emotion. *Brain and Cognition*, 32, 67-82.

Moscovitch, M., Strauss,E., & Olds, J. (1981). Handedness and dichotic listening performance in patients with unipolar endigenous depression who received ECT. *American Journal of Psychiatry,* 133, 988-990.

Myslobdsky, M. S., & Horesh, N. (1978). Bilateral electrodermal activity in depressive patients. *Biological Psychology*, 6, 111-120.

Neubauer, A., Schulter, G., & Pfurtscheller, G. (1988). Lateral eye movements as an indication of hemispheric preference: an EEG validation study. *International Journal of Psychophysiology,* 6, 177-184.

Oyebode, F., Kennedy, S., & Davison, K. (1986). Psychiatric sequelae of subarachnoid haemorrhage. *British Journal of Hospital Medicine*, 36, 106-108.

Paolucci, S., Antonucci, G., Pratesi, L., Traballesi, M., Grasso, M. G., & Lubich, S. (1999). Poststroke depression and its role in rehabilitation of inpatients. *Archive of Physical Medicine and Rehabilitation,* 80, 985-990.

Passero, S., Nardini, M., & Battistini, N. (1995). Regional cerebral blood flow changes following chronic administration of antidepressant drugs. *Progress in Neuropsychopharmacology, and,Biological Psychiatry*, 19, 627-636.

Peele, T, L. (1961). *The neuroanatomic basis for clinical neurology*. New York: McGraw-Hill.

Perini, G. (1986). Emotions and personality in complex partial seizures. *Psychotherapy Psychosomatic,* 45, 141-148.

Perini, G., & Mendius, R. (1984). Depression and anxiety in complex partial seizures. *Journal of Nervous and Mental Disease,* 172, 287-290.

Perris, C. (1974). Averaged evoked responses (AER) in patients with affective disorders. *Acta Psychiatrica Scandinavica,* 255, 89-98.

Philpot, M. P., Banerjee, S., Needham,-Bennett, H., Costa, D. C., & Ell, P. J. (1993). 99mTc-HMPAO single photon emission tomography in late life depression : A pilot study of regional cerebral blood flow at rest and during a verbal fluency task. *Journal of Affective Disorders*, 28, 233-240.

Pine, D. S., Kentgen, L. M., Bruder, G. E., Leite, P., Bearman, K., Ma, Y., & Klein, R. G. (2000). Cerebral laterality in adolescent major depression. *Psychiatry Research*, 93, 135-144.

Pogue- Geile, M. F., & Harrow, M. (1984). Negative and positive symptoms in schizophrenia and depression: A follow- up. *Schizophrenia Bulletin*, 10, 371-387.

Pozzi, D., Golimstock, A., Petracchi, M., Garcia, H., & Starkstein, S. (1995). Quantified electroencephalographic changes in depressed patients with and without dementia. *Biological Psychiatry*, 38, 677-683.

Raine, A. (1991). Are lateral eye-movements a valid index of functional hemispheric asymmetries? *British Journal of Psychology*, 82, 129-135.

Ramos-Brieva, J. A., Olivan, J., Palomares, A., & Vela, A. (1984). Is there right hemisphere dysfunction in major depression? *International Journal of Neuroscience*, 23, 103-109.

Reuter-Lorenz, P., & Davidson, R. J. (1981). Differential contributions of the two cerebral hemispheres for perception of happy and sad faces. *Neuropsychologia*, 19, 609-614.

Riley, W. T., Treiber, F. A., & Woods, M. G. (1989). Anger and hostility in depression. *Journal of Nervous and Mental Disease*, 177, 668- 674.

Robinson, R. G., Lipsey, J. R., Bolla-Wilson, K., Bolduce, P. L., Pearlson, G. D., Rao, K., & Price, T. R. (1985). Mood disorders in left-handed stroke patients. *American Journal of Psychiatry,* 142, 1424-1429.

Roemer, R. A., Shagass, C., Dubin, W., Joffe, R., & Siegal, L. (1992). Quantitative EEG in elderly depressives. *Brain Topography*, 4, 285-290.

Ross, E. (1984). Right hemisphere's role in language, affective behaviour and emotion. *Trends in Neurosciences,* 7, 342-346.

Ross, E. D., & Mesulam, M. M. (1979). Dominant language functions of the right hemisphere ? Prosody and emotional gesturing. *Archives of Neurology*, 36, 144- 148.

Rush, A. J., Schlesser, M. A., Stokely, E., Bonte, F. R., & Altshuller, K. Z. (1982). Cerebrel blood flow in depression and mania. *Psychopharmacology Bulletin*, 18, 6-8.

Russell, J. A. (1995). Facial expressions of emotion: what lies beyond minimal universality ? *Psychological Bulletin*, 118, 379- 391.

Sackeim, H. A., & Decina, P. (1983). Lateralized neuropsychological abnormality in bipolarsand in children of bipolar probands. In P. Flor-Henry, & J. Gruzelier (Eds.), *Laterality and psychopathology* (pp. 103-128). Amsterdam: Elsevier.

Sackeim, H. A., Greenberg, M., Weiman, A., Gur, R. C., Hungerbuhler, J., & Gechwind, N. (1982). Functional brain asymmetry in the ___expression of positive and negative emotions: Lateralization of insults in cases of uncontrollable emotional outbursts. *Archives of Neurology*, 19, 210-218

Sackeim, H. A., & Gur, R. C. (1978). Lateral asymmetry in intensity of emotional ___expression. *Neuropsychologia,* 16, 473-481.

Sackeim, H. A., Prohovnik, I., Moeller, J. R., Brown, R. P., Apter, S., Prudic, J., Devanand, D. P., & Mukherjee, S. (1990). Regional cerebral blood flow in mood disorders. I. Comparison of major depressives and normal controls at rest. *Archives of General Psychiatry*, 47, 60-70.

Safer, M. A., & Leventhal, H. (1977). Ear differences in emotional tone of voice and verbal content. *Journal of Experimental Psychology: Human Perception and Performance*, 3, 75-82.

Saxby, L., & Bryden, M. P. (1984). Left ear superiority in children for processing auditory emotional material. *Developmental Psychology*, 21, 72-80.

Schaffer, C. E., Davidson, R. J., & Saron, C. (1983). Frontal and parietal electroencephalogram asymmetry in depressed and nondepressed subjects. *Biological Psychiatry*, 18, 753-762.

Schneider, S. J. (1983). Multiple measures of hemispheric dysfunction in schizophrenia and depression. *Psychological Medicine*, 13, 287-297.

Schroeder, J., Saver, H., Wilhelm, K. R., Neidermeier, T., & Georgi, P. (1989). Regional cerebral blood flow in endogenous psychoses: A Tc-99m HMPAO-SPECT pilot study. *Psychiatry Research*, 29, 331-333.

Scott, W. D., & Ingram, R. E. (1998). Affective influences in depression: conceptual issues, cognitive consequences, and multiple mechanisms. In W. F. Flack, & J. D. Laird (Eds.), *Emotions in psychopathology* (pp. 200- 215). New York: Oxford University Press.

Sergent, J. (1988). Some theoretical and methodological issues in neuropsychological research. In F. Boller & J. Gradman (Eds.), *Handbook of neuropsychology* (Vol. 1, pp. 69-81). North Holland: Elsevier.

Shackman, A. J. (2000). Anterior cerebral asymmetry, affect, and psychopathology: Commentary on the withdrawal-approach model. In R. J. Davidson (Ed.), *Anxiety, depression and emotion* (pp.109-132). New York: Oxford University Press.

Sheline, Y. I. (2000). 3D MRI studies of neuroanatomic changes in unipolar major depression: the role of stress and medical comorbidity. *Biological Psychiatry*, 48, 791-800.

Sheline, Y. I., Barch, D. M., Donnelly, J. M., Ollinger, J. M., Snyder, A. Z., & Mintun, M. A. (2001). Increased amygdala response to masked emotional faces in depressed subjects resolves with antidepressant treatment: an fMRI study. *Biological Psychiatry*, 50, 651-658.

Shenal, B. V., Harrison, D. W., & Demaree, H. A. (2003). The neuropsychology of depression : A literature review and preliminary model. *Neuropsychological Review*, 13, 33- 42.

Silverstein, M. L., & Meltzer, H. Y. (1983). Neuropsychological dysfunction in the major psychoses. In P. Flor-Henry, & J. Gruzelier (Eds.), *Laterality and psychopathology* (pp. 143-152). Amsterdam: Elsevier.

Sison, C. E., Alpert, M., Fudge, R., Stern R. M. (1996). Constricted expressiveness and Psychophysiological reactivity in schizophrenia. *Journal of Nervous and Mental Disease*, 184, 589- 597.

Smith, G. S., Reynolds, C. F. 3rd, Pollock, B., Derbyshire, S., Nofzinger, E., Dew, M. A., Houck, P. R., Milko, D., Meltzer, C. C., & Kupfer, D. J. (1999). Cerebral glucose metabolic response to combined total sleep deprivation and antidepressant treatment in geriatric depression. *American Journal of Psychiatry*, 156, 683-689.

Sommer, I., Ramsey, N., Kahn, R., Aleman, A., & Bouma, A. (2001). Handedness, language lateralization and anatomical asymmetry in schizophrenia: metaanalysis. *British Journal of Psychiatry,* 178, 344-351.

Spalletta, G., Guida, G., & Caltagirone, C. (2003). Is left stroke a risk-factor for selective serotonin reuotake inhibitor antidepressant treatment resistance? *Journal of Neurology,* 250, 449-455.

Springer, S., & Deutsch, G. (1990). *Left brain, right brain* (3rd ed.). San Francisco: W. H. Freeman.

Starkstein, S. E., Robinson, R. G., Berthier, M. L., Parikh, R. M., & Price, T. R. (1988). Differential mood changes following basal ganglia vs thalamic lesions. *Archive of Neurology*, 45, 725-730.

Stewart, J. W., Bruder, G. E., McGrath, P. J., & Quitkin, F. M. (2003). Do age of onset and course of illness define biologically distinct groups within atypical depression? *Journal of Abnormal Psychology*, 112, 253-262.

Stone, M. A. (1980). Measures of laterality and spurious correlation. *Neuropsychologia,* 18, 339-345.

Strauss, E., & Moscovitch, M. (1981). Perception of facial expressions. *Brain and Language,* 13, 308-332.

Suberi, M., & McKeever, W. F. (1977). Differential right hemisphere memory storage of emotional and nonemotional faces. *Neuropsychologia,* 15, 757-768.

Taylor, M., & Abrams, R. (1983). Cerebral hemisphere dysfunction in the major psychoses. In P. Flor-Henry, & J. Gruzelier (Eds.), *Laterality and psychopathology* (pp. 153-162). Amsterdam: Elsevier.

Tenke, C. E., Bruder, G. E., Toway, J. P., Leite, P., & Sidtis, J. J. (1993). Correspondence between brain ERP and behavioural asymmetries in a dichotic complex tone test. *Psychophysiology,* 30, 62-70.

Terzian, H. (1964). Behavioural and EEG effects of intracarotid amytal injection. *Acta Neurochirurgica,* 12, 230-239.

Thomas, K. M., Drevets, W. C., Whalen, P. J., Eccard, C. H., Dahl, R. E., Ryan, N. D., & Casey, B. J. (2001). Amygdala response to facial expressions in children and adults. *Biological Psychiatry*, 49, 309-316.

Tucker, D. M. (1981). Lateral brain function, emotion, and conceptualization. *Psychological Bulletin,* 89, 19-46.

Tucker, D. M. (1983). Asymmetries of coherence topography: Structural and dynamic aspects of brain lateralization. In P. Flor-Henry, & J. Gruzelier (Eds.), *Laterality and psychopathology* (pp. 349-362). Amsterdam: Elsevier.

Tucker, D. M., Stenslie, C. E., Roth, R. S., & Shearer, S. L. (1981). Right frontal lobe activation and right hemisphere performance: Decrement during depressed mood. *Archives of General Psychiatry,* 38, 169-174.

Vakili, K., Pillay, S. S., Lafer, B., Fava, M., Renshaw, P. F., Bonello-Cintron, C. M. (2000). Hippocampal volume in primary unipolar major depression: a magnetic resonance imaging study. *Biological Psychiatry*, 47, 1087-1090.

Victoroff, J. I., Benson, F., Grafton, S. T., Engel, J. Jr, & Mazziotta, J. C. (1994). Depression in complex partial seizures. Electroencephalography and cerebral metabolic correlates. *Archive of Neurology*, 51, 155-163.

Von Knorring, L. (1983). Interhemispheric EEG differences in affective disorders. In P. Flor-Henry, & J. Gruzelier (Eds.), *Laterality and psychopathology* (pp. 315-326). Amsterdam: Elsevier.

Warren, L. R., Butler, R. W., Katholi, C. R., Crews, E. L., & Halsey, J. H. (1984). Focal changes in cerebral blood flow produced by monetary incentive during a mental mathematics task in normal and depressed subjects. *Brain and Cognition*, 3, 71-85.

Wechsler, A. (1973). The effect of organic brain disease on recall of emotionally charged versus neutral narrative texts. *Neurology,* 23, 130-135.

Weddell, R. A., Miller, J. D., & Trevarthen, C. (1990). Voluntary emotional facial expression in patients with focal cerebral lesions. *Neuropsychologia,* 28, 49-60.

Welsh, T. N., & Elliott, D. (2001). Gender differences in a dichotic listening and movement task: lateralization or strategy? *Neuropsychologia,* 39, 25-35.

Wexler, B. E. (1980). Cerebral laterality and psychiatry: A review of the literature. *American Journal of Psychiatry*, 137, 279-291.

Wexler, B. E., & Halwes, T. (1985). Dichotic listening tests in studying brain behaviour relationships. *Neuropsychologia*, 23, 545-559.

Wexler, B. E., & Heninger, G. R. (1979). Alterations in cerebral laterality during acute psychotic illness. *Archive of General Psychiatry*, 36, 278-284.

Wilbur, M. P., & Roberts-Wilbur, J. (1985). Lateral eye-movement responses to visual stimuli. *Perceptual and Motor Skills*, 61, 167-177.

Yazici, K. M., Kapucu, O., Erbas, B., Varoglu, E., Gulec, C., & Bekdik, C. F. (1992). Assessment of changes in regional cerebral blood flow in patients with major depression using the 99m Tc- HMPAO single photon emission tomography method. *European Journal of Nuclear Medicine,* 19, 1038-1043.

Yecker, S., Borod, J. C., Brozgold, A., Martin, C., Alpert, M., & Welkowitz, J. (1999). Lateralization of facial emotional expression in schizophrenic and depressed patients. *Journal of Neuropsychiatry and Clinical Neuroscience*, 11, 370-379.

Yozawitz, A., Bruder, G. E., Sutton, S., Sharpe, L., Gurland, b., Fleiss, J., & Costa, L. (1979). Dichotic perception: Evidence for right hemisphere dysfunction in affective psychosis. *British Journal of Psychiatry*, 135, 224-237.

Yurgelun-Todd, D. A., Gruber, S. A., Kanayama, G., Killgore, D. S., Baird, A. A., & Young, A. D. (2000). fMRI during affect discrimination in bipolar affective disorder. *Bipolar Disorder*, 2, 237-248.

Zahn, T. P. (1986). Psychophysiological approaches to psychopathology. In M. G. H. Coles, E. Donchin. & S. W. Porges (Eds.), *Psychophysiology: Systems, process, and applications* (pp.508-610). Ney York: The Guilford Press.

In: Depression and Dementia
Editor: Suptendra Nath Sarbadhikari, p. 183-212
ISBN 1-59454-114-0

Chapter 7

RECENT ADVANCES IN THE BIOLOGY OF DEPRESSION: CLINICAL PERSPECTIVES

Shailesh Kumar
Department of Psychiatry
Private bag 3023
Rotorua Hospital, Rotorua
New Zealand
Email: shailesh.kumar@lakesdhb.govt.nz

ABSTRACT

This chapter outlines some of the recent biological advances in our understanding of depression as a mental disorder. Significant advances have been made in the psychosocial aspects of depression especially in the psychological models and interventions for the condition. Whilst they are essential in the treatment of depression, they are beyond the scope of this chapter and will not be discussed in detail. An attempt is made to focus on recent advances only.

INTRODUCTION

Despite significant advances in the detection and management of psychiatric conditions, depression remains an under-diagnosed and under-treated condition. A well- designed study, Depression Research in European Society (DEPRES), investigated 75,000 adults drawn from the general population across Europe. 17% of the subjects were reported to suffer from depression and 43% of them had not consulted a doctor. Among those who had consulted a doctor only 30% received medication for depression and only 10% of patients with major depressive disorder had been prescribed an antidepressant by their primary care physician (Lepine et al, 1997). Similar findings were reported by a more recent study from the USA. While more than 30 million adults in the United States experience major depressive disorder (MDD), most patients still received inadequate treatment (Kessler et al, 2003). According to the criteria used in the study, treatment for MDD was considered "minimally adequate" if patients attended at least four outpatient visits for pharmacotherapy (use of an antidepressant or mood stabilizer for at least 30 days) or at least eight psychotherapy sessions (lasting at least half an hour) with an appropriate mental health professional. The study found that only 21.7% of patients with 12-month MDD received adequate care in the year preceding the survey (Kessler et al, 2003).

This chapter outlines some of the recent biological advances in our understanding of depression as a mental disorder. Significant advances have been made in the psychosocial aspects of depression especially in the psychological models and interventions for the condition. Whilst they are essential in the treatment of depression, they are beyond the scope of this chapter and will not be discussed in detail. An attempt is made to focus on recent advances only.

Prevalence and Burden of Depression: Health Economics and Epidemiology

Interest in depression is growing rapidly for two reasons: a) we are beginning to understand the pervasive presence of depression b) our understanding of burden associated with depression has improved. Depressive disorders are widely prevalent in all societies and countries and tend to be chronic, and disabling. Point prevalence in the USA for depression has been estimated at 3% in general population, 5-9% in women and 2-3% in men (APA 2000). It has also been reported that about 6% of the general American population meet the criteria for major depressive disorder or dysthymia at any time (APA, 2000). 20% of those with major depressive disorder were predicted to have symptoms that persisted beyond 2 years. (Keller et al, 1992). It is noteworthy that the prevalence of sub-threshold depressive disorders is higher than MDD and estimated in the range of 3 to 9%. 10 to 25% of women and 5 -12% of men in the United States will experience MDD in their lifetime (APA, 2000).

Depression appears to be even more prevalent in the general medical population. The prevalence rate rises to 10% among people who contact general health service for any reason and is even higher among patients with chronic conditions (heart diseases, Diabetes, etc) (Ustun and Sartorius, 1995). There is some evidence that the incidence of depression may in fact be on the rise (Sartorius, 2003) This rise could be attributed to several potential factors such as more people survive to an age of higher risk for depression, people with chronic medical conditions have a heightened life expectancy, chronic medical conditions are associated with depressive disorders and more women taking hormonal contraception, which is thought to increase their vulnerability to depression.

The earlier view that depression is a disorder of developed world or Anglo-Saxon cultures has also been challenged. It has been reported in all cultures almost at a similar rate, though presentations may differ. We now know that clinical features such as sad or anxious mood, loss of initiative and interest, reduced sleep, and appetite are independent of culture (Sartorius et al 1980). Features such as guilt, shame and somatization may vary with different cultures (Jenkins 1990). Such differences can partly be attributed to the way in which different cultures adhere to mind body dichotomy –somatic manifestations of depression tends to be less common in cultures with less dichotomous views (Kronmuller & Mundt 2001). Among various somatic features associated with depression, pain would appear to be the commonest symptom presented by patients with depression. Two theories have been put forward to explain why depressed patients often present with pain and other somatic symptoms: a. During depressed state the perception of pain and other bodily sensations may be amplified (Meana, 1998) and b. given that serotonin and norepinephrine are involved in the perception of pain as well as the pathogenesis of depression, there may be a common neuro-chemical pathway for both conditions.

The impact of depression on the health services, individual and society are considerable. Ten years ago, the annual cost of depression in the United States varied between US $ 43.7 – 52.9 billion dollars (Greenberg et al 1993). This estimate included cost incurred due to health care, suicide and work place losses. In the UK the cost of treating depression has been estimated at £887 million and is likely to exceed the cost of treating hypertension and diabetes added together (£439 million and £300 million respectively) (Department of Health, 1996). Overall medical costs doubled in those with depression. It is also known that depressed patients are likely to utilize healthcare services three times more frequently (Katon and Schultzberg 1992) and visit emergency rooms seven times more often than non depressed patients (Johnson, Weissman and Klerman 1992). Consequently we find that 1-1.5 million years are lost per year due to depressive illness in established market economies (Europe, USA, Africa and Latin America). It has been suggested that days lost from work owing to depression exceeds all other disorders (Broadhead et al, 1990).

The burden to society of various diseases has been qualified and quantified using a single standard construct called DALY (Disability Adjusted Life Years) in a World Bank report (Murray & Lopez, 1996). DALY objectively measures years of life lost to premature death and years lived with a disability of specified severity and duration. More than one in every ten years lived with a disability was due to Unipolar Depression. This report stated that in the age group 15-44 years depression was responsible for 10% of all DALY's. It was predicted that DALY due to depression was likely to rise to 15% by the year of 2020 making depression second only to ischaemic heart disease in terms of world-wide disease burden.

Two landmark studies, DEPRES and LIDO have further highlighted the morbidity caused by depression. The Depression research in European society (DEPRES) study reported that people with Major Depression lost four times more working days than non-sufferers (Murray et al 1996). LIDO (Longitudinal Investigation of Depression Outcomes) was a cross-national observational study conducted in six different cities and targeted a cohort of individuals attending primary care services. The relationship between symptom severity, quality of life, level of functioning, cost of treatment and outcome of depression were reported among patients who met the criteria for either major depressive disorder or sub-threshold depression, but had remained untreated for at least three months (Chisholm et al, 2003). Medical co-morbidity was associated with 17-46 % increase in health care costs in five of the six sites. This study confirmed that co-morbidity played a greater contributory role than symptom severity alone in the economic consequences of depression.

At the individual level, depression is associated with significant morbidity and mortality. A US study of over 11,000 outpatients with chronic or non-chronic conditions found that patients with depression had worse physical and social role functioning than patients with no chronic physical conditions. The functioning of patients with depression was worse than that of patients with chronic medical conditions such as Diabetes, Arthritis and back complaints (Wells et al, 1989). High prevalence of concomitant physical conditions such as Arthritis, Hypertension, Backache, Diabetes and Heart problems have also been reported in the depressed population and causes a worsened prognosis for both (Lyons et al 1994). The risk of suicide is a major issue with depression. A study reported that 56% of patients with depression attempted suicide at least once (Goodwin and Jamison, 1990). According to various estimates 10-15% patients with severe depression die by committing suicide (Miles 1977, Winokur and Tsuang, 1975).

Depression has considerable impact on family and work. Marital disharmony, increased divorce rates, disruption of other social roles (transmission of culture, rearing of children and support to family members) is all associated with depression. Similarly, depressive disorders are associated with difficulties in relationships with work colleagues and problems such as absenteeism, decreased productivity and with very high levels of unemployment (Sartorius 2003)

Depression tends to be commoner in boys until adolescence when it rises in the favour of girls. The trend that continues through the rest of life cycle. Women to men ratio being 2:1. Among women, married, divorced, separated and widows are at higher risk compared to their single counter parts. Interestingly enough married men are relatively protected from depression unlike married women.

Classification and Types of Depression

Kraepelin (1913) described clinical features of the depressive episode in manic depression but Leonhard (1957) suggested that this group of mental illness should be further classified in bipolar and unipolar affective disorders. Angst (1966) and Perris (1966) were the first to produce convincing results demonstrating the scientific validity behind such an approach, which was based on longitudinal presentation. Later, other methods of sub-typing were introduced including endogenous/ reactive, psychotic/neurotic depression, primary/secondary depression etc. Each of these approaches has been based on differing philosophies and therefore warrants further discussion.

Endogenous/ Reactive

This classification has been the longest one to dominate in taxonomy of depression. It uses factor analysis and is based on the tenet that depressive disorder can be classified on the basis of aetiology into two groups -endogenous where symptoms are caused by factors inside the individual and reactive by factors outside the individual. The finding compromises internal consistency of this model that a high score on one factor doesn't predict high score on another. Such classification may have some biological basis because Dexamethasone Suppression Test and the impaired growth hormone response with clonidine are commonly reported in endogenous but not in reactive depression.

Retarded/Anxious

Retarded depression is associated with marked psychomotor retardation whereas anxious depression is associated with just psychomotor activity. It was recommended that energising antidepressants such as imipramine were better suited for retarded depression whereas sedating antidepressants such as amitryptiline were preferred for agitated depression (Kielholz 1971). Once again well designed studies have failed to support this classification. Biological markers have been described in support. People with retarded depression have reduced sweating and salivation. Low Homo Vanylic Acid, a dopamine metabolite has also been described in endogenous depression but has been attributed to lowered body movement.

Psychotic/Neurotic

Traditionally speaking psychotic depression has been used to denote a more severe type of depression. Neurotic depression has described milder forms of depression. In an attempt to operationalise criteria psychotic depression is used to describe depression associated with psychotic features mostly nihilistic and hypochondriac delusions being common.

Unipolar/Bipolar

RDC criteria describes unipolar depression as a disorder of least two depressive episodes with a minimum 2 months of normal functioning in between but without a history of hypomania or mania. The presence of the latter warrants a diagnosis of bipolar affective disorder. Some interesting distinctions do exist between the two conditions. The rate of a positive family history is higher in bipolar affective disorder; age of onset is earlier for bipolar affective disorder (i.e. twenties or late adolescence) as opposed to recurrent depressive disorder (in thirties); gender ratio is equal for bipolar but women have a higher prevalence for recurrent depression; episodes tend to be shorter and more frequent in bipolar and the risk of drug-induced hypomania/mania is also higher in bipolar.

Primary /Secondary

Depression that can be attributed to another medical or psychiatric condition is called secondary depression. Depression without any demonstrable cause is considered primary. Psychiatric conditions commonly associated with depression are schizophrenia, schizoaffective disorder, personality disorders, phobic disorders, obsessive compulsive disorder, Briquet syndrome, anti social personality disorder, alcoholism and substance abuse. Hypothyroidism is quoted as one of the commonest factors associated with secondary depression and is thought to be present in up to 52% of people with depression. Certain medications such as Glucocorticoids and anti-hyertensives have been implicated as causes for secondary depression. Similarly medical conditions including diabetes mellitus, ischaemic heart disease, human immune deficiency virus, cancer, chronic pain, fibromyalgia, chronic fatigue syndrome and irritable bowel syndrome have been implicated.

The main criticism of this classification is that secondary depression is too heterogeneous and over inclusive because it incorporates such wide ranging sub-categories. Furthermore, it is imperative in this classification that only biological factors may cause secondary depression whereas a significant proportion of patients experience depression following life events. If we believe that depression in these cases was a result of life events then why not call them "secondary depression" too?

Chronic Major Depression

The term chronic depression is used to denote depression that persists for two years or longer. It is also true, however, that depression by nature, is a chronic and recurrent illness. While untreated episodes typically don't last for more than 6-9 months, more than 40% of patients who recover from an episode of unipolar depression are likely to experience a recurrence after two years, a figure that rises to 60% after five years (Keller & Boland, 1998). Fifteen to twenty percent of patients with depression will have episodes lasting longer than two years (Keller et al. 1992). Up to one third of patients may partially recover from a major depressive episode but the lack of complete remission may persist for two-years or more (Mueller et al 1996). A personality pattern of self-blame, beliefs of inadequacy, low self-esteem, hopelessness and worthlessness and the lack of continuity of treatment are commonly associated with chronicity (APA, 2000). 10-15 % of patients with chronic depression commit suicide increasing the risk thirty fold.

DSM IV (APA, 2000) describes four subtypes of chronic depression:

1. Chronic Major Depressive Disorder: Major depressive disorder of at least two year duration
2. Dysthymic Disorder: depressed mood (not syndromal depression) of at least two year duration and persists most of the time.
3. Dysthymic Disorder with Major Depressive Disorder (Double Depression)- major depression super imposed on dysthymia of at least two year duration
4. Depressive Disorder in partial (incomplete) remission: recurrent episodes of depression without full recovery in between episodes.

Dysthymic Disorder

It is best described as sporadic, persistent and mild depression, which, may occur at the rate of 3% in the general population. Typically it begins at an early age. Onset after 20 years of age is considered late for dysthymia. Depressed mood and depressive symptoms tend to be present for more days than not but euthymic periods of up to two months can occur. More than 50% patients with dysthymia may experience superadded depressive episodes, "double depression" (see above).

ETIOLOGY

Biological Factors

Genetic Factors

Genetic factors tend to play a strong role in the causation of depressive disorders but perhaps not as much as bipolar affective disorder. Heritability has been calculated to be about 0.8-0.9 for bipolar and 0.45 for recurrent depressive disorder (Pliszka, 2003). As a result we see that while morbidity risk of depression is 10-15% for a first degree relative as opposed to 3% in the general population. 50% concordance rate for monozygotic twins and 10-25%

dizygotic twins have been noted. No or little effects of rearing have been suggested by adoption studies. Genetic factors alone can not explain the aetiology of depression. Like all other mental disorders, no single locus has been found, not all offspring or indeed monozygotic twins, develop the illness and it is difficult to explain the late development of the illness despite having a significant genetic loading. It is now commonly accepted that genetic factors interact with environmental factors to produce depression.

Neuro Transmitters in Depression

Monoamine Hypothesis

This was the first neuro-chemical model proposed as an etiological factor for depression. It was based on the view that depression was the result of disturbance in noradrenaline and serotonergic systems. (Bunney & Davis, 1965: Schildkeraut, 1965 & Coppen, 1967). This model remains most influential in our understanding of the neuro chemical basis for depression and was responsible for the discovery of a number of antidepressants including tri-cyclics and MAO inhibitors. Animal and human studies reported that depleting tryptophan, a precursor of serotonin, caused a relapse of depression. Similarly depletion of nor-adrenalin by the inhibition of enzyme tyrosine hydroxylase had a similar effect (Delgardo et al, 1993).

A third monoamine to be investigated in the aetiology of depression was dopamine (DA), known to be associated with the reward and reinforcement. A deficiency of mesolimbic dopamine (DA) has been put forward as the cause behind some of the symptoms of depression (e.g., psychomotor retardation, anhedonia and loss of motivation). A recent study has quantified the amounts of dopaminergic proteins in the depressed amygdala, compared to normal individuals. The study showed that the binding of [(125)I]RTI 55 to DA transporter was significantly lower in the basal and central amygdaloid nuclei, whereas the binding of [(125)I]epidepride to D2/D3 receptors was significantly higher in the basal, central, and lateral amygdaloid nuclei in major depression compared with control subjects. Combining their findings with the previous finding that DA depletion in rats can induce a reduction in the DA transporter and an upregulation of D2/D3 receptors the authors supported the hypothesis that DA deficiency in the mesolimbinc area may cause depression (Klimek et al 2002)

The main difficulty with this model was that depleting either noradrenaline, serotonin or dopamine could not produce depression in patients who had not experience depression before. Researchers had to look at examining the roles of sub-cellular disturbance including receptors, secondary messengers and gene revelation.

Another difficulty in explaining the causation of depression by the deficiency of mono-amines was that even though Specific Serotonin Reuptake Inhibitors could cause an immediate reuptake inhibition, antidepressant effects did not appear for 2-4 weeks. In other words the deficiency state of serotonin could be corrected immediately and yet antidepressant effect would not follow for several weeks. It was suggested that 2-4 weeks was the time taken for desensitization, down regulation of receptors and some neuroplastic changes at the receptor level which are responsible for the antidepressant effect of these drugs (Duman, Malberg & Thome, 1999).

Serotonergic Receptor Physiology in Depression

Three classes and fourteen receptors sub-types have been described for serotonin. Sub-types 1A, 2A and 2C in the prefrontal cortex are associated with depression. (Graeff, 1997: Stahl, 1998).

Serotonergic receptors are located in the raphe nuclei off the mid-brain, pons and medulla. Axons ascend from these sites to the cerebral cortex, basal ganglia, limbic cortex/hippocampus and hypothalamus. Furthermore axons from the raphe nuclei descend to the medulla and spinal cord. Immediately after an SSRI is introduced serotonin transporters are blocked at the dendrites and axon of the serotonergic neurons. With the continued rise of serotonin level in the somato-dendritic area a down regulation of 5-HT1A auto-receptors takes place. A loss of regulation of impulse flow in the neuron follows and serotonin is released from the pre-synaptic axon terminal resulting in the rise of concentration of serotonin at the postsynaptic cleft.

It is noteworthy that with the administration of SSRIs, serotonin concentration rises in all sites where serotonergic receptors are found. Because these receptors are widely distributed throughout the human body, side-effects involving gastrointestinal system, central nervous system and sexual dysfunction are frequently reported. Increased serotonin availability at the 5 HT3 receptors in the brain stem vomiting centre (emetic centre) is thought to cause the gastrointestinal side effects and stimulation of 5HT1 receptors in the vascular system may be associated with headache and migraine. (Harvey, 1997).

Nor-Adrenaline

Nor-adrenergic receptors are concentrated in the locus ceruleus. From this site axons ascend to the prefrontal cortex, cerebellum, thalamus/hypothalamus, limbic system and spinal cord. Of these pathways the one projecting from locus ceruleus to prefrontal cortex is thought to be the most important pathway associated with depression. Nor-adrenergic neurons in the limbic region are responsible for the regulation of mood, emotions, energy and motivation. Alpha 2 and beta 1 subtypes of adrenergic receptors, especially those found in the cortices, are commonly linked with depression. The density of Beta adrenoceptors on the lymphocytes of patients with depression as well as those of the frontal cortex of suicide victims have been reported to be less (Leonard, 1997). This observation has also formed the basis of down regulation of beta-receptor as a marker of antidepressant efficacy (Leonard, 1997).

Inter Relationship between Different Neuro Transmitters

Despite several claims, no one neurotransmitter has been identified as the main or only chemical responsible for causing depression. Some authors have therefore looked at how different neuro-transmitetrs affect mood and other functions associated with depressed affect (Stahl, 1998). There is some evidence to indicate that while all 3 neurotransmitters (dopamine, norepinephrine, and serotonin) affect mood, and that both norepinephrine and serotonin may affect anxiety. Stahl (1998) suggested that dopamine may preferentially regulate motivation, pleasure, and reward, serotonin preferentially regulates impulsivity, sex, appetite, aggression, obsessions and compulsions. Norepinephrine may preferentially regulate vigilance, motivation, alertness and energy. Serotonin and norepinephrine together may influence depression, anxiety, pain, irritability, and cognitive function. This conceptualisation has lead to adopting a "broad spectrum" approach (ie, attacking from both the serotonergic and noradrenergic approach) in the treatment of depression, especially in resistant cases

(Leuchter & Jain, 2002) Therefore, modern psycho-pharmacologists are taking increasing interest in multi receptor activity and the manner in which different receptors interact with each other. For instance dopamine and nor-adrenaline are affected when the frontal cortex nor-adrenaline transporters are blocked by any drug that has this property. Either selectively (antidepressants such reboxetine and desipramine) or non selectively (venlafaxine, duloxetine and tricyclic antidepressants). As a direct corollary we see that these drugs enhance the action of dopamine and nor-adrenaline but only in the frontal cortex. These actions are also associated with improved cognitive functioning (Stahl, 2003). It has been suggested that because very few dopamine transporters are present in the frontal cortex, dopamine is inactivated by nor-adrenaline transporters but not by dopamine transporters in these regions. It is therefore possible to enhance dopamine in frontal cortex by inhibiting nor-adrenaline reuptake. Selective nor-adrenaline reuptake inhibitors are able to increase both dopamine and nor-adrenaline in the frontal cortex without increasing dopamine in sub cortical areas.

Substance P

Substance P (SP) is an 11 amino acid residue molecule and belongs to the group of neuropeptide known as neurokinins (NK). SP and NK receptors are localized in regions of brain involved in the control of depression, anxiety and stress response namely the amygdala, hypothalamus, hippocampus, frontal cortex, raphe ncuclei and locus ceruleus (Saria, 1999). SP affects mood and emesis due to action in the brain and controls nosiception by acting at the spinal cord level. The neuro chemical effects of SP are caused by its binding to and activating of the NK1 receptors. This is the most widely and extensively investigated neurochemical pathway in the brain. Inhibition of SP-NK1 pathway maybe a useful approach to the treatment of depression and associated anxiety (Manthy, 2002).

It has been suggested that pharmacologic or genetic inactivation of NK1 receptors is effective in the regulation of mood and therefore has a potential role in the treatment of depression. Some initial findings of SP-NK1 receptor antagonists (SPA) have been reported in the treatment of refractory depression (Krishnan, 2002). Two important agents in this regard are Aprepitant (a high affinity and selectivity for the human NK1 receptor with no pharmacologic activity against receptors for other neurotransmitters implicated in depression such as nor-epinephrine, serotonin and dopamine) and compound A (high oral bio-availability and brain penetration as well as by high selectivity and affinity for the NK1 receptor) (Krishnan, 2002).

Intra-Cellular Models

The intracellular signal transduction pathways may prove to be the final pathway for antidepressant activity. Two broad classes of such pathways have been described: second messenger system (cAMP, cGMP, inositol phosphate, Ca^{2+} and nitric oxide) and neurotrophin and cytokine receptors acting through a series of tyrosine kinases (Henn, 2001). Chronic antidepressant usage has been shown to cause changes in the expression of subcellular components of the signaling pathways. The stimulation of the adrenoceptor subtypes alpha 2, beta 1 and beta 2 receptors may result in cyclic adenosine monophosphate mediated intracellular protein phosphorylation. This in turn activates transcription factors which modulate gene expression. Alpha 2 adrenoceptors are also found on serotonin terminals and are believed to regulate serotonin release at pre-synaptic terminals (Mongeau, Blier & De-montigny, 1997). This presence has been offered as an explanation for the influence of expression of serotonin receptors as well as the functioning of the serotonergic system by noradrenalin network. Furthermore, adrenergic and serotonergic receptors share common second messenger pathways through conversions at the level of GTP binding proteins or effector molecules (Manji, 1992; Racagni & Brunello, 1999). With regard to neurotrophin and cytokine receptor pathway a neurotrophin termed brain derived neurotrophic factor (BDNF) may play an antidepressant role. This view is based on the finding that all types of antidepressants and ECT cause an upregulation of the expression of BDNF. Furthermore, BDNF are reported to play a significant role in neural plasticity of fully developed brain as well as in spouting of serotonergic and nor adrenergic neurons. Henn (2001) has suggested that changes in neurotrophin levels can lead to subtle structural and functional changes in multiple transmitter neurons which alter the feelings of hopelessness and ultimately depression.

EEG

Sleep disturbance is a very common feature of depression and has ignited interest in poylsomnographic research. Clinically, early morning wakening, sleep interruption, shortened & intermittent sleep, which is not restful or refreshing, are frequently reported. These problems are associated with reduction in the total amount of slow wave and a shortened REM latency to 40 minutes as opposed to normal 90 minutes (Kupfer and Foster, 1978). REM preponderance during the latter half of sleep and reduction in time spent in slow wave, as well as in slow wave density have also been reported. In a recent review Sarbadhikari and Chakrabarty (2001) have suggested that clinical remission in patients with depression is often reflected in the reorganisation of electrophysiological changes in brain.

Functional Neuroimaging Studies

Functional neuroimaging methods such as functional magnetic resonance imaging (fMRI) and positron emission tomography (PET) have been used to correlate the clinical features of depression, the neurofunctional changes in the brains of people with depression and their underlying brain circuitry. Two major brain areas have been implicated in major depression – the prefrontal cortex/anterior cingulated and the hippocampus. It has been well known that patients with depression often show neuropsychological deficits in executive functions such as lack of concentration, attention deficits, mood-congruent memory biases and lack of motivation. Other symptoms such as a pervasive lack of positive affect, negative mood states, anxiety symptoms affect cognitive functions indirectly, for example through memory functions. Neuroimaging studies have shown abnormalities in regions of the medial and the lateral prefrontal cortex, the limbic system and basal ganglia and most importantly the medial prefrontal cortex (especially the dorsal and ventral part of the anterior cingulate and the medial orbitofrontal cortex). Neuroimaging studies have shown neuromodulatory influences on these regions are mediated by dopaminergic and serotonergic neuronal inputs both widely exploited in the treatment of depression (Erk et al 2002). It has been recently suggested by Schatzberg (2002) that a smaller hippocampus could be associated with a higher glucocorticoid levels during stressful times leading to cognitive disturbance outlined above whereas an excess of glucocorticoid could cause atrophy of specific brain regions. This finding has regenerated interest in the glucocorticoids in the aetiology of depression even though they have been known to play a significant role for several decades.

Cortisol and Glucocorticoid Receptors

Hypothalamic Pituitary Adrenal (HPA) axis has been long implicated in the aetio-pathogenesis of depression based on findings such as increased level of cortisol in plasma, urine and cerebrospinal fluid, exaggerated cortisol responses to ACTH and enlarged pituitary and adrenal glands. (Owens & Nemeroff, 1993). A recent review has highlighted the role of two specialised Gluocorticoid Receptors: the high affinity type I receptor (MR) and the low affinity type II receptor (GR) because cortisol, the final product of the HPA axis acts on these receptors. (McQuade & Young, 2000). The number of GR is thought to be modulated by tricyclic antidepressants by an increase in GR mRNA (Pepin et al, 1989), which may indeed result in an increase in receptor protein – an effect not shown by SSRI's (McQuade & Young, 2000). These findings have prompted interest in five types of future therapeutic targets for depression that can modulate the effects of hypercortisolaemia and/or the mechanism underlying it (McQuade & Young, 2000). Dehydroepiandrosterone (with antiglucocorticoid properties) Steroid Synthesis inhibitors (to lower the raised levels of cortisol) corticotrophin – release hormone antagonist (to counteract the over secretion of CRH in mood disorders), Type II CR agonist (by activating the GR mediated negative feedback mechanism that regulated cortisol levels) Type II GR antagonists (by blocking a detrimental effects of the raised levels of circulating cortisol and their ability to up regulate Type II GR). These opportunities are still in an early phase and more research is needed before their wide use can be advocated.

TREATMENT: PHILOSOPHY, GOALS AND OPTIONS

Biological Treatment of Depression

Pharmacological: Antidepressants

Antidepressants appear to be more widely investigated than other methods of treatment for depression. Due to a possible lack of commercial interest psychotherapies have not been rigorously evaluated over the past fifty years, a period that has seen a sharp rise in a collective effort to find newer and better antidepressants. It is however also true that psychological methods of treating depression have improved significantly during this period. Research therapists tend to follow manuals and are generally better trained in their respective schools of psychotherapy. It is not always possible to achieve the purist approach of academic researchers investigating psychotherapies in clinical setting where clinicians tend to be more eclectic in their approaches. This may be a possible factor why we don't see the same efficacy of psychotherapy in clinical settings as described in the literature. Furthermore, in comparison to psychotherapy, it is easier to be trained in the use of antidepressants for doctors and therefore doctors have tended to use antidepressants widely in the treatment of depression.

The monoamine oxidase inhibitors (MAOIs) were the first group of anti depressants to be introduced on the market in the 1950s. The tricyclic antidepressants (TCAs) were introduced in the 1960s. The selective serotonin reuptake inhibitors (SSRIs) (fluoxetine, sertraline, paroxetine, fluvoxamine, citalopram, escitalopram) have been introduced since the 1980s. Research interest was diverted in the last decade to finding other pure re-uptake inhibitors or anti-depressants that worked on more than one site. Examples of the latter grpup include nefazodone, mirtazapine, venlafaxine and more recently duloxetine (a serotonin-norepinephrine reuptake inhibitor)

Tricyclic Antidepressants (TCAs)

TCA's have proven to be very efficacious in the treatment of depression for 30 years but their widespread usage has fallen because of multiple side effects as well as lethality in cases of overdose. There is some evidence to suggest that tricyclics are more efficacious in the treatment of severe depression. This differential effect could be due to the effects of TCAs on the nor-adrenergic system which appears to be the predominant pathway in severe depression. In a study of depressed patients with melancholia (Paroxetine 1990) treated with either clomipramine (a TCA with "dual" action) or with paroxetine (an SSRI that is mostly serotonergic), both agents were effective over a 6-week period. Interestingly, patients on paroxetine were still fairly symptomatic with an average score of 14 on the HAM-D. On the other hand, patients treated with clomipramine had an average score of 8, which is closer to achieving full remission. Therefore it is possible that drugs such as clomipramine, amitriptyline and possibly imipramine by virtue of being dual reuptake inhibitors (acting on serotonin and nor-adrenergic system) may be more effective than mono system specific reuptake inhibitors (desipramine, nortriptyline and tetracyclic maprotiline). (Thase, 2003).

MAOIs

These have been used as antidepressants for over 40 years and have strong efficacy but are limited in usage because of safety and tolerability concerns. They play an important role in treatment resistant or severe depression. (Thase, 2003) and may be making a comeback.

SSRIs

These antidepressants have become popular in the last decade and because they work on serotonergic system only, their side effect profile is much better. They are not as lethal as tricyclics or MAO inhibitors in cases of overdose.

Multi-Action Agents

Medication such as venlafaxine and mirtazapine act directly on serotonin and noradrenalin systems and are better tolerated that tricylics. Most of the evidence on the comparative benefit of multi-action agents gives promising results by having greater abilities to achieve remission but report on acute phase treatment only. Mirtazapine, even though not a reuptake inhibitor and has a different mechanism of action, compares favorably with venlafaxine (Guelfi et al 2001).

In a meta-analyses of trials comparing venlafaxine with SSRIs and placebos in depressed patients, venlafaxine emerged to be not only better than SSRIs and placebo but produced improvement in 2 weeks as opposed to 4 weeks for the SSRI group (Thase et al 2001). The review reported a remission rate of 45% for venlafaxine; 35% for SSRIs, and 25% for placebo. A recent study (Detke et al 2002) compared duloxetine vs placebo and 20 mg paroxetine. It reported duloxetine at 40 mg had a 35% remission rate compared with a 30% remission rate with placebo and 37% with paroxetine. However, when the dosage was increased to 80 mg, duloxetine had a 50% remission rate. Information on the safety profile of these drugs in long term use is still limited.

Mechanism of Action of Antidepressants

An increase in the firing rate of serotonergic receptors as well as an increase in serotonin concentration, mostly in the intra-synaptic region, have been put forward as the main mechanisms of action of several antidepressants. Furthermore, Tri-Cyclic antidepressants (TCAs), Selective Serotonin Reuptake Inhibitor (SSRI) and Mono Amine Oxidase Inhibitor (MAOI) appear to share a delay in onset of action or 2-4 weeks.

SSRI

These antidepressants include a structurally diverse group of compounds which have a common property of selectively blocking the reuptake of serotonin (5HT). It is worth noting that they do not block dopamine or nor-adrenaline. They also have some other but less potent pharmacologic action. Despite the fact that SSRIs reach the brain within minutes or hours of administration and the effects on serotonin reuptake can be measured immediately, their therapeutic effect is delayed by 2-4 weeks.

In order to explain the lag in onset of antidepressant effects, the neurobiological changes seen at the 5 HTsynapse level need to be examined. Serotonin reuptake inhibition in the hippocampal region causes over activation of inhibitory 5-HT1A auto receptors resulting in the reduction of the generation of action potential in these nerve terminals. As a result, serotonin release in postsynaptic terminal areas is reduced. Continuous SSRI exposure leads to elevated serotonin concentrations in the cell body area, 5-HT1A auto receptors become desensitized and the firing of serotonin neurons is normalized. 5HT1B auto receptors (which control the amount of serotonin by electrical impulse) also become desensitized after 2-3 weeks of SSRI administration. This desensitization occurs in the presence of reuptake blockade in terminal areas so serotonin neuro transmission is enhanced (Blier, 2001). The enhanced serotonergic transmission leads to receptor down regulation which is the proposed final pathway for anti-depressant activity.

Multi-Action Agents

Post hoc analysis of antidepressant activity has suggested that multi-action agents (drugs that work on more than one receptor site such as mirtazapine and venlafaxine) have an early onset of action compared to other antidepressants such as SSRIs. It is possible that this phenomenon could be due to early restoration of sleep and a reduction in anxiety rather than a specific early antidepressant effect (Nieremberg, 2001). Mirtazapine is not an inhibitor of serotonin reuptake but it blocks the alpha 2 adrenoceptor on the cell bodies on noradrenergic and serotonergic nerve terminals in the fore brain. To be more specific, it blocks the inhibitory alpha 2 adrenoceptor on serotonin terminals in the locus ceruleus and on noradrenergic terminals in the raphe nuclei throughout the brain (Nieremberg, 2001). However, the only head to head comparison of mirtazapine and venlafaxine indicated that there was no significant difference in the time of onset of action (Guelfi, 1999).

Choice of Antidepressants

More than 20 antidepressants are available worldwide. They are broadly classified as

1. Early antidepressants:
    a. Mono Amine Oxidase Inhibitor (MAOI) Phenelzine, Isocarboxazid, Tranylcypromine and Selegiline
    b. Tri Cyclic Antidepressants – Tertiary Amines (Amitryptiline, Doxepin,

Imipramine and Trimipramine) Secondary Amines (Desipramine, Nortryptiline Protryptiline)
   c. Tetra Cyclic Antidepressants (Amoxapine, Maprotiline)
2. Newer antidepressants:
   a. Selective Serotonin Reuptake Inhibitor (SSRI) Fluoxetine, Paroxetine, Sertraline, Citalopram, Escitalopram
   b. Receptor blockers e.g. Mianserin and Trazodone
   c. Selective Nor Adrenergic Inhibitors (SNRI) e.g. Reboxetine
   d. Multi site agents: Venlafaxine, Duloxetine

Given the plethora of choice psychiatrists tend to chose antidepressants on the basis of past response, medication interaction, short and long-term side effects, patient preference, likelihood of adherence, co-morbidity and costs. Goals of treating depression are not only to relieve the symptoms of depression and reduce the risk of relapse but to also restore normal social functioning and minimise the adverse affects associated with antidepressant therapy.

Most studies have found that the older TCAs and the relatively new SSRIs are at their best comparable. There is no data to suggest that one drug is more efficacious than another. Efficacy of SSRIs is well documented but they have distinct adverse event profile including gatro-intestinal events, sexual dysfunction, headaches and anxiety, which may lead to non-compliance. Some authors have suggested that SSRIs tend to lose efficacy following long-term treatment (Harvey, 1997). The relatively short acting antidepressants including paroxetine and citalopram have been associated with a "discontinuation syndrome" characterised by anxiety, irritability, sleep problems, nausea, vomiting, diarrhoea, vertigo, light headedness.

There is emerging evidence that noradenergic antidepressants (Venlaflaxine, Mirtazapine and Milnacipran) may be more effective than SSRI in treating severe depression because it is important to correct nor-adrenaline deficiency in chronic and severe depression cases (Montgomery, 1997). Reboxetine is the first selective Nor Adrenergic Reuptake Inhibitor (SNRI) that selectively inhibits NA re-uptake. It acts differently to the nor-adrenergic TCAs (e.g. desipramine) which predominantly inhibit the noradrenergic re-uptake transporter and also have a considerable affinity for other receptors. Reboxetine has negligible invitro affinity for serotonin and dopamine uptake sites and for adrenergic, histaminergic receptors and only weak affinity for muscarinic receptors. (Riva et al, 1989). Side effects associated with reboxetine include tremor, tachycardia and urinary hesitancy which are expected on the basis of its neurotransmitter activity (Riva et al, 1989). It has recently been reported that reboxetine may be associated with better outcome and social functioning than fluoxetine (Dubini et al, 1997).

Social functioning with antidepressant therapy is receiving attention. One study comparing Fluoxetine with Clomipramine and Amitriptyline reported that though the symptoms responded similarly in the three groups, both TCA's were significantly more effective than Fluoxetine in improving the general health perception and social functioning of patients. Recent studies indicate Reboxetine treatment improves social functioning while still maintaining effective symptom relief but it is unclear whether the improved response with reboxetine is due to better treatment adherence or specific effect on social functioning. It is worth highlighting in this regard that while a greater improvement in social functioning with reboxetine is being flagged as an evidence that it is a better class of antidepressant, it is not clear at this stage whether improvement in social functioning is due to some specific neurochemical effect on social functioning by antidepressants or a reflection of a general overall improvement in depression or indeed whether either serotonin or noradrenaline have a dominant effect in the area of social functioning.

Side Effects of Antidepressants

Common side effects of SSRIs include gastrointestinal effects, sexual dysfunction (mainly decreased libido and delayed ejaculation), insomnia, or sedation. TCAs have become unpopular due to their broad range of side effects including sedation, weight gain, postural hypotension, anticholnergic side effects such as blurred vision, dry mouth, urinary retention, impotence and cardiac side effects such as tachycardia, palpitations, arrhythmia etc. They may be lethal in overdose largely due to their cardio-toxic side effects. Mirtazapine, causes sedation and weight gain. Hypoamnic switch (hypomanic or manic episodes precipitated by antidepressants) is a particularly significant side effect of all antidepressants and is more likely to happen in patients with bipolar affective disorder (especially bipolar II) and rapid cycling mood disorders. The newer antidepressant medications appear to be associated with less medication-induced switching to a manic episode when compared with the TCA and MAOI agents. Bupropion has a lower rate of switching to mania but is significant for having anxiogenic effects, causing insomnia, and is contraindicated in patients with a seizure or eating disorder. Venlafaxine may be more likely to cause hypoamnic switch, has many of the side effects of the SSRIs and has hypertensive effects especially in higher dosage. Finally , newer antidepressants appear to be safer in terms of overdose lethality than the TCA or MAOI antidepressants.

Length of Treatment with Antidepressants

Current evidence does not support the notion that once patients have recovered from an acute depressive episode the dose of antidepressant medication can be reduced. Frank et al (1993) reported that halving the dose of Imipramine significantly increased the risk of relapse. Similarly it is also recognized that either withdrawing or tapering maintenance therapy too soon may worsen the outcome of depressive disorder. Patients should continue on the same dose of antidepressants for two cycles of recurrent depressive disorder. This period may span over 4-6 years. A small but very well designed double-blind study investigated the risk of recurrence after three and a half years of treatment with Imipramine. Patients were randomly assigned to continue for a further two years of full dose maintenance therapy or to switch to placebo. Only 5% of patients in the Imipramine group experienced recurrence compared to 70% in the placebo group. It would appear that even three and a half years of antidepressant therapy was inadequate to prevent a subsequent recurrence in these patients after the withdrawal of maintenance therapy.

The above view is countered by another school which believes long-term treatment with antidepressant drugs may worsen the course of depression in certain patients (Fava, 2003). The long-term use of antidepressant drugs may increase a biochemical vulnerability to depression and worsen the long-term outcome and symptomatic expression of the illness. This may decrease both the likelihood of subsequent responses to pharmacologic treatment and the duration of symptom-free periods. This observation has evolved because despite our improved ability to detect and treat depression the long-term outcome of the condition has not markedly changed. This paradoxical effect could be explained by patients receiving inadequate treatment in general practice, patients not complying with treatment or medical co morbidity worsening the outcome. (Fava et al, 2001: Schneider et al, 2000 & Michoulon et al, 2001). Tolerance to antidepressant drugs, resistance to antidepressant drugs and switching to sub-clinical bipolar conditions have been put forward as likely explanation for this trend (Fava 2003).

Non Pharmacological Methods of Treating Depression

Electroconvulsive Therapy (ECT)

ECT has remained the gold standard of treatment efficacy for severe or refractory depression particularly if it is associated with life threatening situations, suicide risk or refusal to eat or drink. While it may be extremely effective in the acute treatment, the risk of relapse is quite high following ECT if medication is not started. The mechanism of action of ECT is not properly understood. Essentially the electrical stimulus used in ECT is powerful enough to induce seizures to a point that activation of the whole brain takes place. A single ECT session produces some highly characteristic changes in the electrical activity in the brain such as initial spike and slow wave discharges, followed by slow waves, and finally flattened EEG. Repeated ECT results in an increasing number of slow waves in the EEG that may last for a month or longer in some cases. The clinical benefit from ECT may be attributed to changes in various neurotransmitter systems. Post synaptic 5-HT1A receptors are sensitized by repeated ECT, but auto-receptors situated in the pre-synaptic neurons are not changed. Similarly ECT may also increase sensitivity to 5-HT of 5-HT3 receptors in the hippocampus, resulting in an increase in the release of neurotransmitters such as glutamate and gamma-aminobutyric acid. Working on other neurotransmitters ECT decreases the auto-receptor functions in noradrenergic and dopaminergic neurons in the locus coeruleus and substantia nigra respectively. This results in an increase in the release of noradrenaline and dopamine. It has been suggested that 5-HT1A-receptor sensitization may be important for explaining the effectiveness of ECT by inducing a decrease in the number of 5-HT2A receptors that are usually elevated in depressive patients. Furthermore 5-HT3-receptor sensitization by ECT may facilitate multiple neurotransmitter release which could play an important role in the treatment of treatment refractory depression (Ishihara and Sasa 1999).

Repetitive Transcranial Magnetic Stimulation

Repetitive transcranial magnetic stimulation (rTMS) is a non-invasive method that has been introduced as a treatment alternative for depression in the last decade. Very strong, pulsed magnetic fields are delivered to the cortices of the patient through a hand held coil sitting on the head. The magnetic pulse induces an electric current in the underlying tissue, capable of depolarizing neurons. A recent systematic review (Martin et al, 2003) (search date 2002, 14 trials) reported that the quality of studies comparing rTMS with *sham* in patients with depression was low. While there was some effect in favour of rTMS after 2 weeks of treatment, the improvement was not significant at the end of 2 weeks follow up. The review concluded that current trials of rTMS were of low quality and provided insufficient evidence to favour rTMS in the treatment of depression.

Vagus Nerve Stimulation

An electronic device called the Neurocybornetic Prosthesis (NCP®) system, originally developed for the treatment of refractory epilepsy has been tried in the treatment of refractory depression. The prosthesis offers electrical stimulation of the left vagus nerve and works very similar to an implanted cardiac pacemaker (Matthews & Elijamel, 2003). A bipolar electrode placed on the left vagus nerve and connected subcutaneously to a pulse generator on the anterior left chest wall stimulates the vagus nerve (DeGiorgio, et al 2001). The initial experience with vagal nerve stimulation in the treatment of depression appears encouraging but this is entirely based on open studies and data on long term efficacy is awaited. VNS may play a significant role in the treatment of less chronic and/or refractory patient population where ECT/drug treatment have failed or is contraindicated.

Phototherapy

Phototherapy is another noninvasive treatment that has been particularly used for patient in the last two decades with a seasonal pattern to their mood disorder. It can be used alone or in conjunction with medication. This method generally involves patients sitting for one or two hours once or twice daily with their eyes open in front of a lamp emanating bright white light (2,500 – 10,000 lux) but not ultra violet rays. The success rate of phototherapy is highly variable and may range from 30-70% but it does tend to have a much quicker onset of action then antidepressants. The efficacy of phototherapy for prophylactic purposes is not known (Vanderholzer & Berger, 2001).

Non Biological Methods of Treating Depression

Psychotherapy

Multiple randomized control trials have shown comparative response rates between psychotherapies and antidepressant medications. Cognitive, behavioural and interpersonal therapy have been subjected to well designed randomized control trials and therefore majority of evidence available in literature is based on these relatively newer methods of treatment.

Combining Antidepressants with Psychotherapy

There is a widely held view that adding antidepressants to psychotherapies tends to improve the outcome of depression. There is however limited evidence to support this. A recent systematic review of 27 studies (N=667) of five RCT's and 22 open label trials reported an overall mean response rate of 62.2% for combination strategies which is comparable to the response rate with different antidepressants. The review concluded that there was limited evidence, mostly in uncontrolled studies, that supported the efficacy of combining antidepressant treatment with psychotherapy, in the management of treatment resistant depression (Lam et al, 2002).

Special Challenges in the Treatment of Depression

The treatment of depression is always fraught with difficulties. Even seemingly simple cases can be complicated by factors such as non compliance, co-morbid psychiatric disorders, personality disorders, drug abuse and physical problems- which all lead to poorer outcomes. There are a number of situations where the treatment of depression may be more complex than others:

Psychotic Depression

Current consensus guidelines support the concurrent usage of antipsychotic and antidepressants rather than the previous approach of using antidepressants alone in the belief that with the alleviation of depression nihilistic delusions and hallucinations improve. An equivalent of 400 mg of chlorpromazine for antipsychotics is recommended. Atypicals should be preferred given the increased risk of tardive dyskinesia in the presence of affective symptoms.

Atypical Depression is a term often used to describe depression with atypical or reverse biological features such as over sleeping (instead of insomnia) over eating (instead of lack of appetite), carbohydrate craving, leaden paralysis or severe form of fatigue (instead of psychomotor agitation), rejection sensitivity and a reactive mood. Most authorities recommend use of a MAO inhibitor but SSRI and bupropion have also been tried with varied success.

Treatment Resistant Depression

Treatment resistant depression (TRD) is commonly defined as depression where two adequate trials (an appropriate dosage used for an adequate length of time usually eight weeks) of different antidepressants have failed. TRD is a significant problem in clinical practice because only 60-70% patients will respond to antidepressants. The remaining patients may be left with a non-responsive depression or significant residual depressive symptoms. Before making a diagnosis of TRD it is important to confirm adherence to treatment because up to two third patients may not take the medication as prescribed. Comorbid psychiatric disorders (e.g. anxiety disorders, OCD, eating disorders and somatisation disorders); comorbid substance abuse and personality disorder are associated with the risk of TRD. Other risk factors for TRD include diagnosis of dysthymia, old age, female sex, low family income and dysfunctional interpersonal relationship. A recent review has recommended the following augmentation strategies for the treatment of TRD (Shelton, 2003)

Lithium

A vast majority of studies on treatment of resistant depression have evaluated lithium as an augmentation agent and these have been favourable.

Thyroid Hormone

TCAs augmented with thyroid hormones have been evaluated and have shown consistent improvement in resistant cases. Studies on thyroid augmentation with SSRI's of MAO inhibitors are lacking.

Antipsychotics

Conventional and atypical antipsychotics have been evaluated as augmentation agents. There is some evidence to suggest that risperidone and olanzapine when combined with an SSRI's such as paroxetine or fluoxetine may be effective. It is worth noting that the risk of tardive dyskinesia will increase in cases of psychotic depression if patients are receiving concomitant antipsychotics.

Cognitive Therapy

When used as an adjunct to antidepressant medication CBT significantly improves the outcome in TRD.

Other strategies such as adding pindolol or psycho stimulants such as dextroamphetamine or methyl-phenidate have been suggested but their effectiveness remain controversial.

Course and Prognosis

Depression is often a chronic and recurring disorder and modern pharmacotherapy appears to have made little impact on its course and prognosis. An excellent naturalistic study of the course of depression was undertaken as part of the National Institute of Mental Health Collaborative Programme on the psychobiology of depression (Lavori et al 1994). The study reported that many patients become depressed again despite adequate long-term pharmacotherapy and the advantages of maintenance antidepressants may diminish after six months of wellness. Furthermore, patients who develop a recurrence after the second depressive episode are at risk of developing more episodes. The risk of recurrence in one year is estimated at 33% rising to 50% in five years and 70% in a lifetime (Thase, 1992). One may also have to consider that depressive relapse and recurrence rates may be substantially higher in clinical than research population. This issue becomes more important if one considers the fact that psychosocial impairment may continue even after a full recovery from a depressive episode for up to a period of five years (Coryell, et al, 1993). Similarly the risk of suicide may remain increased compared with the rest of the population for at least three years following an acute depressive episode.

Several studies have attempted to identify risk factors for recurrence of depressive disorder and most of them have reported that the risk of future depression increases with recurrence. Having two prior depressive episodes is reported to convey an 80% risk of recurrence, and the risk rises rapidly to 90% with three episodes. Other risk factors associated with chronicity include age of onset, either before the age of 21 or after the age 60, female gender and a seasonal pattern (between 10-20% of patients with recurrent depression may have a seasonal pattern) (Ternan, *et al* 1988). Certain personality types (e.g. those with a tendency to neuroticism) may be more prone to depression), a poor level of social support, no self-esteem and self-confidence have also been reported to be associated with an increased risk of relapse (Lara et al, 1997, Dew et al 1997).

In most cases the length of individual episode range from 3- 13 months and tend to be longer in the elderly (Kronmuller & Mundt 2001). If one compares the average duration of depressive episodes today with that described by Kraepelin (1913), nearly a century ago, which was 6-8 months one could conclude that modern pharmacotherapy has not lead to a significant reduction in the suffering of patients affected. Similarly, while 70-92% may recover from a first episode 63-76% of patients relapse in 10-20 years. Relapses tend to be more frequent in bipolar affective disorder.

More recently, patients appear to be experiencing depression at a younger age. Median age of onset for depression was described as 30-40 years in earlier studies but now days this is often quoted as 20-30 years. Unlike schizophrenia, where age of onset in women appears to be later (Hafner et al, 1989), the age of onset does not differ between genders. A bimodal peak in the incidence of depression was seen in the Economic Catchment Area study which noted a second small peak in the age group of 50-60. It is commonly known that with increasing age, the interval between depressive episodes decreases.

DEPRESSION IN SPECIFIC POPULATIONS

Depression and Women

A number of studies across the world have reported a much higher prevalence of depressive disorders within women when compared to men. This ration may vary from 1.6 (Lebanon, Taiwan) to 3.1 (West Germany). (Weissman et al, 1996). Possible explanations include women tend to seek help more often than men, biological differences between men and women in brain structures or reproductive functions or differences in coping mechanisms. Furthermore depressive symptoms in women commonly occurs in relation to changes in the reproductive system such as the premenstrual period, pregnancy, the post-partum period and the peri-menopause. (Kornstein, 2001).

Women tend to present with reverse vegetative symptoms such as an increased appetite, weight gain, hyper somnolence, reverse diurnal variation (mood being worse in the evenings), predominantly irritable mood. Furthermore women are more likely to report anger, somatisation, anxiety and psychomotor retardation as well as greater functional impairment in family and marital roles. (Kornstein, 2001). Similarly, women tend to have a chronic and recurrent depressive illness compared to men. Their episodes tend to be longer and more frequent than men. Women also tend to experience more co-morbid anxiety disorder, eating disorder and other psychiatric disorder than men. Depressed men on the other hand tend to have co-morbid alcohol and substance abuse. (Kornstein, 2001). A recent meta-analysis of gender differences and treatment response to imipramine reported that 62% of men were responders compared with 51% of women, ($P < .001$) (Hamilton et al 1996). Similar findings have been reported by other studies which have found that women tend to have a poorer response to treatment compared to men for depressive conditions although differential response to medication may exist. A recent study from New Zealand has reported that melancholic men forty years or older showed a superior response to nortryptiline whereas melancholic women in the age group 18-24 responded better to fluoxetine (Joyce et al 2003).

Manifestation of Depression Across the Reproductive Cycle

Pre Menstrual Syndrome (PMS)

Criteria for PMS are looser than that of Pre Menstrual Dysphoric Disorder in DSM IV. This is reflected in the reported prevalence of the two conditions- 40% Vs 2-10% respectively. Despite a considerable overlap between the clinical features of PMS or PMDD with depression and clinical response with antidepressants, there is evidence to suggest that the two conditions are widely different. SSRIs have been most extensively tried but their use is only recommended in the luteal phase of the menstrual cycle. Other evidence in this regard include lower dosage of SSRI is used and it produces a quicker onset compared to depression. Furthermore, noradrenergic antidepressants are not effective in the treatment of PMS/PMDD.

Premenstrual mood changes and depressive symptomatology may appear in several ways in relation to the premenstrual period: symptoms may become worse, new symptoms may appear or impulsive episodes, including suicidal attempts, may become more frequent. DSM-IV criteria requires the presence of a minimum of five of the following symptoms with at least one being mood symptom: low mood, irritability, anxiety/tension, mood swings, fatigue, sleep changes, appetite changes, decreased interest, difficulty concentrating, feeling overwhelmed or out of control and, physical symptoms (eg, bloating, breast tenderness, water retention etc). These symptoms must cause functional impairment and for at least prospective two cycles daily changes must occur. Several authors recommend treatment of depressive symptoms throughout the menstrual cycle. Recent studies have evaluated fluoxetine (Freeman, et al 1999, Steiner et al, 1995), clomipramine (Sunblad et al, 1993) and sertraline (Freeman et al 1999, Halbreich et al, 2000) in the treatment of PMDD and have reported a superiority of these drugs over placebo or other drugs. Because most women prefer not to take medication during their symptom free follicular phase, the trend these days is to treat PMDD only during the luteal phase of the cycle.

Pregnancy

Contrary to earlier belief, pregnancy is no longer seen to offer any protective effects against depression. The risk of a major depressive episode maybe five times greater in pregnant women compared to general population (O'Hara et al, 1990). It is often a challenge to diagnose depression during pregnancy because many symptoms of depression such as fatigue, sleep problems, erratic appetite are invariably present during pregnancy. Medical disorders overlap (Anaemia, gestational diabetes, thyroid disturbance) and compound the diagnosis. Cognitive features of depression (anhedonia, guilt, hopelessness and suicidal ideation or intent) if present are strong indicators of clinical depression.

No psychotropic drugs are recommended for use during pregnancy. A decision, however, often has to made weighing the risks of not treating versus treating depression in pregnant mothers. Untreated depression is associated with the risks of poor prenatal care, substance use, suicide, obstetric complications, post-partum depression and a risk of infanticide during the post-partum period. Maternal depression adversely affects the foetus, Pre-term birth, low birth weight, intrauterine growth retardation and lower Apgar scores have been reported in depressed mothers and are attributed to problems with uterine circulation or uterine irritability. Similarly depressed mothers are likely not to take care of themselves and their physical health may suffer due to problems with appetite and self care. Depression during pregnancy is also associated with disruption in family life and may have deleterious effects on development.

Treatment with antidepressants in pregnant mothers maybe associated with three types of risks:

Organ Malformation

There is insufficient evidence to suggest that any of the current antidepressants may cause organ malformation. It is however important to weigh the benefits of antidepressant medication during pregnancy and they should be used as a last resort with close follow up.

Neonatal Toxicity withdrawal syndromes have been described soon after birth because all antidepressants are highly lipid soluble, cross the placental barrier and foetal concentrations drop dramatically after birth. Jitteriness, irritability and seizures have been desribed with antidepressants. Clomipramine withdrawal is known to have caused bowel obstruction and urinary retention. Similarly SSRI may lead to poor neonatal adaptation, respiratory distress, and feeding problems.

Long Term Behavioural Sequala

Again these are not described in detail despite the fact that antidepressants have been around for more than fifty years.

Post-Partum Depression

Post partum depression is a significant problem because it affects 10-20% of women giving birth and 25% may still be depressed on child's first birthday. Diagnosing and treating postpartum depression is vital because it not only affects the mother but has adverse effects on child development. A depressed mother is likely to be unresponsive to a baby's cries, may be withdrawn or over-intrusive, or even hostile to the baby. They are likely to play less with babies. Symptoms and signs of major depressive episode occurring within four weeks of delivery are considered diagnostic of post-partum depression. SSRIs are considered to be the treatment of choice for severe or moderate cases whereas CBT is effective for mild to moderate cases. In severe cases where an early onset of antidepressant action is required ECT is preferred. Even though being highly lipid soluble agents all antidepressants are secreted in small quantities in breast milk and their concentration is negligible in infant serum.

Menopause

Previously it was believed that menopause was associated with a high prevalence of depression in women. It was suggested that as women lost their reproductive ability it affected their sense of identity and self-esteem, resulting into depression. This view has not been supported by prospective studies (Kornstein, 2001). Minor mood symptoms associated with peri-menopause may often respond to estrogen therapy. Once a major depressive episode sets in estrogen alone may not be effective. Limited available data suggests that SSRIs should be considered as the first line treatment for mood disorders in women across the spectrum.

Diagnosing and Treating Depression in the Elderly

The population of elderly is steadily growing globally with improved health conditions and life expectancy. Co-morbid medical conditions such as cerebral vascular accidents, dementia and psycho-social factors such as bereavement and isolation tend to be commoner in the elderly. These circumstances are known predictors of depression. Consequently a second peak in the incidence of depression is seen globally in the elderly population. This problem is so significant that a separate category of late onset depression has been described in the context of the elderly. Compared with patients with early onset depression, patients with late onset depression are less likely to have a family history of depression and are more likely to have cognitive impairment, cerebral atrophy, grey matter changes, medical co-morbidity and higher mortality (NIH, 1992). There may be a considerable overlap between dementia and depression as both have marked similarity in clinical presentations such as lack of energy, loss of interest, sleep disturbance.

Given the frequent reporting of orthostatic hypotension and cerebral vascular accidents, MAOI's and TCA's are not considered to be drug of first choice for depression in the elderly. SSRI's appear to be better tolerated in the elderly. Similarly they are more prone to develop all adverse side effects of MAOI inhibitors and SSRI's. Hyponatraemia, weight loss and balance problems are often reported in the elderly population. Each of these side effects are associated with medication non-compliance and relapse. Starting at a low dose and titrating slowly is essential in the treatment of depression in the elderly.

Depression in Children

Depression in children is being increasingly recognised as a significant problem. Epidemiological studies based on general populations show a point prevalence of 10 to 15 percent for depressive symptoms in children and adolescents (Smucker et al., 1986). The prevalence of syndromal depression is lower than that of symptoms but is still considerable. Among all children between the ages of 9 to 17 years the prevalence of MDD has been estimated at 5 percent (Shaffer et al., 1996). As outlined above, depression is more commonly observed in adolescent girls than adolescent boys (girls: boys=2:1). At a prepubertal stage boys outnumber girls in the prevalence of depression.

It is important to make a distinction between depression presenting as a symptom versus a depressive syndrome in children and adolescent population and to understand that the presentation of depression in children and adolescents is different from adults. For instance often depressed children and adolescents may present with a failure to make expected weight gains, as opposed to actual weight loss, as is the case with adults. Similarly, irritability, aggression and physical complaints (i.e. stomach pains, headaches) may often be presenting features of depression in children and adolescent. Sadness or a depressed mood is uncommon as the presenting complaint in children. Younger children may show a loss of interest in activities they previously enjoyed. Self-criticism, referential thinking, feeling unloved, pessimism, hopelessness and thoughts of suicide may be occasionally present. It is noteworthy that these symptoms may be present in the absence of depression in children.

Major depressive disorder is a serious condition characterized by one or more major depressive episodes and the same diagnostic criteria used in adults are applied to children. In children and adolescents, an episode may last from 7 to 9 months (Birmaher et al., 1996a, 1996b). Full blown depressive episodes have several similar features as adults including indecisiveness, attention and concentration difficulties, lack of energy or motivation; self neglect and disturbed sleep patterns. On the other hand psychotic features in children and adolescent are infrequent, and when they occur, auditory hallucinations are more common than delusions (Ryan et al., 1987; Birmaher et al., 1996a, 1996b). Separation anxiety or social phobic symptoms are commonly associated with depression in depressed children and adolescents (Kolvin et al., 1991; Birmaher et al., 1996a, 1996b).

Intervention

CBT has been tried extensively in this population. The maladaptive thinking style of depression is targeted and negative automatic thoughts are challenged and substituted with positive thoughts in this treatment modality. Similarly by having positive activities and behaviours that are likely to increase reward from their environment, children are likely to enjoy a sense of accomplishment, which in turn is known to have a therapeutic effect. Psycho-education of the family and the child/adolescent is integral to management. Educational needs of the child should not be overlooked and attention should be paid to establishing therapeutic relationship based on mutual trust and respect.

SSRIs rather than tricyclic antidepressants are the drugs of choice for treating depression in this age group. A recent open trial of fluoxetine for inpatient adolescents with major depression reported fluoxetine produced greater reduction in depression scores than imipramine (Strober et al., 1999). Furthermore, fluoxetine was well tolerated. This is a significant finding because side effects for TCAs especially sedation and weight gain may be unacceptable to younger people.

Conclusions

At a time when we have either conquered or controlled most of other illnesses depression is emerging as a significant health problem. There is considerable evidence that depression is growing and it is predicted that it will continue to do so in the near future causing significant mortality and morbidity.

Significant advances have been made in the biology of depression both regarding the etiology and treatment. Genetic, neurochemical, neuro anatomical, neuro humoral and electrophysiological factors have been put forward as aetiological factors. Antidepressants, ECT and Light therapy are the main biological methods of treatment while vagal nerve stimulation (VNS) and transcranial magnetic stimulation (TMS) are being evaluated.

Selective serotonergic reuptake inhibitors offered a significant advance in our understanding of how modern antidepressant medication can be found. Selective noradrenergic reuptake inhibitors have been added as another powerful weapon in the collection of modern psycho pharmacologist. These drugs are thought to be better not only because they may have an earlier onset of action compared to older drugs but also because they may help with social functioning. Treatment of depression may be particularly challenging in cases where refractory depression develops, atypical features of depression are present or in patients with chronic depression. Special consideration needs to be made for treating depression in women at different phases in their reproductive life, in the elderly and in children. It is possible that treating depression aggressively may improve the future course and prognosis.

References

Angst J (1966) Zur Atiologie und Nosologie endogener depressiver Psychosen. *Eine genetische, soziologische und klinische Studie*. Springer, Berlin.

APA (American Psychiatric Association). (2000) *Diagnostic and Statistical Manual of Mental Disorders, Fourth Edition, Tenth Revision.* Washington, DC: American Psychiatric Association;

Birmaher, B., Ryan, N. D., Williamson, D. E., Brent, D. A., & Kaufman, J. (1996). Childhood and adolescent depression: A review of the past 10 years. Part II. *Journal of the American Academy of Child and Adolescent Psychiatry, 35,* 1575–1583.

Birmaher, B., Ryan, N. D., Williamson, D. E., Brent, D. A., Kaufman, J., Dahl, R. E., Perel, J., & Nelson, B. (1996). Childhood and adolescent depression: A review of the past 10 years. Part I. *Journal of the American Academy of Child and Adolescent Psychiatry. 35*: 1427–1439.

Blier, P (2001) Pharmacology of rapid onset antidepressant strategies. *Journal of Clinical Psychiatry: 62(suppl 15):*12-17.

Broadhead, W., Blaxer, D., George, L., et al (1990) Depression, disability days and days lost from work in a prospective epidemiological study. *Journal of the American Medical Association, 264,* 2524-2528

Bunney, WE, Davis, JM. (1965) Norepinephrine in depressive reactions. *Arch Gen Psychiatry. 13:*483-494

Chisholm, D; Diehr, P; Knapp, M; Patrick, D, Treglia, M And Simon G (2003) Depression status, medical comorbidity and resource costs : vidence from an international study of major depression in primary care (LIDO), *British Journal of Psychiatry 183*: 121-131.

Coppen A.(1967) The biochemistry of affective disorders. *Br J Psychiatry 113*:1237-1264

Coryell W, Scheftner W, Keller M, et al.(1993) The enduring psychosocial consequences of mania and depression. *Am J Psychiatry 150*:720-727

Dubini A, Bosc M, Polin V. (1997) Noradrenaline-selective versus serotonin-selective antidepressant therapy: differential effects on social functioning. *J Psychopharmacol. 11*(4 Suppl):S17-23

DeGiorgio, C.M, Amar, A & Apuzzo, M.L.J (2001) *Surgical anatomy, implantation technique, and operative complications in vagus nerve stimulation* (eds SC Schacter & D Schmidt) London, Martin Dunitz.

Delgado PL, Miller HL, Salomon RM, et al.(1993) Monoamines and the mechanism of antidepressant action: affects of catecholamine depletion on mood of patients treated with antidepressants. *Psychopharmacol Bull 29*:389-396

Department of Health (1996) *NHS Executive Report: Burdens of Disease. Leeds*: Department of Health

Detke MJ, Lu Y, Hayes JR, Demitrack MA.(2002) Duloxetine, 60 mg once daily, for major depressive disorder: a randomized double-blind placebo-controlled trial. *J Clin Psychiatry. 63:*308-315.

Dew MA, Reynolds CF, Houck PR et al.(1997) Temporal profiles of the course of depression during treatment. *Arch Gen Psychiatry 54*:1016-1024

Duman RS, Malberg J, Thome J.(1999) Neural plasticity to stress and antidepressant treatment. *Biol Psychiatry 46*:1181-1191

Erk, S., Henrik Walter, H and Spitzer H. (2002) Functional Neuroimaging of Depression. Kaschka (ed): *Perspectives in Affective Disorders. Adv Biol Psychiatry*. Basel, Karger, vol 21, pp 63–69

Fava GA, Mangelli L, Ruini C. (2001) Assessment of psychological distress in the setting of medical disease. *Psychother Psychosom 70*:171-175

Fava, G.A. (2003) Can long-term treatment with antidepressant drugs worsen the cause of depression. *Journal of Clinical Psychiatry; 64*;123-133.

Frank E, Kupfer DJ, Perel JM, et al. (1993) Comparison of full-dose versus half-dose pharmacotherapy in the maintenance treatment of recurrent depression. *J Affect Disord 27*:139-145

Freeman EW, Rickels K, Sondheimer SJ, et al. (1999) Differential response to antidepressants in women with premenstrual syndrome/premenstrual dysphoric disorder: a randomized controlled trial. *Arch Gen Psychiatry 56*:932-939

Goodwin F, Jamison K (1990) Manic depressive illness. Oxford University Press. London.

Graeff FG. (1997) Serotonergic systems. *Psychiatr Clin North Am 20:*723-739.

Greenberg PE, Stiglin LE, Finkelstein SN, et al.(1993) The economic burden of depression in 1990. *J Clin Psychiatry 54*:405-419.

Guelfi JD, Ansseau M, Timmerman L, Korsgaard S. (2001) Mirtazapine versus venlafaxine in hospitalized severely depressed patients with melancholic features. *J Clin Psychopharmacol. 21*:425-431

Guelfi JD. (1999) Efficacy and tolerability of mirtazapine versus venlafaxine in hospitalized severely depressed patients with melancholia. *Int J Neuropsychopharmacol 3 (suppl 1)*:S245-S246

Hafner H, Riecher A, Maurer K, Loffler W, Munk-Jorgensen P, Stromgren E (1989) How does gender influence age at first hospitalisation for schizophrenia? *Psychological Medicine. 19*: 903-918

Halbreich U, Bergeron R, Stout A, et al. (May 17 2000) Intermittent luteal phase dosing of sertraline is effective in premenstrual dysphoric disorder. *In: New Research Abstracts of the 153rd Annual Meeting of the American Psychiatric Association;* Chicago, Ill. Abstract NR506:195

Hamilton JA, Grant M, Jensvold MF. (1996) Sex and treatment of depression: when does it matter? In: Jensvold MF, Halbreich U, Hamilton JA, eds. Psychopharmacology and Women: Sex, Gender, and Hormones. Washington, DC: *American Psychiatric Press*; 241-257

Harvey BH. (1997) The neurobiology and pharmacology of depression. *South Afr Med J 87:*540-552

Henn F (2001) Neurobiology of Affective Disorders. In Contemporary Psychiatry. *Specific Psychiatric Disorders (vol3)*. Eds F Henn, N Sartorius, H Helmchen and H Lauter. Springer Berlin. Pp 268-277.

Ishihara K, and Sasa M (1999) Mechanism underlying the therapeutic effects of electroconvulsive therapy (ECT) on depression. *Jpn J Pharmacol ; 80*:185-9

Jenkins JH, Kleinman A, Good BJ (1990) Cross cultural studies of depression. In Becker J, Kleinman A (eds) *Advances in mood disorders*. Erlbaum, Hillsdale.

Joyce PR, Mulder RT, Luty SE, McKenzie JM and Rae AM (2003) A differential response to nortryptiline and fluoxetine in melancholic depression: the importance of age and gender. *Acta Psychiatrica Scandinavica. 108*:20-23

Johnson J. Weissman MM, Klerman GL. (1992) Service utilization and social morbidity associated with depressive symptoms in the community. *JAMA 267*:1478-1483.

Katon W, Schulberg H. (1992) Epidemiology of depression in primary care. *Gen Hosp Psychiatry 14:*237-247.

Keller MB, Lavori PW, Mueller TI, Endicott J, Coryell W, Hirschfeld RM, Shea T. (1992) Time to recovery, chronicity, and levels of psychopathology in major depression. A 5-year prospective follow-up of 431 subjects. *Arch Gen Psychiatry.. 49*:809-16.

Keller MB, Boland RJ. (1998) Implications of failing to achieve successful long-term maintenance treatment of recurrent uni-polar major depression. *Biol Psychiatry 44*:348-360

Kessler, RC; Berglund, P; Demler, O; Jin, R; Koretz, D; Merikangas, KR; Rush AJ, Walters, EE; Wang, PS, (2003) The Epidemiology of Major Depressive Disorder: Results From the National Comorbidity Survey Replication (NCS-R). *JAMA.;289*:3095-3105.

Kielholz P (1971) *Diagnose und Therapie der Depression fur den Praktiker.* Lehmann, Munich.

Klimek V, Schenck J, Han H, Stockmeier C, Ordway G. (2002) Dopaminergic abnormalities in amygdaloid nuclei in major depression: a postmortem study. *Biol Psychiatry ;52(7)*:740

Kolvin, I., Barrett, M. L., Bhate, S. R., Berney, T. P., Famuyiwa, O. O., Fundudis, T., & Tyrer, S. (1991). The Newcastle Child Depression Project. Diagnosis and classification of depression. *British Journal of Psychiatry. Supplement, 11*, 9–21.

Kornstein, S.G. (2001) The evaluation and management of depression in women across the lifespan. *Journal of Clinical Psychiatry: 62 (suppl 24)*;11-17.

Kraepelin E (1913) Psychiatrie. *Ein Lehrbuch fur Studierende und Arzte, vol3 Klinische Psychiatrie, part 2.* Barth Leipiz.

Krishnan, K.R.R (2002) Clinical experience with substance P receptors (NK1 antagonist) in depression. *Journal of Clinical Psychiatry. 63 (suppl 11)* 25-29.

Kronmuller KT and C Mundt (2001) Depressive episodes. In Contemporary Psychiatry. *Specific Psychiatric Disorders (vol3).* Eds F Henn, N Sartorius, H Helmchen and H Lauter. Springer Berlin. Pp183-207.

Kupfer DJ and Foster FG (1978) EEG sleep and depression. In Williams RL, Karacan I and Frazier SH (eds) *Sleep disorders , diagnosis and treatment.* Wiley, New York, pp 163-204

Lam, R.W., Dante, D.C.W., Cohen, N.L. & Kennedy, S.H. (2002) Combining antidepressants for treatment resistant depression; a review. *Journal of Clinical Psychology; 63*; 686-693.

Lara ME, Leader J, Klein DN. (1997) The association between social support and course of depression: is it confounded with personality? *J Abnorm Psychol 106*:478-482

Lavori, P Keller MB, Scheftner W et al.(1994) Recurrence after recovery in unipolar MDD: an observational follow up study of clinical predictors and somatic treatment as a mediating factor. *Int J Meth Psychiatr Res: 4*:211:229

Leonard BE.(1997) Noradrenaline in basic models of depression. *Eur Neruropsychopharmacol 7* (suppl 1): S11-S16

Leonhard (1957) *The classification of endogenous psychoses. English translation of the 8th German edition of Aufteiling der endogenen psychosen* by R Berman. Irvington, New York (1979)

Lepine JP., Gastpar M., Mendlewicz J., Tylee A. (1997). Depression in the community - The first Pan-European study DEPRES (Depression Research In European Society). *Int. Clin. Psychopharmacol. 12*:19-29.

Leuchter A, Jain R.(October 28-31 2002) Addressing both the emotional and physical symptoms: beyond serotonin, two are better than one in treating depression. *Program and abstracts of the 15th Annual US Psychiatric Congress;* Las Vegas Nevada. Symposium 26-0.

Lyons RA, Lo SV, Littlepage BN (1994) Comparative health status of patients with 11 common illnesses in Wales. *J Epidemiol Community Health. 48*:388-90

McQuade, R & Young A.H (2000) future therapeutic targets in mood disorders: the glucocorticoid receptor. *Br. J. Psychiatry. 177*:390-395.

Manji HK. (1992) G proteins: implications for psychiatry. *Am J Psychiatry 149*:746-760

Manthy, P.W. (2002) Neurobiology of the substance P and the NK1 receptor. *Journal of Clinical Psychiatry, 63* (suppl:6-10)

Martin JL, Barbanoj MJ, Schlaepfer TE, Thompson E, Perez V, Kulisevsky J.(2003) Repetitive transcranial magnetic stimulation for the treatment of depression. Systematic review and meta-analysis. *Br J Psychiatry. 182*:480-91

Matthews, K & Eljamel, M.S (2003) Vagus Nerve Stimulation and refractory depression. Please can you switch me on doctor. *Br J Psychiatry. 183*: 181-183.

Meana M. (1998) The meeting of pain and depression: comorbidity in women. *Can J Psychiatry. 43*:893-899.

Michoulon D, McColl Vuolo R, Howarth S, et al, (2001) Management of major depression in the primary care setting. *Psychother Psychosom 70*:103-107

Miles C(1977) Conditions predisposing to suicide: a review. *J N Mental Disorder. 164*: 231-246

Mongeau R, Blier P, de Montigny C. (1997) The serotonergic and noradrenergic systems of hippocampus: their interactions and the effects of antidepressant treatments. *Brain Res Rev 23:* 145-195

Mueller TI, Keller MB, Leon AC, Solomon DA, Shea MT, Coryell W, Endicott J (1996) Recovery after 5 years of unremitting major depressive disorder. *Arch Gen Psychiatry. 53*:794-9

Murray CJ, Lopez AD. (1996) *The Global Burden of Disease: A Comprehensive Assessment of Mortality and Disability From Diseases, Injuries and Risk Factors in 1990 and Projected to 2020.* Cambridge, Mass: Harvard School of Public health on behalf of the World Health Organisation and the World Bank;

Murray, CJL. The global burden of disease. In: Murray CJL, Lopex AD, (1996) eds. *Global Burden of Disease and Injury Series, vol 1*, Boston, Mass: The Harvard School of Public Health; 201-293

Nieremberg, A.,. (2001) Do some antidepressants work faster than others? *Journal of Clinical Psychiatry. 62 (suppl 15)*; 22-25.

NIH Consensus Development Panel on Depression in Late Life. (1992) Diagnosis and treatment of depression in late life. *JAMA; 268*:1018-1024

O'Hara MW, Zekoski EM, Phllips LH, et al. (1990) Controlled prospective study of postpartum mood disorders: comparison of childbearing and non-childbearing women. *J Abnorm Psychol* 13-15

Owens, M.J. & Nemeroff, C.B. (1993) The Role of CRF in the Pathophysiology of Affective Disorders: *Laboratory and Clinical Studies (vol.172).* New York: John Wiley & Sons.

Paroxetine: a selective serotonin reuptake inhibitor showing better tolerance, but weaker antidepressant effect than clomipramine in a controlled multicenter study. Danish University Antidepressant Group. *J Affect Disord*. 1990;18:289-299.

Pepin, M.C., Beaulieu, S. & Bardern, N. (1989) Antidepressants regulate glucocorticoid receptor messenger RNA concentrations in primary neuronal cultures. Brain Research. *Molecular Brain Research, 6,* 77- 83.

Perris C (1966) A survey of bipolar and unipolar recurrent depressive psychoses. *Acta Psychiatrica Scandinavica. 194 (suppl)* 1-189

Pliszka, SR (2003) *Neuroscience for the mental health clinician.* New York, Guildford Press pp 203.

Racagni G, Brunello N. (1999) Physiology to functionality: the brain and neurotransmitter activity. *Int Clin Psychopharmacol 14 (suppl 1)*: S3-S7

Riva M, Brunello N, Rovescalli AC, et al. (1989) Effect of reboxetine, a new antidepressant drug, on the central noradrenergic system: behavioural and biochemical studies. *J Drug Dev 1*:243-253

Ryan, N. D., Puig-Antich, J., Ambrosini, P., Rabinovich, H., Robinson, D., Nelson, B., Iyengar, S., & Twomey, J. (1987). The clinical picture of major depression in children and adolescents. *Archives of General Psychiatry, 44*, 854–861.

Sarbadhikari, SN,. Chakrabarty K (2001) Chaos in the brain: a short review alluding to epilepsy, depression, exercise and lateralization. *Medical Engineering & Physics 23*: 445-455..

Saria A. (1999) the tachykinin NK1 receptor in the brain: pharmacology and putative functions. *Eur J Pharmacol 375*:51-60

Schatzberg AF (2002) Major depression: Causes or Effects? *Am J Psychiatry. 159* : 1077-1079

Sartorius N, Jablensky A, Gulbinat W and Ernberg (1980) WHO collaborative study: assessment of depressive disorders. *Psychol Med. 10*: 743-749.

Sartorius N. (2003) Physical symptoms of depression as a public health concern. J Clin *Psychiatry. 64 (Suppl 7):*3-4

Schildkraut JJ. (1965) The catecholamine hypothesis of affective disorders: a review of supporting evidence. *Am J Psychiatry 122*:509-522

Schneider G, Kruse A, Nehen HG, et al. (2000) The prevalence and differential diagnosis of subclinical depressive syndromes in inpatients 60 years of older. *Psycother Psychosom 69:*251-260

Shaffer, D., Gould, M. S., Fisher, P., Trautment, P, Moreau, D., Kleinman, M., & Flory, M. (1996). Psychiatric diagnosis in child and adolescent suicide. *Archives of General Psychiatry, 53,* 339–348.

Shelton RC. (2003) The use of antidepressants in novel combination therapies.
*J Clin Psychiatry. 64 (Suppl 2):*14-8

Smucker, M. R., Craighead, W. E., Craighead, L. W., & Green, B. J. (1986). Normative and reliability data for the Children's Depression Inventory. *Journal of Abnormal Child Psychology, 14*, 25–39.

Stahl SM. (1998) Basic psychopharmacology of antidepressants, part 1 : antidepressants have seven distinct mechanisms of action. *J Clin Psychiatry 59 (suppl 4):*5-14

Stahl, S.M. (2003). Neuro transmission of cognition, part two, selective NRI's are smart drugs; exploiting regionally selective actions on both dopamine and norapeniphrine to enhance cognition. *Journal of Clinical Psychiatry. 64*:110-111.

Steiner M, Steinberg S, Stewart D, et al. (1995) Fluoxetine in the treatment of premenstrual dysphoria. Canadian Fluoxetine/Premenstrual Dysphoria Collaborative Study. *N Engl J Med 332:*1529-1534

Strober, M., DeAntonio, M., Schmidt-Lackner, S., Pataki, C., Freeman, R., Rigali, J., & Rao, U. (1999). The pharmacotherapy of depressive illness in adolescents: An open-label comparison of fluoxetine with imipramine-treated historical controls. *Journal of Clinical Psychiatry, 60*, 164–169

Sunblad C, Hedberg MA, Eriksson E. (1993) Clomipramine administered during the luteal phase reduces the symptoms of premenstrual syndrome: a placebo-cotnrolled trial. *Neuropsychopharmacology* 9:133-145

Ternan, M. On the question of mechanism in phototherapy: considerations of clinical efficacy and epidemiology. *J Biol Rhythms 1988; 2*:47-53.

Thase ME, Entsuah AR, Rudolph RL. (2001) Remission rates during treatment with venlafaxine or selective serotonin reuptake inhibitors. *Br J Psychiatry. 178*:234-241.

Thase ME. (1992) Long-term treatments of recurrent depressive disorders. *J Clin Psychiatry 53 (9, suppl)*:32-44

Thase, M.E. (2003) Effectiveness of antidepressants; comparative remission rates. *Journal of Clinical Psychiatry: 64(suppl 2)*; 3-7.

Ustun TB and Sartorius N (1995) *Mental illness in general health care: An international study*. Wiley Chicester.

Vanderholzer, U & Berger, M (2001) Other methods of somatic therapy for depression. *In Contemporary Psychiatry. Specific Psychiatric Disorders (vol3).* Eds F Henn, N Sartorius, H Helmchen and H Lauter. Springer Berlin. Pp 337-346.

Weissman MM, Bland R, Canino GJ, et al. (1996) Cross-national epidemiology of major depression and bipolar disorder. *JAMA 276*:293-299

Wells KB, Stewart A, Hays RD, Burnam MA, Rogers W, Daniels M, Berry S, Greenfield S, Ware J. (1989) The functioning and well-being of depressed patients. Results from the Medical Outcomes Study *JAMA. 262*:914-9.

Winokur G and Tsuang M (1975) The Iowa 500: suicide in mania, depression and schizophrenia. *Am J Psychiatry. 132*: 650-651

In: Depression and Dementia
Editor: Suptendra Nath Sarbadhikari, p. 213-244
ISBN 1-59454-114-0

Chapter 8

NONLINEAR DYNAMICAL ANALYSIS: ITS APPLICATIONS TO EEG RECORDINGS IN DEMENTIAS

Jaeseung Jeong*
Center for Neurodynamics and the Department of Physics,
Korea University, Seoul 136-701, South Korea

ABSTRACT

Nonlinear dynamical analysis (NDA) has been extensively applied to a variety of physiological data for the last two decades. One of its major contributions is to the electroencephalogram (EEG) in patients with dementias, particularly Alzheimer's disease (AD). The hallmark of nonlinear EEG abnormalities in demented patients is the globally decreased complexity of EEG patterns and a prominent decrease in information transmission among cortical areas quantified by information-theoretic measures like mutual information. These findings might be associated with functional disconnections among cortical areas resulting from death of cortical neurons, axonal pathology, cholinergic deficits etc, and thus decreased nonlinear processes underlying cortical dynamics in dementias. While the average diagnostic accuracy of EEG for dementias using conventional analyses is currently about 80%, it has been shown that NDA of EEG recordings might contribute to the improvement of the accuracy of differential diagnosis of dementias and early detection in the preclinical stage. This article introduces the concepts and algorithms of NDA and focuses on primary findings of EEG abnormalities in dementia patients obtained from NDA. We suggest that NDA provides not only potentially valuable diagnostic information but also a deeper understanding of neuropathological mechanisms underlying dementias in ways that are not possible by conventional spectral analyses.

Keywords: Dementias; Alzheimer's disease; electroencephalography; nonlinear; complexity; diagnosis.

---

* Address correspondence to: Jaeseung Jeong, Ph.D. Center for Neurodynamics, Department of Physics, Korea University, Sungbuk-gu, Anham-dong 5-1, Seoul, South Korea 136-701, phone: +82-2-3290-4288, fax: +82-2-3290-3534, email: jsjeong@complex.korea.ac.kr

INTRODUCTION

Dementia is one of the most common disorders among the elderly population. The prevalence rate of dementia in persons aged 65 years or over has been reported to be about 3.6-10.3% in Western countries and 1.8-10.8% in Asian countries since the mid-1980s (Lee et al., 2002; Ritchie and Lovestone, 2002). The prevalence increases prominently with age, so that dementia affects up to 50% of all Americans aged 80 years or over (Vicioso, 2002). Among several subtypes of dementia, Alzheimer's disease (AD) is the most frequent cause of dementia. Approximately 50-60% of patients with dementia over 65 are clinically related to AD. In 2002, 4.3 million individuals are estimated to be with AD in the United States (Lahiri et al., 2002). This number is projected to increase to 15 million by 2050, and consequently the personal and social ramifications of the disease will be more significant. Thus, early detection and effective treatment of AD are critical issues in dementia research.

Since Hans Berger, the discoverer of EEG signals firstly observed pathological EEG sequences in a historically verified AD patient (Berger, 1931, 1932), a large number of studies on the EEG of dementias have been performed. The hallmark of EEG abnormalities in demented patients, in particular AD patients, is a slowing of the rhythms and a decrease in coherence among different brain regions. An increase in theta and delta activity and a decrease in alpha and beta activity are observed (Coben et al., 1983, 1985; Giaquinto and Nolfe, 1986; Brenner et al., 1986), and a reduced coherence of the alpha and beta bands is frequently found (Leuchter et al., 1987; Dunkin et al., 1994; Locatelli et al., 1998). Furthermore, these abnormalities are correlated with the severity of the disease (Hughes et al., 1989; Kowalski et al., 2001). For the last two decades, the EEG has been utilized as a useful tool for diagnosing dementias (for review, Rosen 1996; Jonkman, 1997).

Recently, nonlinear dynamical analysis (NDA) has been developed in the field of nonlinear dynamics and chaos theory to explore complex dynamics of physiological processes. In particular, the application of NDA to EEG recordings has been shown to provide valuable information on the cortical dynamics underlying the EEGs. One of major contributions of NDA is to the EEG in patients with dementias. Nonlinear abnormalities of the EEG in AD are characterized by the decreased complexity of EEG patterns and lowered functional connectivity among cortical areas. These results indicate decreased nonlinear processes and coupling interactions underlying the EEG in AD. Many studies have provided a growing body of evidence that NDA of brain electrical activity in demented patients is capable of offering potentially valuable diagnostic information and a better understanding of the neuropathological mechanism of dementias.

In this review, we focus on EEG abnormalities in AD among several subtypes of dementias, because EEG changes of AD patients have been intensively studied. This article firstly introduces the concepts and algorithms of NDA, and then summarizes main findings about EEG abnormalities in AD patients obtained from NDA as well as linear methods. Clinical neurophysiology of AD underlying these EEG abnormalities is also considered. The EEG as a tool for differential diagnosis and early detection of dementias and as a measure of functional connectivity among cortical regions is intensively discussed. A large part of this chapter was previously published in Jeong (2002, 2004).

Concepts and Algorithms of NDA

The fundamental assumption of NDA is that EEG signals are generated by nonlinear deterministic processes with nonlinear coupling interactions between neuronal populations. Nonlinear deterministic systems may show a sensitive dependence on initial conditions, implying that different states of a system, being arbitrarily close initially, can become exponentially separated in sufficiently long times. This behavior is called deterministic chaos. These systems behave very irregular and complex, similar to stochastic systems. Given the highly nonlinear nature of neuronal interactions at multiple levels of spatial scales, it is quite natural to apply nonlinear methods to the EEG.

Complex dynamical systems like the brain commonly involve a large number of interrelated variables that are impossible to measure directly. Thus, the major problem is how to analyze multi-dimensional dynamics knowing only a few variables that can be measured. Takens (1981) has shown that, if we measure any single variable with sufficient accuracy for a long period of time, it is possible to reconstruct the underlying dynamic structure of the entire system from the behavior of that single variable using delay coordinates and the embedding procedure. Based on this theorem, now we can extract information as to the underlying cortical dynamics by analyzing a bunch of the trajectories (i.e. the attractor) reconstructed from the time series (i.e. EEG). This procedure is referred to as the inverse problem. The geometric and dynamical properties of the trajectories in the phase space are quantified by nonlinear measures.

The first step of the embedding procedure in nonlinear EEG analysis is to transform the one-dimensional EEG data into multidimensional phase space. The concept of phase space is central to the analysis of nonlinear dynamics. In a hypothetical system governed by n variables, the phase space is n-dimensional. Each state of the system corresponds to a point in the phase space whose n coordinates are the values assumed by the governing variables for this specific state. If the system is observed for a long period of time, the sequence of points in the phase space forms a trajectory. This trajectory fills a subspace of the phase space, called the system's attractor. The reconstruction of the attractor in the phase space is carried out through the technique of delay coordinates (Kantz and Schreiber, 1997). To unfold the projection back to a multivariate state space that is a representation of the original system, the delay coordinates $y(t) = [x_j(t), x_j(t+\tau), x(t+2\tau), ..., x_j(t+(d-1)\tau)]$ from a single time series x_j is used, where $y(t)$ is a point of the trajectory in the phase space at time t, $x_j(t+i\tau)$ is the coordinates in the phase space corresponding to the time-delayed values of the time series, τ is the time delay between the points of the time series considered, and d is the embedding dimension (Fig. 1).

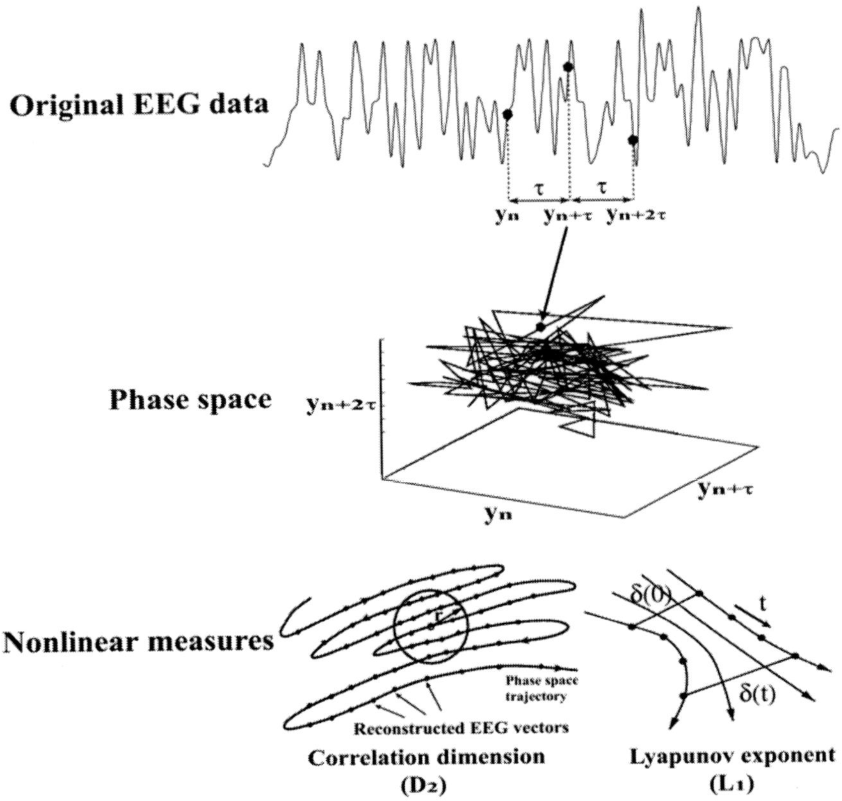

Fig. 1 A schematic diagram of nonlinear dynamical analysis of the EEG. The first step is to transform the EEG data into multidimensional phase space using delay coordinates. Nonlinear measures like the first positive Lyapunov exponent and correlation dimension are estimated from the attractor in the phase space reconstructed from the EEG data.

The choice of an appropriate time delay τ and embedding dimension d is important for the success of reconstruction with finite data. For the time delay τ, the first zero-crossing time of the auto-correlation or the first local minimum of the average mutual information of the EEG is often utilized. Mutual information measures linear and nonlinear dependence of two variables, while the autocorrelation estimates linear dependence. It has shown that the mutual information provides a more reliable delay time than does autocorrelation (Fraser and Swinney, 1986). The optimal embedding dimension can be obtained using the method developed by Kennel et al. (1992). The algorithm of this method is based on the idea that in the passage from dimension *d* to dimension *d+1*, one can differentiate between points on the orbit that are true neighbors and those which are false. A false neighbor is a point in the data set that is a neighbor solely because we are viewing the orbit (the attractor) in too small an embedding space ($d < d_{min}$). When a large enough embedding space has been achieved ($d \geq d_{min}$), all neighbors of every orbit point in the multivariate phase space will be true neighbors. A properly fixed value ranging 5 to 20 or minimum value obtained from the Kennel's method is often used for the embedding dimension in the NDA.

The geometric and dynamical properties of the trajectories in the phase space can be quantified by nonlinear measures. An important measure is the dimensionality of the attractor, referred to as the correlation dimension (D_2) or dimensional complexity. The D_2 reflects the number of independent variables that are necessary to describe the dynamics of the system. For instance, the D_2 of the attractor is zero in the case of steady-state behavior, and the D_2 of the periodic attractor is one. In chaotic states, the D_2 usually takes on non-integer values. The larger the D_2 of the attractor, the more complicated the behavior of the nonlinear system. The D_2 is therefore a measure of complexity of the process being investigated and characterizes the distribution of points in the phase space. The D_2 of the EEG is generally considered to be a reflection of the complexity of the cortical dynamics underlying EEG recordings (Röschke and Aldenhoff, 1991).

The D2 of the attractors from the EEG is commonly evaluated using the Grassberger-Procaccia Algorithm (GPA) (Grassberger and Procaccia, 1983). This algorithm determines the D2 by counting the relative number of pairs of points in the phase-space that are separated by a distance less than r:

$$D2 = \lim_{r \to 0} \lim_{N \to \infty} \frac{\log C(r, N)}{\log r} \tag{1}$$

where the correlation integral C(N, r) is defined by

$$C(r) = \frac{1}{N^2} \sum_{\substack{i,j=1 \\ i \neq j}}^{N} \theta(r - |\vec{y}_i - \vec{y}_j|) \tag{2}$$

where y_i and y_j are the points of the trajectory in the phase space, N is the number of data points in the phase space, the distance r is a radius around each reference point y_i and θ is the Heaviside function, defined as 0 if $y<0$, and 1 if $y \geq 0$. For small r, the correlation integral exhibits the scaling property: $C(N, r) \propto r^{D2}$. For fractal attractor the local scaling exponent is constant which region is called a scaling region. If this plateau is convincing enough, this scaling exponent (i.e. the slope of the $C(r)$ on a log-log plot) can be used as an estimate of the D_2.

As another measure of complexity, Lyapunov exponents estimate the mean exponential divergence or convergence of nearby trajectories of the attractor in the phase space. This reflects the sensitive dependence on the initial. A system possessing at least one positive Lyapunov exponent is chaotic. Lyapunov exponents are usually ordered in a descending fashion from L_1 (the highest value) to L_n (the lowest value), where n is equal to the dimensionality of the phase space. Positive L_1 of a time series indicates the presence of chaos in the underlying dynamics of the time series. The larger the positive L_1 of the attractor, the more complicated the behavior of the nonlinear system. While the D_2 is a static, geometric measure, the L_1 is relatively a dynamic measure conditions (Fell et al., 1993).

The L_1 of time series is usually computed using the Wolf algorithm (Wolf et al., 1985). The Wolf algorithm calculates the initial vector distance $\delta(0)$ of two nearby points and evolves its length $\delta(t)$ at a certain propagation time t. If the vector length between the two points becomes too large, a new reference point is chosen with properties minimizing the replacement length and the orientation change. Then, the two points are evolved again, and so on. After m propagation steps, the first positive Lyapunov exponent, L_1, results from the sum over the logarithm of the ratios of the vector distances divided by the total evolving time:

$$L_1 = \frac{1}{m}\sum_{i=1}^{m}\frac{\ln\frac{\delta_i(t)}{\delta_i(0)}}{t\cdot\ln 2}(bits/s) \tag{3}$$

where t is the evolving time, $\delta(0)$ and $\delta(t)$ are the initial and the final separations between the points in the fiducial trajectory and in the nearest-neighbor trajectory separated in time t, respectively. The graphical presentation of the nonlinear methods is given in Fig. 1. The overall scheme of the nonlinear dynamical analysis is shown in Fig. 2.

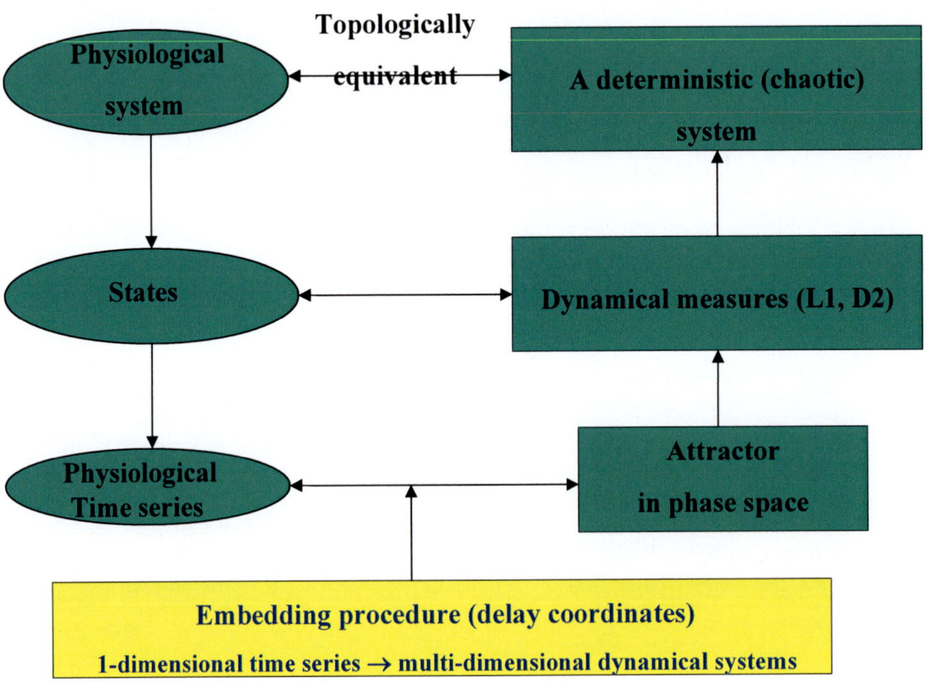

Figure 2. Overall scheme of the nonlinear dynamical analysis

The surrogate data method is often used to help detect nonlinear deterministic structure within the data. Surrogate data can be constructed by phase randomization of the original signals. In this way, surrogate data are produced whose linear properties such as power spectrum and histogram are unchanged, whereas nonlinear properties that may be present are destroyed. Statistical differences of nonlinear measures between the original data and its surrogate data indicate the presence of nonlinear structure in the original data. The detailed algorithm for generating the surrogate data is presented in the paper of Schreiber and Schmitz (2000). More detailed algorithms of NDA are present in other review papers (Pritchard and Duke, 1992; Cerutti et al., 1996; Kantz and Schreiber, 1997; Schreiber, 1999; Abarbanel and Rabinovich, 2001; Faure and Korn, 2001). C-code programs estimating nonlinear measures are available in the website developed by Hegger and his colleagues (1999).

Clinical Neurophysiology of AD

The neuropathology of AD is characterized by widespread neuronal cell loss, neurofibrillary tangles, and senile plaques in the hippocampus, entorhinal cortex, neocortex and other brain regions (Selkoe, 1994). Senile plaques are extracellular aggregates of amyloid β-peptides, and neurofibrillary tangles are the aggregation of tau proteins. Hyperphosphorylated tau, produced by an imbalance between protein phosphorylation and dephosphorylation due to a decrease in the activity of protein phosphatase-2A which regulates the activities of tau kinases, is the major protein subunit of neurofibrillary tangles (Iqbal et al., 2002; Smith et al., 2002). Tangles are found mainly in the limbic structures, particularly hippocampal and parahippocampal regions, whereas extensive diffuse and neuritic amyloid plaques form preferentially throughout the neocortex (Price and Morris, 1999; Price et al., 2001). Reduced brain weight, cortical atrophy, and ventricular enlargement are also prominent in the brains of AD patients. The size of the hippocampus and of the temporal horn of the lateral ventricle is associated with the number of neurofibrillary tangles in the hippocampus (DeCarli et al., 1990), whereas cortical atrophy is correlated with the amount of senile plaques in the cortex afflicted by AD (Davis et al., 1995).

AD frequently takes a typical clinical course reflecting the underlying expanding neuropathology (Förstle and Kurz, 1999; Bianchetti and Trabucchi, 2001; Storey et al., 2002). In the preclinical stage of AD, no reliable and valid symptoms are detected to allow a very early diagnosis before the manifestation of irreversible cognitive deficits. In the mild stage, an impairment of learning and memory is usually notable. The declarative recent memory is predominantly affected with early loss of memory for everyday events. Semantic difficulties with word generation and a deterioration of object naming are also prominent. In the moderate dementia stage, language difficulties become more obvious as word finding difficulties, paraphasia, and the circumstantialities increase (Förstle and Kurz, 1999). Deficits in other cognitive abilities, such as judgment, abstract or logical reasoning, planning, and organizing, appear during the progression of the disease (Bianchetti and Trabucchi, 2001). One third of AD patients at this stage develop illusionary misidentifications and other delusional symptoms arose from cognitive deficits (Reisberg et al., 1996). Aimless and restless activity, like wandering and hoarding, is commonly observed (Devanand et al., 1997). In the late stage of illness, almost all cognitive functions are severely damaged, and motor functions including chewing and swallowing are profoundly disturbed. The average duration of survival of AD patients is 5 - 8 years after clinical diagnosis (Bracco et al., 1994).

Linear EEG Abnormalities in AD

Slowing of EEG in AD

Computerized EEG spectral analysis has shown a decrease in the mean frequency with an increase in delta and theta power and a parallel decrease in alpha and beta power in AD patients compared with those of normal elderly subjects (Stigsby et al., 1981; Coben et al., 1983, 1985; Visser et al., 1985; Brenner et al., 1986; Giaquinto and Nolfe, 1986; Coben et al., 1990; Maurer and Dierks, 1992; Szelies et al., 1992; Schreiter-Gasser et al., 1993; Ihl et al., 1993; Bennys et al., 2001), even during rapid eye movement (REM) sleep (Petit et al., 1992;

1993; Montplaisir et al., 1996; Hassainia et al., 1997). It is generally thought that the earliest changes are an increase in theta activity and a decrease in beta activity, which are followed by a decrease in alpha activity. Delta activity increases later during the course of the disease. Patients with severe dementia exhibit a decrease in alpha and an increase in delta activity (Stigsby et al., 1981; Coben et al., 1985; Penttilä et al., 1985; Hier et al., 1991), whereas patients with mild dementia show a decrease in beta and an increase in theta activity (Coben et al., 1983, 1985). Topographic analysis revealed that an increase in slow activity is prominent in the left temporal area of AD patients (Breslau et al., 1989; Rice et al., 1990). Studies in which different methods were used on the same population demonstrated that an estimated diagnostic accuracy of spectral and visual EEG analyses is approximately 80% (Brenner et al., 1988; Hooijer et al., 1990). It is of clinical interest to find that the EEG abnormality is associated with cognitive deficits. A good correlation are found between EEG spectral measures and cognitive deterioration scores, such as the Folstein (Mini-mental) score (Brenner et al., 1986; Leuchter et al., 1987; Filipovitch et al., 1989; Leuchter et al., 1993; Elmståhl et al., 1994; Schreiter-Gasser et al., 1994; Stijers et al., 1997), the global deterioration score (Helkala et al., 1991; Prichep et al., 1994; Passero et al., 1995), and a composite neuropsychological test score (Penttilä et al., 1985).

EEG in AD as a Potential Predictor

Whether the EEG is a potential predictor of the progression of dementia is of most clinical importance (for a review, see Jelic, 1999). Although Berg et al. (1984) reported that spectral measures of the EEG are not predictive of the progression to moderate or severe dementia, many studies support the possibility of early detection of AD using EEG recordings (Helkala et al., 1991; Prinz et al., 1992; Schreiter-Gasser et al., 1994; Claus et al., 1998, 2000; Petrosian et al., 2001). Current EEG studies on mild cognitive impairment (MCI) have especially aimed toward the detection of preclinical AD. MCI is a clinical condition by objective memory disturbances in the absence of other cognitive deficits (Petersen et al., 1999) or more generally characterized by all cognitive changes observed in ageing that are insufficient to meet dementia criteria (Burns and Zaudig, 2002; Nestor et al., 2004). EEG studies found that theta power (Zappoli et al., 1995; Jelic et al., 1996; Grunwald et al., 2001) as well as other EEG parameters (Jelic et al., 1996, 2000; Elmståhl and Rosén, 1997; Huang et al., 2000) differs significantly between healthy and MCI subjects, although these EEG parameters for MCI subjects were mostly intermediate between those of controls and dementia subjects with considerable overlap. A recent study found significant theta power differences during haptic tasks between healthy controls and MCI subjects (Grunwald et al., 2002), suggesting that activation paradigms in EEG studies can increase the sensitivity for cases at risk of developing AD.

EEG in AD as a Differential Diagnostic Indicator

The EEG as an effective tool for differential diagnosis of AD from other dementias has been extensively studied. Particularly, the possibility of differential diagnosis of AD from vascular dementia (VaD) using the EEG has been much investigated. Although neuroimaging analysis of hippocampal atrophy has been proved very effective in detecting AD (de Leon et al., 1989; Scheltens et al., 1992; Jack et al., 1992; Erkinjuntti et al., 1993), the main criteria for distinguishing AD from VaD are usually the case history and neuropsychiatric examination. It is controversial about a diagnostic value of the EEG differentiating AD from VaD (Harrison et al., 1979; Ettlin et al., 1989; Robinson et al., 1994). A number of studies failed to find any significant difference of EEG measures between in AD and VaD (Soininen et al., 1982; Ettlin et al., 1989; Robinson et al., 1994). In contrast, the uneven distribution of EEG abnormalities is clearly observed in VaD patients using multi-channel EEG mapping, offering 63% classification accuracy (Saletu et al., 1991). A higher incidence of focal abnormalities and more preservation of occipital alpha activity are found in VaD patients than those of AD patients (Soininen et al., 1982; Erkinjuntti et al., 1988; Giannitrapani et al., 1991; Rosen et al., 1993; Sloan and Fenton, 1993).

On the other hand, the EEG is very useful for distinguishing AD patients from patients with senile depression with an accuracy of about 70-85% (Brenner et al., 1988; Reynolds et al., 1988; Brenner et al., 1989; Hooijer et al., 1990; Moe et al., 1993; Boerman et al., 1994). Patients with histologically verified fronto-temporal cortical atrophy exhibit normal EEG patterns or a moderate, diffuse increase in relative theta power (Johannesson et al., 1977, 1979) and the absence of an increase in slow EEG activities and a decrease in fast activities (Lindau et al., 2003). Demented patients with Parkinson's disease have a decrease in relative alpha power in comparison with age- and sex-matched non-demented Parkinsonian patients and healthy subjects (Neufeld et al., 1994a). A more detailed diagnostic value of the EEG for AD is presented in other reviews (Rosen, 1996; Jonkman, 1997).

Pathogenesis of EEG Slowing in AD

What is the pathophysiological origin of the EEG slowing in AD? A major promising candidate is the cholinergic deficit. AD is thought to be a syndrome of neocortical disconnection, in which profound cognitive losses arise from the disrupted structural and functional integrity of long corticocortical tracts (Leuchter et al., 1992). Senile plaques and neurofibrillary tangles of AD prominently involve the origins and terminations of long cortico-cortical association fibers (Pearson et al., 1985; Rogers and Morrison, 1985; Esiri et al., 1986; Lewis et al., 1987). The brain of AD patients exhibits a significant reduction in markers of cholinergic transmission (Bartus et al., 1982; Coyle et al., 1983; Collerton, 1986). Since several studies demonstrated that acetylcholine (ACh) and the basal forebrain system maintain desynchronized EEG activity (Kanai and Szerb, 1965; Celesia and Jasper, 1966; Cuculic et al., 1968; Spehlmann and Norcross, 1982; Metherate et al., 1992), a loss of cholinergic innervation of the neocortex might play a critical role in the EEG slowing of AD.

The critical role of the cholinergic deficit in the EEG slowing in AD is also supported by EEG studies using scopolamine (for a review, see Ebert and Kirch, 1998). Scopolamine is a non-selective muscarine receptor antagonist that blocks the stimulation of post-synaptic receptors. After the scopolamine administration, an increase in delta and theta power and/or a decrease in alpha and beta power are detected in healthy subjects (Bartus et al., 1982; Sannita et al., 1987; Buzsaki et al., 1988; Sloan et al., 1992; Neufeld et al., 1994b; Ebert et al., 2001).

The hypothesis that basal forebrain neurons are severely affected in AD and result in a cerebral cholinergic deficit that underlies the memory loss and other cognitive symptoms, so-called the cholinergic hypothesis, has been the stimulus for a great deal of effort in experimental pharmacology and a large number of clinical trials, and has served as the rationale for the development of drugs currently approved for AD treatment. Until now, four drugs for AD which have been approved for prescription use by US Food and Drug Administration all belong to the drug category of Acetylcholinesterase (AChE) inhibitors. Although they do not halt progression of the disease, all have been shown to improve memory and cognitive functions in patients with mild and moderate AD (Lahiri et al., 2002). There are a lot of studies reporting that these drugs result in a significant decrease in the mean absolute power of theta activity (Kogan et al., 2001), decreases in the mean alpha and delta power (Reeves et al., 2002), and a lesser EEG deterioration (Adler and Brassen, 2001; Rodriguez et al., 2002), in AD patients. These significant effects of cholinergic drugs on the EEG suggest that EEG abnormalities of AD patients are highly associated with a decline in memory and cognitive function by cholinergic deficits.

However, solely the cholinergic dysfunction is not sufficient to produce cognitive and electrophysiological symptoms of AD. Davis and his colleagues (1999) found that patients with the early stages of AD who are already experiencing the characteristic symptoms of AD at death show no evidence of deficiency of either choline acetyltransferase (ChAT) or AChE activity. This work suggests that the AD symptoms, at least in the early stages, are not primarily caused by a loss of cholinergic transmission, even though there is a large body of evidence that such deficits do occur as the disease progresses. Most surprisingly, elevated ChAT activity suggesting upregulation of cholinergic systems is found in the frontal cortex and hippocampus of individuals with MCI (DeKosky et al., 2002). There is now increasing evidence for the hypothesis that cholinergic neurons in MCI are not normally regulated (Sarter and Bruno, 1999, 2002). Although the number of cholinergic terminals is either unchanged or even increased in MCI, their trophic factor regulation is disrupted (Chen et al., 1997; Sarter and Bruno, 1999; Sarter and Turchi, 2002). These recent findings suggest a more subtle dysregulation of basal forebrain neurons rather than substantial cell death in the basal forebrain early in AD.

Decreased EEG Coherence in AD

Coherence analysis of the EEG has been used to estimate the degree of functional connectivity among cortical areas. EEG coherence is defined as the square of the cross-spectrum of the electrodes divided by the product of the power spectra of the individual electrodes. It is often estimated separately for each of the frequency bands and for specific pairs of electrodes, such as F3-C3, or averaged over all electrode pairs for each frequency band as a global measure of connectivity. Decreased coherence reflects reduced functional connections between cortical areas beneath the electrodes or reduced common modulation of two areas by a third.

EEG coherence analysis in AD has been applied to examine whether the cognitive decline is associated with changes in functional connections between cortical regions and whether different types of dementia are related to specific changes. A well-established feature in AD is a decrease in coherence of the alpha and beta bands in various types of dementia between both close and distant channels, suggesting functional disconnections among cortical regions (O'Conner et al., 1979; Leuchter et al., 1987; 1992; Besthorn et al., 1994; Dunkin et al., 1994; Sloan et al., 1994; Locatelli et al., 1998). This deceased coherence of fast bands is significantly correlated with cognitive impairment (Dunkin et al., 1994; Jelic et al., 1996). This might result from a loss of long cortico-cortical association fibers, because long-distance anatomical connections between different cortical regions are obviously required for functional interactions. In this view, the decreased EEG coherence in AD patients supports the hypothesis that AD is a neocortical disconnection syndrome.

In addition to anatomical disconnections of long cortico-cortical fibers, changes in synaptic couplings among cortical neurons might be of importance. A decrease in synaptic couplings can reduce long-distance functional connections even when the anatomical connections are intact. A distinct feature of AD is a loss of acetylcholine, an excitatory neurotransmitter of the cerebral cortex. Synaptic blockade of the cholinergic system by the application of scopolamine, an anticholinergic drug, reduces the EEG coherence in humans (Kikuchi et al., 2000). If the decreased EEG coherence in AD is simply due to a loss of cortical neurons, it would be difficult to explain why all frequencies are not equally affected (Stam et al., 2003). In patients with the most severe cognitive impairment, coherence of slow EEG rhythms is unaffected (Besthorn et al., 1994), or reduced (Knott et al., 2000b), or rather increased (Locatelli et al., 1998; Comi et al., 1998). An increase in the slow band power in AD patients is associated with a cortical loss of choline acetyltransferase (Reinikainen et al., 1988; Soininen et al., 1992). Anticholinergic drugs in healthy subjects induce an increase in coherence of slow bands (Sloan et al., 1992). In addition, an animal study (Villa et al., 2000) showed that a loss of acetylcholine results in a decrease in high-frequency couplings and an increase in low-frequency couplings. Thus, it is possible that the decrease in EEG coherence of AD results from both anatomical disconnections among different cortical regions and reduced cholinergic coupling interactions between cortical neurons.

NONLINEAR EEG ABNORMALITIES IN AD

Decreased Complexity of EEG in AD

A number of studies offer growing evidence that NDA of brain electrical activity in AD patients is capable of providing potentially useful diagnostic information (for a review, see Jeong, 2002). Woyshville and Calabrese (1994) demonstrated, using single-channel EEGs, that AD patients have reduced values of the correlation dimension (D_2) in the occipital EEG compared with those of healthy subjects, and that, within AD patients, autopsy-confirmed AD patients have more reduced D_2 values than probable AD patients. The D_2 reflects the number of independent variables that are necessary to describe the dynamics of the system. In nonlinear EEG analysis, the D_2 is considered to be a reflection of the complexity of the cortical dynamics underlying EEG recordings. Thus, reduced D_2 values of the EEG in AD patients indicate that brains injured by AD exhibit a decrease in the complexity of brain electrical activity. Besthorn et al. (1995) and Jeong et al. (1998) used multi-channel EEG recordings and a time-delay embedding method to show that AD patients have lower D_2 values than those of age-approximated healthy subjects in almost all electrodes. Using a spatial embedding method, Stam et al. (1995) and Yagyu et al. (1997) found markedly reduced spatio-temporal brain activity in AD patients in comparison with that in normal controls. All these findings indicate globally decreased complexity of brain electrical activity in AD patients.

Pathophysiological implications of the decreased EEG complexity in AD are not clear. A decrease in dynamical complexity of the EEG in AD patients might arise from neuronal death, deficiency of neurotransmitters like acetylcholine, and/or loss of connectivity of local neuronal networks. The reduction of the dimensionality in AD is possibly an expression of the inactivation of previously active networks. Also, a loss of dynamical brain responsivity to stimuli might be responsible for the decrease in the EEG complexity of AD patients. Pritchard et al. (1991, 1993) found that AD patients do not have D_2 differences between in eyes-open and eye-close conditions, whereas normal subjects have prominently increased eyes-open D_2 values compared with eyes-closed D_2 values. These results suggest that AD patients exhibit a loss of brain responsivity to changing environmental stimuli. Therefore, given that EEG patterns reflect cortical activity (information processing) of the brain, the reduced EEG complexity in AD suggests the deficient information processing of the cortex due to the inactivation of previously active networks or a loss of dynamical brain responsivity to external stimuli.

Using the first positive Lyapunov exponents (L_1), Stam et al. (1995) and Jeong et al. (1998) demonstrated the decreased complexity of brain activity in AD patients compared with that of age-matched healthy subjects. The L_1 describes the divergence of trajectories starting at nearby initial states. While the D_2 is a static, geometric measure, the L_1 is relatively a dynamic measure. It is true that both D_2 and L_1 are used as a measure of complexity in NDA, but the L_1 of the EEG can be often interpreted as a measure of flexibility of information processing of the brain (Fell et al., 1995). The flexibility is understood as the facility of the central nervous system to reach different states of information processing from similar initial states (Röschke and Aldenhoff, 1991). In this context, decreased L_1 values in AD patients indicate a drop in the flexibility of information processing of the AD brains.

The surrogate data method has been applied to investigate nonlinearity of the EEG in AD patients. Surrogate data are constructed by phase randomization of original EEG signals (Schreiber and Schmitz, 2000). In this way, linear properties (e.g. power spectrum) of the surrogate data are unchanged, but their nonlinear structure that may be present is destroyed. Therefore, statistical differences of a nonlinear measure between the original data and their surrogate data indicate the presence of nonlinearity in the original data. Both normal subjects and AD patients exhibit significant D_2 differences between original and their surrogate EEG data (Stam et al., 1995; Jelles et al., 1999b), indicating the presence of nonlinearity in the EEG. Besides, Jelles et al. (1999b) found smaller differences between original and the surrogate EEG data in AD patients than in healthy subjects. This indicates that the decrease in the EEG complexity of AD patients may be attributable to decreased nonlinear neurodynamics underlying the EEG, which might be associated with the cognitive decline. In another study, Jelles et al. (1999a) detected no change in the nonlinear structure between healthy subjects and patients with mild AD. This suggests that linear dynamics of the EEG changes first in the course of AD followed by changes in nonlinear dynamics.

Nonlinear Measures as a Diagnostic Tool of AD

Nonlinear measures are quite efficient as a diagnostic indicator of AD. Pritchard et al. (1994) assessed the classification accuracy of the EEG using nonlinear measures and a neural-net classification procedure in addition to linear methods. The combination of linear and nonlinear analysis improves the classification accuracy of the AD/control status of subjects up to 92%. Besthorn et al. (1997) reported that the D_2 correctly classified AD and normal subjects with an accuracy of 70%. Good correlations are found between nonlinear measures and the severity of the disease (Besthorn et al., 1995; Yagyu et al., 1997), a slowing of EEG rhythms (Besthorn et al., 1995), and neuropsychological performance (Ikawa et al., 2000). Furthermore, the global entropy can quantify EEG changes induced by drugs (Pezard et al., 1998), suggesting a possibility that nonlinear measures is capable of quantifying the effect of drugs on the course of the disease. Taken together, we believe that nonlinear measures are a potentially useful indicator for diagnosis of AD, assessment of neuropsychological deficits, and pharmacological treatment evaluations.

There are a few studies on differential and early diagnosis of AD using nonlinear methods. AD patients exhibit lower L_1 values than those of Parkinson patients (Stam et al., 1994, 1995) and lower D_2 and L_1 values than those of patients with VaD (Jeong et al., 2001a). VaD patients appear to have an uneven distribution of the D_2 values over the regions relative to AD patients and normal controls, even though the statistics did not confirm this. In the early stage of AD, nonlinear EEG abnormalities in AD patients, i.e. the decreased complexity and increased predictability, are observed mainly in frontal and temporal areas (Jelles at al., 1999a). It is of importance to determine whether NDA can provide additional information helpful for differential and early diagnosis of AD in future.

Reduced Degrees of Functional Connectivity in AD Brains

Recently, the mutual information (MI) (Jeong et al., 2001b) and synchronization method (Stam et al., 2003) have been applied to the EEG in AD patients. While coherence measures only linear dependencies in electrical activity across different brain regions, MI and synchronization analyses take into account both linear and nonlinear dependencies. MI analysis showed that the interdependencies between different electrodes are reduced in AD patients in comparison with those in normal controls, particularly over frontal and antero-temporal regions (Jeong et al., 2001b). A decrease in the MI between distant electrodes and between inter-hemispheric electrodes is prominently found in AD patients. Stam et al. (2003) found a significant loss of EEG synchronization in the beta band and its correlation with MMSE scores in subjects with MCI as well as AD. Since the MI and synchronization of the EEG reflect linear and nonlinear functional connections among cortical regions, a decrease in these measures in AD suggests an impairment of information transmission among cortical regions.

Table 1. Summary of main findings of EEG studies on nonlinear dynamics in AD patients

Authors (year)	Sample	Analysis methods	Main findings
Pritchard et al. [1991, 1993]	ADs, young controls, elderly controls	D_2	A loss of dynamical brain responsivity to stimuli in AD patients
Pritchard et al. [1994]	14 ADs, 25 controls	D_2 and neural network	The addition of the D_2 improves the classification accuracy of the AD/control status of subjects up to 92%.
Woyshville and Calabrese [1994]	6 probable ADs, 6 autopsy-confirmed ADs, 8 controls	D_2	Lower D_2s in ADs than those of controls. Lower D_2s in autopsy-confirmed ADs than those of probable ADs
Stam et al. [1994]	15 demented patients, 17 Parkinson patients, 20 controls	D_2, spatial embedding	Lower D_2s in demented patients than those of controls and Parkinson patients. A positive correlation of D_2 with beta power, and a negative correlation with delta and theta power.
Besthorn et al. [1995]	50 ADs, 42 controls	D_2	Lower D_2 values in AD patients than in controls
Stam et al. [1995]	9 demented patients, 13 Parkinson patients, 9 controls	K_2, L_1, D_2, spatial embedding, surrogate data method	The presence of nonlinear structure in the EEG. Lower D_2 and L_1 in demented patients than those of controls. Higher L1 in Parkinson patients than in demented patients.
Besthorn et al. [1997]	50 ADs, 42 controls	D_2, back propagation neural network, PCA	The D2 correctly classified AD/normal subjects in about 70%. A maximum of 86.6% correct classifications is reached using PCA.
Yagyu et al. [1997]	21 ADs, 29 mild cognitive impairment, 29 subjective memory complaint	D_2, spatial embedding	Lower D_2s in AD patients than those of mild cognitive impairments and subjective memory complaints. A positive correlation between D_2 and cognitive performance (MMSE and WAIS-R scores).
Pezard et al. [1998].	12 ADs	Entropy	A significant effect of the drug (an experimental molecule: S 12024-2) are found compared with placebo. An increase in entropy for the highest dose (200mg)
Jeong et al. [1998]	12 ADs, 12 controls	D_2, L_1, optimal embedding dimension method	Lower D_2 and L_1 values in AD patients than in controls.
Jelles et al. [1999a]	24 probable ADs, 22 controls	D_2, surrogate data method	Lower D_2 in AD patients than in controls. D_2 differences between original and surrogate data are significant in both groups. Smaller differences between original and surrogate data are found in AD patients.

Table 1. Summary of main findings of EEG studies on nonlinear dynamics in AD patients (Continued)

Authors (year)	Sample	Analysis methods	Main findings
Jelles et al. [1999b]	42 controls, 7 ADs	D_2, nonlinear prediction, surrogate data method	Lower D_2 and higher predictability in demented subjects than in normal subjects. Major differences between demented and healthy subjects are not due to nonlinearity
Ikawa et al. [2000]	24 ADs.	D_2, neuropsychological tests	Significant correlations between D_2 and neuropsychological test scores
Jeong et al. [2001a]	12 ADs, 12 VaDs, 14 controls	D_2, L_1	Lower D_2s and L_1s in VaD patients than in AD patients, and controls in some channels. An uneven distribution of D_2s and L_1s in VaD patients.
Jeong et al. [2001b]	15 ADs, 15 controls	Mutual information	Lower MIs in AD patients than in controls, in particular over frontal and antero-temporal regions, in distant electrodes in the right hemisphere, and between interhemispheric electrodes.

AD, Alzheimer's disease; VaD, Vascular dementia; D_2, correlation dimension; K_2, Kolmogorove entropy; L_1, the first positive Lyapunov expoenent; PCA, principal component analysis; MI, mutual information.

In fact, clear evidence for the presence of the nonlinear couplings in long cortico-cortical fibers is rarely found. Villa et al. (2000) detected indirect evidence for the existence of nonlinear, functional cortico-cortical interactions. They used bispectral analysis to measure the shift of phase-coupled frequencies (somewhat analogous to frequencies of resonance) in multiple local field potentials in the rat temporal cortex. After the application of the immunotoxin 192 IgG-saporin, which provokes a selective loss of NGFr-positive basal forebrain cholinergic neurons similar to the loss of its integrity in the AD brain, a decrease in choline acetyltransferase activity and an increase of the phase coupling in low frequencies are found. This indicates a decrease in functional cortico-cortical interactions, and suggests that nonlinear coupling is present among long cortico-cortical fibers. Since neurodynamics includes many highly nonlinear processes (McKenna et al., 1994), MI analysis or other methods capable of measuring nonlinear dependencies among multichannel signals should be utilized to quantify both linear and nonlinear coupling interactions among cortical areas. The investigation of nonlinear interactions among cortical areas and their functional role will be, therefore, a critical issue in multi-channel analysis.

DISCUSSION

Significance of EEG Recordings in AD

There are several reasons why intensive research has been performed on the EEG in AD. One reason is that AD is a cortical dementia in which EEG abnormalities are more frequently shown. Subcortical dementias exhibit relatively normal EEG patterns compared with cortical dementias (Verma et al., 1987). The EEG abnormalities in AD directly reflect anatomical and functional deficits of the cerebral cortex damaged by the disease. Thus, the investigation of EEG dynamics is expected to provide with fruitful clues about the neuropathology of AD. Another reason is that coherence analysis of the EEG in AD allows non-invasive assessment of synaptic dysfunction. The synaptic plasticity is critical for brain functions, particularly learning and memory. A number of evidence suggest that disturbances of synaptic connections may underlie numerous neurological and psychiatric disorders including AD (Masliah and Terry, 1993), schizophrenia (Feinberg, 1983), epilepsy (Sutula, 1990), and Parkinsonism (Donnan et al., 1991). A decrease in functional connectivity and its correlation with the degree of dementia suggest that EEG coherence studies of AD may help understand the association between synaptic plasticity and cognitive performance (Cook and Leuchter, 1996). In addition to these reasons, it is of physical interest to investigate nonlinear EEG dynamics in AD to understand the role of nonlinearity in brain functions. Nonlinear dynamical analysis of the EEG has revealed that a decreased complexity of EEG patterns and reduced functional connections in AD are likely due to decreased nonlinear cell-dynamics and/or nonlinear couplings among cortical areas as well as linear couplings (Jelles et al., 1999b; Villa et al., 2000; Jeong et al., 2001b). Therefore, NDA of the EEG in dementias might provide potentially valuable diagnostic information about the progress of the disease that cannot be assessed by conventional analyses and a deeper understanding of the neuropathological mechanisms of dementias.

Limitations of NDA

With an increasing body of evidence for the usefulness of NDA in AD patients, there are several limitations on NDA to solve. First of all, the fundamental assumption of NDA that the EEG generates by a deterministic process is still disputable. Much research has proven the nonlinear, deterministic character of cortical dynamics. The EEG has a finite non-integer correlation dimension (D_2) and a positive value of averaged local Lyapunov exponents, indicating the presence of deterministic chaos in the EEG (Babloyantz, 1985; Soong and Stuart, 1989; Kowalik, 2000). The surrogate data method capable of detecting nonlinear determinism within a time series also revealed that EEG recordings have a nonlinear structure (Pritchard et al., 1995; Rombouts et al., 1995; Elhers et al., 1998; Jelles et al., 1999b; Stam et al., 1999; Kowalik, 2000). These findings support the hypothesis that brain oscillators are governed by nonlinear, deterministic processes. In contrast, there have been several studies reporting that the EEG may not be produced by a low-dimensional chaotic system (Theiler et al., 1992, Rapp et al., 1993; Theiler and Rapp, 1996; Pritchard et al., 1995). They demonstrated that filtered noise can mimic low-dimensional chaotic attractors as the EEG data do. Recently, more direct methods have been applied to detect nonlinear determinism within the EEG (Jeong et al., 1999, 2002a, b) to show that the EEG might not be generated by a low-dimensional deterministic process. Despite no compelling evidence for deterministic nature of the EEG, a large number of studies have shown that nonlinear dynamical methods allow characterization of different physiological and pathological brain states (for intensive reviews, see Wackermann, 1999; Le Van Quyen et al, 2001; Sarbadhikari and Chakrabarty, 2001). Therefore, nonlinear measures are meaningful only when they are used as a relative measure of complexity to quantify an irregular behavior of the brain, instead of being used as an absolute measure to differentiate between periodic, chaotic and stochastic dynamics.

Another limitation of NDA is that the absolute values of nonlinear measures depend sensitively on algorithms used or parameters in the algorithms, such as the embedding dimension, the time delay, the number of data point, and the cut-off noise level. Thus, in order to diagnose AD accurately, a large pool of sample data for autopsy-confirmed AD patients and the age- and sex-matched healthy controls and other patient groups are needed to compare their nonlinear measures with the algorithm and the parameters fixed. Furthermore, a large number of data points are required to reconstruct the whole attractor (i.e. entire dynamics of the system) in the phase space and thus to obtain reliable results. Unfortunately, the data length required for reliable results in principle is beyond the experimental possibility for physiological data.

Thirdly, given that nonlinear measures like the D_2 or L_1 reflect nonlinear dynamics of the attractor in the phase space reconstructed from the EEG, the physiological implications of the changes in these measures in pathological brain states are not clear. For example, the D_2 of the EEG indicates the number of parameters pertaining to the underlying cortical dynamics, but it does not provide any information on the physiological correspondence of each parameter. This shortcoming appears to limit the usefulness of NDA. Furthermore, the number of the degree of freedom revealed by the D_2 estimation of the EEG in AD is about 6 – 10 (Jeong, 2002), which is too high to develop a mathematical model to produce the EEG in AD patients. Although there have been several studies attempting to build up empirical, dynamical models based on raw EEG data and information obtained from NDA (Kadtke, 1995; Kadtke and Kremliovsky, 1996, 1997), mathematical theory and analysis methods for high-dimensional, physiological systems should be further developed and established (Cremers and Hubler, 1981; Crutchfield and McNamara, 1987).

Finally, it is noteworthy that nonlinear dynamics of the EEG is possibly influenced by many physiological factors including age (Meyer-Lindenberg, 1996; Anokhin et al., 1996, 2000), sex (Anokhin et al., 2000) and intelligence (Anokhin et al., 1999; Lutzenberger et al., 1992), as well as by the severity of the disease. Although the effect of normal aging on EEG dynamics is somewhat disputable (Visser, 1991; Dustman et al., 1993; Angeleri et al., 1997), the effect of these factors should be considered with caution during analysis to obtain reliable results and to have appropriate interpretations.

AD as a Dynamical Disease

Nonlinear dynamics and chaos theory suggest that Alzheimer's disease can be a dynamical disease which is characterized by changes in the qualitative dynamics of physiological processes, leading to abnormal dynamics and disease (Mackey and Milton, 1987; Belair et al., 1995). Ageing and age-related diseases often accompany a wide-ranging loss of physiological complexity from molecular to cellular, and from tissue to organismic levels (Kyriazis, 2003). The disruptions of fractal and nonlinear physiological properties leads to an increase in regularity and stochasticity (i.e. an increase in uncorrelated true randomness), a situation encountered during ageing and age-related diseases (Lipsitz and Goldberger, 1992; Toussaint and Schneider, 1998; Goldberger et al., 2002a,b). An underlying dysfunction of several individual subsystems, such as synaptic and receptor alterations and other molecular changes, might result in a loss of complex properties seen in ageing or AD brains (Narayanan et al., 2001; Yates, 2002). The deceased EEG complexity in AD might reflect a loss of physiological complexity at molecular or cellular level with wide-ranging cognitive changes. Interestingly, Nakayama et al. (2001) demonstrated that morphological patterns of senile plaques are very fractal. Therefore, it is significant to monitor alterations in EEG complexity in AD as the disease progresses, and furthermore, to reverse this loss and reinstate physiological complexity by applying multiple external physiological stimuli (Dokoumetzdis et al, 2001; Lipsitz, 2002).

Perspectives and Future Directions

EEG abnormalities of AD patients have been extensively studied for several decades. The role of the EEG in diagnosis and clinical evaluations of AD becomes more significant. One of the most critical issues of EEG studies on AD is improvement of the accuracy of differential diagnosis of AD and early detection in the preclinical stage. As mentioned earlier, the diagnostic accuracy of the EEG based on a broad survey of the literature is currently about 80%. One of proposed ideas for increasing the diagnostic accuracy is to use structural and functional neuroimaging methods, such as computed tomography (CT), magnetic resonance imaging (MRI), single photon emission computed tomography (SPECT), positron-emission tomography (PET), and functional magnetic resonance imaging (fMRI), in combination with the EEG. This multimodal approach has been found predominant for diagnosing dementias (for reviews, Scheltens and Korf, 2000; DeCarli, 2001; Jagust, 2001; Kumari et al., 2002; Albert, 2003; Kantarci and Jack, 2003; Petrella et al., 2003). For example, the combination of EEG and PET variables results in approximately 90% overall correct classification with a specificity of 100% (Jelic et al., 1999). EEG and MRI measurements of the hippocampus obtain the highest scores of abnormalities in patients with probable AD (Jonkman, 1997). Furthermore, CT- and MRI-based measurements of hippocampal atrophy provide a useful early marker of AD (Scheltens, 1999). These neuroimaging techniques can offer not only supplementary information for diagnosis of AD, but also an opportunity to explore structural, functional, and biochemical changes in the brain leading to new insights into the pathogenesis of AD.

The possible usefulness of the EEG in early detection of AD can be fully evaluated by examining EEG alterations in subjects having risk factors for AD. Particularly, EEG studies on MCI might facilitate the ability to diagnose AD at a very early stage, preferably before dementia symptoms are apparent. Although structural volumetric MRI, PET, and SPECT are currently most commonly used neuroimaging modalities in MCI studies, quantitative EEGs also have potential to become a valuable tool in early diagnosis of AD (Wolf et al., 2003). There is growing evidence from prospective studies that increased theta activity, decreased alpha and beta activity, and slowed mean frequency may be predictors of dementia in subjects with MCI (Elmståhl et al., 1997; Huang et al., 2000; Jelic et al., 2000) On the other hand, recent studies investigated whether or not genetic heterogeneity of ε4 allele of apolipoprotein E (APOE), a major biological risk factor for late onset AD, affected the EEG in AD patients (Lehtovirta et al., 1996, 2000; Jelic et al., 1997; Riekkinen et al., 1997; Alvarez et al., 1999). Jelic et al. (1997) found that AD patients homozygous for the APOE ε4 allele have reduced right and left temporoparietal, right temporofrontal, and left occipitoparietal coherence, indicating that APOE ε4 seems to be associated with selective decreases in functional connectivity as assessed by EEG coherence. Additionally, we expect that novel methods for EEG analysis will help improve the accuracy of early detection of AD (Musha et al., 2002; Stam et al., 2003).

Another important issue is to quantify the severity of the disease using the EEG to provide demented patients and their families with a more reliable prediction of the disease's course and appropriate clinical treatments and to facilitate planning for necessary social resources. Long-term follow-up studies of the EEG in subjects with MCI are quite necessary. Besides, quantitative changes of EEG dynamics in AD patients with treatment of drugs should be investigated.

Finally, the use of new mathematical methods is required to explore the abnormal cortical dynamics underlying the EEG in AD. Nonlinear dynamical methods might provide a useful tool to help in understanding brain electrical activity in terms of the collective dynamics of neurons, as well as improvement of the accuracy of differential and early diagnosis of AD. While spectral analysis of the EEG in AD patients has been intensively performed, many critical issues relating to nonlinear dynamics of the EEG in AD are rarely investigated. For instance, the association between nonlinear EEG dynamics and cognitive performance, longitudinal changes in nonlinear dynamics of the EEG during the progression of the disease, drug effects on nonlinear neurodynamics, and nonlinear functional connectivity among cortical areas afflicted by AD should be further examined. EEG studies on these issues using nonlinear dynamical methods might contribute to a deeper understanding of pathophysiology of AD in ways that are not possible by conventional spectral analysis.

ACKNOWLEDGEMENTS

This study was supported by Creative Research Initiatives of the Korean Ministry of Science and Technology.

REFERENCES

Abarbanel HD, Rabinovich MI. Neurodynamics: nonlinear dynamics and neurobiology. *Curr Opin Neurobiol* 2001;11:423-430.

Adler G, Brassen S. Short-term rivastigmine treatment reduces EEG slow-wave power in Alzheimer patients. *Neuropsychobiology* 2001;43;273-276.

Albert MS. Detection of very early Alzheimer disease through neuroimaging. *Alzheimer Dis Assoc Disord* 2003;17 Suppl 2:S63-S65.

Alvarez XA, Mouzo R, Pichel V, Perez P, Laredo M, Fernandez-Novoa L, Corzo L, Zas R, Alcaraz M, Secades JJ, Lozano R, Cacabelos R. Double-blind placebo-controlled study with citicoline in APOE genotyped Alzheimer's disease patients. Effects on cognitive performance, brain bioelectrical activity and cerebral perfusion. *Methods Find Exp Clin Pharmacol* 1999;21:633-644.

Angeleri F, Angeleri VA, Foschi N, Giaquinto S, Nolfe G, Saginario A, Signorino M. Depression after stroke: an investigation through catamnesis. *J Clin Psychiatry* 1997;58:261-265.

Anokhin AP, Birbaumer N, Lutzenberger W, Nikolaev A, Vogel F. Age increases brain complexity. *Electroencephalogr Clin Neurophysiol* 1996;99:63-68.

Anokhin AP, Lutzenberger W, Birbaumer N. Spatiotemporal organization of brain dynamics and intelligence: an EEG study in adolescents. *Int J Psychophysiol* 1999;33:259-273.

Anokhin AP, Lutzenberger W, Nikolaev A, Birbaumer N. Complexity of electrocortical dynamics in children: developmental aspects. *Dev Psychobiol* 2000;36:9-22.

Babloyantz A, Salazar JM, Nicolls C. Evidence of chaotic dynamics of brain activity during the sleep cycle. *Phys Lett A* 1985;111:152-156.

Bartus RT, Dean RL 3rd, Beer B, Lippa AS. The cholinergic hypothesis of geriatric memory dysfunction. *Science* 1982;217:408-414.

Belair J, Glass L, An Der Heiden U, Milton J. Dynamical disease: Identification, temporal aspects and treatment strategies of human illness. *Chaos* 1995;5:1-7.

Bennys K, Rondouin G, Vergnes C, Touchon J. Diagnostic value of quantitative EEG in Alzheimer's disease. *Neurophysiol Clin* 2001;31:153-160.

Berg L, Danziger WL, Storandt M, Coben LA, Gado M, Hughes CP, Knesevich JW, Botwinick J. Predictive features in mild senile dementia of the Alzheimer type. *Neurology* 1984;34:563-569.

Berger H, Über das Elektrenkephalogramm des Menschen. Dritte Mitteilung. *Arch Psychiatr Nervenkr* 1931:94:16-60.

Berger H. Dritte Mitteilung ber das Elektrenkephalogramm des Menschen. Fűnfte Mitteilung. *Arch Psychiatr Nervenkr* 1932:98:231-254.

Besthorn C, Forstl H, Geiger-Kabisch C, Sattel H, Gasser T, Schreiter-Gasser U. EEG coherence in Alzheimer disease. *Electroencephalogr Clin Neurophysiol* 1994;90:242-245.

Besthorn C, Sattel H, Geiger-Kabisch C, Zerfass R, Forstl H. Parameters of EEG dimensional complexity in Alzheimer's disease. *Electroencephalogr Clin Neurophysiol.* 1995;95:84-89.

Besthorn C, Zerfass R, Geiger-Kabisch C, Sattel H, Daniel S, Schreiter-Gasser U, Forstl H. Discrimination of Alzheimer's disease and normal aging by EEG data. *Electroencephalogr Clin Neurophysiol* 1997;103:241-248.

Bianchetti A, Trabucch M. Clinical aspects of Alzheimer's disease. *Aging Clin Exp Res* 2001;13:221-230.

Boerman RH, Scheltens P, Weinstein HC. Clinical neurophysiology in the diagnosis of Alzheimer's disease. *Clin Neurol Neurosurg* 1994;96:111-8.

Bracco L, Gallato R, Grigoletto F, Lippi A, Lepore V, Bino G, Lazzaro MP, Carella F, Piccolo T, Pozzilli C. Factors affecting course and survival in Alzheimer's disease: a 9-year longitudinal study. *Arch Neurol* 1994;51:1213-1219.

Brenner RP, Ulrich RF, Spiker DG, Sclabassi RJ, Reynolds CF 3rd, Marin RS, Boller F. Computerized EEG spectral analysis in elderly normal, demented and depressed subjects. *Electroencephalogr Clin Neurophysiol* 1986;64:483-492.

Brenner RP, Reynolds CF 3rd, Ulrich RF. Diagnostic efficacy of computerized spectral versus visual EEG analysis in elderly normal, demented and depressed subjects. *Electroencephalogr Clin Neurophysiol* 1988;69:110-117.

Brenner RP, Reynolds CF 3rd, Ulrich RF. EEG findings in depressive pseudodementia and dementia with secondary depression. *Electroencephalogr Clin Neurophysiol.* 1989;72:298-304.

Breslau J, Starr A, Sicotte N, Higa J, Buchsbaum MS. Topographic EEG changes with normal aging and SDAT. *Electroencephalogr Clin Neurophysiol* 1989;72:281-289.

Burns A, Zaudig M. Mild cognitive impairment in older people. *Lancet* 2002;360:1963-1965.

Buzsaki G, Bickford RG, Armstrong DM, Ponomareff G, Chen KS, Ruiz R, Thal LJ, Gage FH. Electric activity in the neocortex of freely moving young and aged rats. *Neuroscience* 1988;26:735-744.

Celesia GG, Jasper HH. Acetylcholine released from cerebral cortex in relation to state of activation. *Neurology* 1966;16:1053-1063.

Cerutti S, Carrault G, Cluitmans PJ, Kinie A, Lipping T, Nikolaidis N, Pitas I, Signorini MG. Non-linear algorithms for processing biological signals. *Comput Methods Programs Biomed* 1996;51:51-73.

Chen KS, Nishimura MC, Armanini MP, Crowley C, Spencer SD, Phillips HS. Disruption of a single allele of the nerve growth factor gene results in atrophy of basal forebrain cholinergic neurons and memory deficits. *J Neurosci* 1997;17:7288-7296.

Claus JJ, Ongerboer de Visser BW, Walstra GJ, Hijdra A, Verbeeten B Jr, van Gool WA. Quantitative spectral electroencephalography in predicting survival in patients with early Alzheimer disease. *Arch Neurol* 1998;55:1105-1111.

Claus JJ, Ongerboer De Visser BW, Bour LJ, Walstra GJ, Hijdra A, Verbeeten B Jr, Van Royen EA, Kwa VI, van Gool WA. Determinants of quantitative spectral electroencephalography in early Alzheimer's disease: cognitive function, regional cerebral blood flow, and computed tomography. *Dement Geriatr Cogn Disord* 2000;11:81-89.

Coben LA, Danziger WL, Berg L. Frequency analysis of the resting awake EEG in mild senile dementia of Alzheimer type. *Electroencephalogr Clin Neurophysiol* 1983;55:372-380.

Coben LA, Danziger W, Storandt M. A longitudinal EEG study of mild senile dementia of Alzheimer type: changes at 1 year and at 2.5 years. *Electroencephalogr Clin Neurophysiol* 1985;61:101-112.

Coben LA, Chi D, Snyder AZ, Storandt M. Replication of a study of frequency analysis of the resting awake EEG in mild probable Alzheimer's disease. *Electroencephalogr Clin Neurophysiol* 1990;75:148-154.

Collerton D. Cholinergic function and intellectual decline in Alzheimer's disease. *Neuroscience* 1986;19:1-28.

Comi GC, Fornara C, Locatelli T, Medaglini S, Cursi M, Minicucci F, Leocani L, Franceschi M. EEG coherence in Alzheimer and multi-infarct dementia. *Arch Gerontol Geriatr* 1998;suppl 6:91-98.

Cook IA, Leuchter AF. Synaptic dysfunction in Alzheimer's disease: clinical assessment using quantitative EEG. *Behav Brain Res* 1996;78:15-23.

Coyle JT, Price DL, DeLong MR. Alzheimer's disease: a disorder of cortical cholinergic innervation. *Science* 1983;219:1184-1190.

Cremers J, Hubler A. Construction of differential equations from experimental data. *Z. Naturforsch* 1981;42A:797-802.

Crutchfield JP, McNamara BS. Equations of motion from a data series. *Complex systems* 1987;1:417-452.

Cuculic Z, Bost K, Himwich HE. An examination of a possible cortical cholinergic link in the EEG arousal reaction. *Prog Brain Res* 1968;28:27-39.

Davis PC, Gearing M, Gray L, Mirra SS, Morris JC, Edland SD, Lin T, Heyman A. The CERAD experience, Part VIII: Neuroimaging-neuropathology correlates of temporal lobe changes in Alzheimer's disease. *Neurology* 1995;45:178-179.

Davis KL, Mohs RC, Marin D, Purohit DP, Perl DP, Lantz M, Austin G, Haroutunian V. Cholinergic markers in elderly patients with early signs of Alzheimer disease. *JAMA* 1999;281:1401-1406.

de Leon MJ, George AE, Stylopoulos LA, Smith G, Miller DC. Early marker for Alzheimer's disease: the atrophic hippocampus. *Lancet* 1989;2:672-673.

DeCarli C, Kaye JA, Horwitz B, Rapoport SI. Critical analysis of the use of computer-assisted transverse axial tomography to study human brain in aging and dementia of the Alzheimer type. *Neurology* 1990;40:872-883.

DeCarli C. The role of neuroimaging in dementia. *Clin Geriatr Med* 2001;17:255-279.

DeKosky ST, Ikonomovic MD, Styren SD, Beckett L, Wisniewski S, Bennett DA, Cochran EJ, Kordower JH, Mufson EJ. Upregulation of choline acetyltransferase activity in hippocampus and frontal cortex of elderly subjects with mild cognitive impairment. *Ann Neurol* 2002;51:145-155.

Devanand DP, Jacobs DM, Tang MX, Del Castillo-Castaneda C, Sano M, Marder K, Bell K, Bylsma FW, Brandt J, Albert M, Stern Y. The course of psychopathologic features in mild to moderate Alzheimer disease. *Arch Gen Psychiatry* 1997;54:257-263.

Dokoumetzidis A, Iliadis A, Macheras P. Nonlinear dynamics and chaos theory: concepts and applications relevant to pharmacodynamics. *Pharm Res* 2001;18:415-426.

Donnan GA, Woodhouse DG, Kaczmarczyk SJ, Holder JE, Paxinos G, Chilco PJ, Churchyard AJ, Kalnins RM, Fabinyi GC, Mendelsohn FA. Evidence for plasticity of the dopaminergic system in parkinsonism. *Mol Neurobiol* 1991;5:421-433.

Dunkin JJ, Leuchter AF, Newton TF, Cook IA. Reduced EEG coherence in dementia: state or trait marker? *Biol Psychiatry* 1994;35:870-879.

Dustman RE, Shearer DE, Emmerson RY. EEG and event-related potentials in normal aging. *Prog Neurobiol* 1993;41:369-401.

Ebert U, Kirch W. Scopolamine model of dementia: electroencephalogram findings and cognitive performance. *Eur J Clin Invest* 1998;28:944-949.

Ebert U, Grossmann M, Oertel R, Gramatte T, Kirch W. Pharmacokinetic-pharmacodynamic modeling of the electroencephalogram effects of scopolamine in healthy volunteers. *J Clin Pharmacol* 2001;41:51-60.

Ehlers CL, Havstad J, Prichard D, Theiler J. Low doses of ethanol reduce evidence for nonlinear structure in brain activity. *J Neurosci* 1998;18:7474-7486.

Elmståhl S, Rosen I, Gullberg B. Quantitative EEG in elderly patients with Alzheimer's disease and healthy controls. *Dementia* 1994;5:119-124.

Elmståhl S, Rosen I. Postural hypotension and EEG variables predict cognitive decline: results from a 5-year follow-up of healthy elderly women. *Dement Geriatr Cogn Disord* 1997;8:180-187.

Erkinjuntti T, Larsen T, Sulkava R, Ketonen L, Laaksonen R, Palo J. EEG in the differential diagnosis between Alzheimer's disease and vascular dementia. *Acta Neurol Scand* 1988;77:36-43.

Erkinjuntti T, Lee DH, Gao F, Steenhuis R, Eliasziw M, Fry R, Merskey H, Hachinski VC. Temporal lobe atrophy on magnetic resonance imaging in the diagnosis of early Alzheimer's disease. *Arch Neurol* 1993;50:305-310.

Esiri MM, Pearson RC, Powell TP. The cortex of the primary auditory area in Alzheimer's disease. *Brain Res* 1986;366:385-387.

Ettlin TM, Staehelin HB, Kischka U, Ulrich J, Scollo-Lavizzari G, Wiggli U, Seiler WO. Computed tomography, electroencephalography, and clinical features in the differential diagnosis of senile dementia: a prospective clinicopathologic study. *Arch Neurol* 1989;46:1217-1220.

Faure P, Korn H. Is there chaos in the brain? I. Concepts of nonlinear dynamics and methods of investigation. *CR Acad Sci III* 2001;324:773-793.

Feinberg I. Schizophrenia: caused by a fault in programmed synaptic elimination during adolescence? *J Psychiatr Res* 1982-83;17:319-334.

Fell J, Roschke J, Bechmann P. Deterministic chaos and the first positive Lyapunov exponent: a nonlinear analysis of the human electroencephalogram during sleep. *Biol Cybern* 1993;69:139-146.

Fell J, Rochke J, Beckmann P. Nonlinear analysis of sleep EEG data in schizophrenia: calculation of the principal Lyapunov exponent. *Psychiatry Research* 1995;56:257-269.

Filipovitch S, Gueguen B, Derouesne C, Ancri D, Bourdel MC, Plancon D. Dementia of Alzheimer type: some features of the posterior cerebral electrical activity. *Psychiatry Res* 1989;29:409-410.

Förstl H, Kurz A. Clinical features of Alzheimer's disease. *Eur Arch Psychiatry Clin Neurosci* 1999;249:288-290.

Fraser AM, Swinney HL. Independent coordinates for strange attractors from mutual information. *Phys Rev A* 1986;33:1134-1140.

Giannitrapani D, Collins J, Vassiliadis D. The EEG spectra of Alzheimer's disease. *Int J Psychophysiol* 1991;10:259-269.

Giaquinto S, Nolfe G. The EEG in the normal elderly: a contribution to the interpretation of aging and dementia. *Electroencephalogr Clin Neurophysiol* 1986;63:540-546.

Goldberger AL, Amaral LA, Hausdorff JM, Ivanov PCh, Peng CK, Stanley HE. Fractal dynamics in physiology: alterations with disease and aging. *Proc Natl Acad Sci USA* 2002a;99 Suppl 1:2466-2472.

Goldberger AL, Peng CK, Lipsitz LA. What is physiologic complexity and how does it change with aging and disease? *Neurobiol Aging* 2002b;23:23-26.

Grassberger P, Procaccia I. Measuring the strangeness of strange attractors. *Physica D* 1983;9:189-208.

Grunwald M, Busse F, Hensel A, Riedel-Heller S, Kruggel F, Arendt T, Wolf H, Gertz HJ. Theta-power differences in patients with mild cognitive impairment under rest condition and during haptic tasks. *Alzheimer Dis Assoc Disord* 2002;16:40-48.

Harrison MJ, Thomas DJ, Du Boulay GH, Marshall J. Multi-infarct dementia. *J Neurol Sci* 1979;40:97-103.

Hassainia F, Petit D, Nielsen T, Gauthier S, Montplaisir J. Quantitative EEG and statistical mapping of wakefulness and REM sleep in the evaluation of mild to moderate Alzheimer's disease. *Eur Neurol* 1997;37:219-224.

Hegger R, Kantz H, Schreiber T. Practical implementation of nonlinear time series methods: The TISEAN package. Chaos 1999;9:413-435. *http://www.mpipks-dresden.mpg.de/~tisean/TISEAN_2.1/index.html*

Helkala EL, Laulumaa V, Soikkeli R, Partanen J, Soininen H, Riekkinen PJ. Slow-wave activity in the spectral analysis of the electroencephalogram is associated with cortical dysfunctions in patients with Alzheimer's disease. *Behav Neurosci* 1991;105: 409-415.

Hier DB, Mangone CA, Ganellen R, Warach JD, Van Egeren R, Perlik SJ, Gorelick PB. Quantitative measurement of delta activity in Alzheimer's disease. *Clin Electroencephalogr* 1991;22:178-182.

Hooijer C, Jonker C, Posthuma J, Visser SL. Reliability, validity and follow-up of the EEG in senile dementia: sequelae of sequential measurement. *Electroencephalogr Clin Neurophysiol* 1990;76:400-412.

Huang C, Wahlund L, Dierks T, Julin P, Winblad B, Jelic V. Discrimination of Alzheimer's disease and mild cognitive impairment by equivalent EEG sources: a cross-sectional and longitudinal study. *Clin Neurophysiol* 2000;111:1961-1967.

Hughes JR, Shanmugham S, Wetzel LC, Bellur S, Hughes CA. The relationship between EEG changes and cognitive functions in dementia: a study in a VA population. *Clin Electroencephalogr* 1989;20:77-85.

Ihl R, Dierks T, Froelich L, Martin EM, Maurer K. Segmentation of the spontaneous EEG in dementia of the Alzheimer type. *Neuropsychobiology* 1993;27:231-236.

Ikawa M, Nakanishi M, Furukawa T, Nakaaki S, Hori S, Yoshida S. Relationship between EEG dimensional complexity and neuropsychological findings in Alzheimer's disease. *Psychiatry Clin Neurosci* 2000;54:537-541.

Iqbal K, Alonso Adel C, El-Akkad E, Gong CX, Haque N, Khatoon S, Pei JJ, Tsujio I, Wang JZ, Grundke-Iqbal I. Significance and mechanism of Alzheimer neurofibrillary degeneration and therapeutic targets to inhibit this lesion. *J Mol Neurosci* 2002;19:95-99.

Jack CR Jr, Petersen RC, O'Brien PC, Tangalos EG. MR-based hippocampal volumetry in the diagnosis of Alzheimer's disease. *Neurology* 1992;42:183-188.

Jagust WJ. Neuroimaging in dementia. *Neurol Clin* 2000;18:885-902.

Jelic V, Shigeta M, Julin P, Almkvist O, Winblad B, Wahlund LO. Quantitative electroencephalography power and coherence in Alzheimer's disease and mild cognitive impairment. *Dementia* 1996;7:314-323.

Jelic V, Julin P, Shigeta M, Nordberg A, Lannfelt L, Winblad B, Wahlund LO. Apolipoprotein E epsilon4 allele decreases functional connectivity in Alzheimer's disease as measured by EEG coherence. *J Neurol Neurosurg Psychiatry* 1997;63:59-65.

Jelic V. Early diagnosis of Alzheimer's disease: focus on quantitative EEG in relation to genetic, biochemical and neuroimaging markers. *PhD thesis,* 1999.

Jelic V, Wahlund L-O, Almkvist O, Johansson S-E, Shigeta M, Winblad B, Nordberg A. Diagnostic accuracies of quantitative EEG and PET in mild Alzheimer's disease. *Alzheimer's reports* 1999;2:291-298.

Jelic V, Johansson SE, Almkvist O, Shigeta M, Julin P, Nordberg A, Winblad B, Wahlund LO. Quantitative electroencephalography in mild cognitive impairment: longitudinal changes and possible prediction of Alzheimer's disease. *Neurobiol Aging* 2000;21:533-540.

Jelles B, Strijers RL, Hooijer C, Jonker C, Stam CJ, Jonkman EJ. Nonlinear EEG analysis in early Alzheimer's disease. *Acta Neurol Scand* 1999a;100:360-368.

Jelles B, van Birgelen JH, Slaets JP, Hekster RE, Jonkman EJ, Stam CJ. Decrease of non-linear structure in the EEG of Alzheimer patients compared to healthy controls. *Clin Neurophysiol* 1999b;110:1159-1167.

Jeong J, Kim SY, Han SH. Non-linear dynamical analysis of the EEG in Alzheimer's disease with optimal embedding dimension. *Electroencephalogr Clin Neurophysiol* 1998;106:220-228.

Jeong J, Kim MS, Kim SY. Test for low-dimensional determinism in electroencephalogram. *Phys Rev E* 1999;60:831-837.

Jeong J, Chae JH, Kim SY, Han SH. Nonlinear dynamic analysis of the EEG in patients with Alzheimer's disease and vascular dementia. *J Clin Neurophysiol* 2001a;18:58-67.

Jeong J, Gore JC, Peterson BS. Mutual information analysis of the EEG in patients with Alzheimer's disease. *Clin Neurophysiol* 2001b;112:827-835.

Jeong J. Nonlinear dynamics of EEG in Alzheimer's disease. *Drug Dev Res* 2002;56:57-66.

Jeong J. EEG dynamics in patients with Alzheimer's disease. *Clin Neurophysiol* 2004;115:1490-1505.

Jeong J, Gore JC, Peterson BS. Detecting determinism in short time series, with an application to the analysis of a stationary EEG recording. *Biol Cybern* 2002a;86:335-342.

Jeong J, Gore JC, Peterson BS. A method for determinism in short time series, and its application to stationary EEG. *IEEE Trans Biomed Eng* 2002b;49:1374-1379.

Johannesson G, Brun A, Gustafson I, Ingvar DH. EEG in presenile dementia related to cerebral blood flow and autopsy findings. *Acta Neurol Scand* 1977;56:89-103.

Johannesson G, Hagberg B, Gustafson L, Ingvar DH. EEG and cognitive impairment in presenile dementia. *Acta Neurol Scand* 1979;59:225-240.

Jonkman EJ. The role of the electroencephalogram in the diagnosis of dementia of the Alzheimer type: an attempt at technology assessment. *Neurophysiol Clin* 1997;27:211-219.

Kadtke J. Classification of highly noise signals using global dynamical models. *Phys Lett A* 1995;203:196-202.

Kadtke J, Kremliovsky M. Classifying complex, deterministic signals. In: Iurii Aleksandrovich Kravtsov, editor. *Predictability of complex dynamical systems.* Berlin, Heidelberg: Springer, 1996:78-102.

Kanai T, Szerb JC. Mesencephalic reticular activiating system and cortical acetylcholine output. *Nature* 1965;2-5:80-82.

Kantarci K, Jack CR Jr. Neuroimaging in Alzheimer disease: an evidence-based review. *Neuroimaging Clin N Am* 2003;13:197-209.

Kantz H, Schreiber T. *Nonlinear time series analysis. Cambridge nonlinear science series* 7, Cambridge University press, Cambridge, 1997.

Kennel MB, Brown R, Abarbanel HDI. 1992. Determining embedding dimension for phase-space reconstruction using a geometrical construction. *Phys Rev A* 1992;45:3403-3411.

Kikuchi M, Wada Y, Koshino Y, Nanbu Y, Hashimoto T. Effects of scopolamine on interhemispheric EEG coherence in healthy subjects: analysis during rest and photic stimulation. *Clin Electroencephalogr* 2000;31:109-115.

Knott V, Mohr E, Mahoney C, Ilivitsky V. Electroencephalographic coherence in Alzheimer's disease: comparisons with a control group and population norms. *J Geriatr Psychiatry Neurol* 2000b;13:1-8.

Kogan EA, Korczyn AD, Virchovsky RG, Klimovizky SSh, Treves TA, Neufeld MY. EEG changes during long-term treatment with donepezil in Alzheimer's disease patients. *J Neural Transm* 2001;108:1167-1173.

Kowalik ZJ. Nonlinear mechanisms of cortical oscillations. *Neurol Neurochir Pol* 2000;34(2 Suppl):53-65.

Kowalski JW, Gawel M, Pfeffer A, Barcikowska M. The diagnostic value of EEG in Alzheimer disease: correlation with the severity of mental impairment. *J Clin Neurophysiol* 2001;18:570-575.

Kumari V, Mitterschiffthaler MT, Sharma T. Neuroimaging to predict preclinical Alzheimer's disease. *Hosp Med* 2002;63:341-345.

Kyriazis M. Practical applications of chaos theory to the modulation of human ageing: nature prefers chaos to regularity. *Biogerontology* 2003;4:75-90.

Lahiri DK, Farlow MR, Greig NH, Sambamurti K. Current drug targets for Alzheimer's disease treatment. *Drug Dev Res* 2002;56:267-281.

Le Van Quyen M, Martinerie J, Navarro V, Baulac M, Varela FJ. Characterizing neurodynamic changes before seizures. *J Clin Neurophysiol* 2001;18:191-208.

Lee DY, Lee JH, Ju YS, Lee KU, Kim KW, Jhoo JH, Yoon JC, Ha J, Woo JI. The prevalence of dementia in older people in an urban population of Korea: the Seoul study. *J Am Geriatr Soc* 2002;50:1233-1239.

Lehtovirta M, Partanen J, Kononen M, Soininen H, Helisalmi S, Mannermaa A, Ryynanen M, Hartikainen P, Riekkinen P Sr. Spectral analysis of EEG in Alzheimer's disease: relation to apolipoprotein E polymorphism. *Neurobiol Aging* 1996;17:523-526.

Lehtovirta M, Partanen J, Kononen M, Hiltunen J, Helisalmi S, Hartikainen P, Riekkinen P Sr, Soininen H. A longitudinal quantitative EEG study of Alzheimer's disease: relation to apolipoprotein E polymorphism. *Dement Geriatr Cogn Disord* 2000;11:29-35.

Leuchter AF, Spar JE, Walter DO, Weiner H. Electroencephalographic spectra and coherence in the diagnosis of Alzheimer's-type and multi-infarct dementia: a pilot study. *Arch Gen Psychiatry* 1987;44:993-998.

Leuchter AF, Newton TF, Cook IA, Walter DO, Rosenberg-Thompson S, Lachenbruch PA. Changes in brain functional connectivity in Alzheimer-type and multi-infarct dementia. *Brain* 1992;115:1543-1561.

Leuchter AF, Cook IA, Newton TF, Dunkin J, Walter DO, Rosenberg-Thompson S, Lachenbruch PA, Weiner H. Regional differences in brain electrical activity in dementia: use of spectral power and spectral ratio measures. *Electroencephalogr Clin Neurophysiol* 1993;87:385-393.

Lewis DA, Campbell MJ, Terry RD, Morrison JH. Laminar and regional distributions of neurofibrillary tangles and neuritic plaques in Alzheimer's disease: a quantitative study of visual and auditory cortices. *J Neurosci* 1987;7:1799-1808.

Lindau M, Jelic V, Johansson SE, Andersen C, Wahlund LO, Almkvist O. Quantitative EEG abnormalities and cognitive dysfunctions in frontotemporal dementia and Alzheimer's disease. *Dement Geriatr Cogn Disord* 2003;15:106-114.

Lipsitz LA. Dynamics of stability: the physiologic basis of functional health and frailty. *J Gerontol A Biol Sci Med Sci* 2002;57:B115-B125.

Lipsitz LA, Goldberger AL. Loss of 'complexity' and aging. Potential applications of fractals and chaos theory to senescence. *JAMA* 1992;267:1806-1809.

Locatelli T, Cursi M, Liberati D, Franceschi M, Comi G. EEG coherence in Alzheimers disease. *Electroenceph clin Neurophys* 1998;106:229-237.

Lutzenberger W, Birbaumer N, Flor H, Rockstroh B, Elbert T. Dimensional analysis of the human EEG and intelligence. *Neurosci Lett* 1992;143:10-14.

Mackey MC, Milton JG. Dynamical diseases. *Ann N Y Acad Sci* 1987;504:16-32.

Masliah E, Terry R. The role of synaptic proteins in the pathogenesis of disorders of the central nervous system. *Brain Pathol* 1993;3:77-85.

Maurer K, Dierks T. Functional imaging procedures in dementias: mapping of EEG and evoked potentials. *Acta Neurol Scand Suppl* 1992;139:40-46.

McKenna TM, McMullen TA, Shlesinger MF. The brain as a dynamic physical system. *Neuroscience* 1994;60:587-605.

Metherate R, Cox CL, Ashe JH. Cellular bases of neocortical activation: modulation of neural oscillations by the nucleus basalis and endogenous acetylcholine. *J Neurosci* 1992;12:4701-4711.

Meyer-Lindenberg A. The evolution of complexity in human brain development: an EEG study. *Electroencephalogr Clin Neurophysiol* 1996;99:405-411.

Moe KE, Larsen LH, Prinz PN, Vitiello MV. Major unipolar depression and mild Alzheimer's disease: differentiation by quantitative tonic REM EEG. *Electroencephalogr Clin Neurophysiol* 1993;86:238-246.

Montplaisir J, Petit D, McNamara D, Gauthier S. Comparisons between SPECT and quantitative EEG measures of cortical impairment in mild to moderate Alzheimer's disease. *Eur Neurol* 1996;36:197-200.

Musha T, Asada T, Yamashita F, Kinoshita T, Chen Z, Matsuda H, Uno M, Shankle WR. A new EEG method for estimating cortical neuronal impairment that is sensitive to early stage Alzheimer's disease. *Clin Neurophysiol* 2002; 113:1052-1058.

Nakayama H, Kiatipattanasakul W, Nakamura S, Miyawaki K, Kikuta F, Uchida K, Kuroki K, Makifuchi T, Yoshikawa Y, Doi K. Fractal analysis of senile plaque observed in various animal species. *Neurosci Lett* 2001;297:195-198.

Nestor PJ, Scheltens P, Hodges JR. Advances in the early detection of Alzheimer's disease. *Nat Med* 2004;10 Suppl: S34-41.

Neufeld MY, Blumen S, Aitkin I, Parmet Y, Korczyn AD. EEG frequency analysis in demented and nondemented parkinsonian patients. *Dementia* 1994a;5:23-28.

Narayanan K, Collins JJ, Hamner J, Mukai S, Lipsitz LA. Predicting cerebral blood flow response to orthostatic stress from resting dynamics: effects of healthy aging. *Am J Physiol Regul Integr Comp Physiol* 2001;281:R716-R722.

Neufeld MY, Rabey MJ, Parmet Y, Sifris P, Treves TA, Korczyn AD. Effects of a single intravenous dose of scopolamine on the quantitative EEG in Alzheimer's disease patients and age-matched controls. *Electroencephalogr Clin Neurophysiol* 1994b;91:407-412.

O'Conner JL, Allen MB, Mahesh VB. Evaluation of in vitro incubation systems for the study of gonadotropin release. *Endocr Res Commun* 1979;6:15-36.

Passero S, Rocchi R, Vatti G, Burgalassi L, Battistini N. Quantitative EEG mapping, regional cerebral blood flow, and neuropsychological function in Alzheimer's disease. *Dementia* 1995;6:148-156.

Pearson RC, Esiri MM, Hiorns RW, Wilcock GK, Powell TP. Anatomical correlates of the distribution of the pathological changes in the neocortex in Alzheimer disease. *Proc Natl Acad Sci USA* 1985;82:4531-4534.

Penttilä M, Partanen JV, Soininen H, Riekkinen PJ. Quantitative analysis of occipital EEG in different stages of Alzheimer's disease. *Electroencephalogr Clin Neurophysiol* 1985;60:1-6.

Petersen RC, Smith GE, Waring SC, Ivnik RJ, Tangalos EG, Kokmen E. Mild cognitive impairment: clinical characterization and outcome. *Arch Neurol* 1999;56:303-308.

Petit D, Montplaisir J, Lorrain D, Gauthier S. Spectral analysis of the rapid eye movement sleep electroencephalogram in right and left temporal regions: a biological marker of Alzheimer's disease. *Ann Neurol* 1992;32:172-176.

Petit D, Lorrain D, Gauthier S, Montplaisir J. Regional spectral analysis of the REM sleep EEG in mild to moderate Alzheimer's disease. *Neurobiol Aging* 1993;14:141-145.

Petrella JR, Coleman RE, Doraiswamy PM. Neuroimaging and early diagnosis of Alzheimer disease: a look to the future. *Radiology* 2003;226:315-36.

Petrosian AA, Prokhorov DV, Lajara-Nanson W, Schiffer RB. Recurrent neural network-based approach for early recognition of Alzheimer's disease in EEG. *Clin Neurophysiol* 2001;112:1378-1387.

Pezard L, Martinerie J, Varela FJ, Bouchet F, Guez D, Derouesne C, Renault B. Entropy maps characterize drug effects on brain dynamics in Alzheimer's disease. *Neurosci Lett* 1998;253:5-8.

Price JL, Ko AI, Wade MJ, Tsou SK, McKeel DW, Morris JC. Neuron number in the entorhinal cortex and CA1 in preclinical Alzheimer disease. *Arch Neurol* 2001;58:1395-1402.

Price JL, Morris JC. Tangles and plaques in nondemented aging and "preclinical" Alzheimer's disease. *Ann Neurol* 1999;45:358-368.

Prichep LS, John ER, Ferris SH, Reisberg B, Almas M, Alper K, Cancro R. Quantitative EEG correlates of cognitive deterioration in the elderly. *Neurobiol Aging* 1994;15:85-90.

Prinz PN, Larsen LH, Moe KE, Vitiello MV. EEG markers of early Alzheimer's disease in computer selected tonic REM sleep. *Electroencephalogr Clin Neurophysiol* 1992;83:36-43.

Pritchard WS, Duke DW. Measuring chaos in the brain: a tutorial review of nonlinear dynamical EEG analysis. *Int J Neurosci* 1992;67:31-80.

Pritchard WS, Duke DW, Coburn KL. Altered EEG dynamical responsivity associated with normal aging and probable Alzheimer's disease. *Dementia* 1991;2:102-105.

Pritchard WS, Duke DW, Coburn KL, Moore NC, Tucker KA. Altered EEG dynamical responsivity associated with Alzheimer's disease: replication and extension. In: Jansen BH, Brandt ME, editors. *Proceedings of the second annual conference on nonlinear dynamical analysis of the EEG*. Singapore: World Scientific, 1993;165-168.

Pritchard WS, Duke DW, Coburn KL, Moore NC, Tucker KA, Jann MW, Hostetler RM. EEG-based, neural-net predictive classification of Alzheimer's disease versus control subjects is augmented by non-linear EEG measures. *Electroencephalogr Clin Neurophysiol* 1994;91:118-130.

Pritchard WS, Duke DW, Krieble KK. Dimensional analysis of resting human EEG II: Surrogate data testing indicates nonlinearity but not low-dimensional chaos. *Psychophysiology* 1995;32:486-491.

Rapp PE, Albano AM, Schmah TI, Farwell LA. Filtered noise can mimic low-dimensional chaotic attractors. *Phys Rev E* 1993;47:2289-2297.

Reeves RR, Struve FA, Patrick G. The effects of donepezil on quantitative EEG in patients with Alzheimer's disease. *Clin Electroencephalogr* 2002;33:93-96.

Reinikainen KJ, Riekkinen PJ, Paljarvi L, Soininen H, Helkala EL, Jolkkonen J, Laakso M. Cholinergic deficit in Alzheimer's disease: a study based on CSF and autopsy data. *Neurochem Res* 1988;13:135-146.

Riekkinen P Jr, Soininen H, Partanen J, Paakkonen A, Helisalmi S, Riekkinen P Sr. The ability of THA treatment to increase cortical alpha waves is related to apolipoprotein E genotype of Alzheimer disease patients. *Psychopharmacology (Berl)* 1997;129:285-288.

Reisberg B, Auer SR, Monteiro I, Boksay I, Sclan SG. Behavioral disturbances of dementia: an overview of phenomenology and methodologic concerns. *Int Psychogeriatr* 1996;8 Suppl 2:169-180

Reynolds CF 3rd, Kupfer DJ, Houck PR, Hoch CC, Stack JA, Berman SR, Zimmer B. Reliable discrimination of elderly depressed and demented patients by electroencephalographic sleep data. *Arch Gen Psychiatry* 1988;45:258-264.

Rice DM, Buchsbaum MS, Starr A, Auslander L, Hagman J, Evans WJ. Abnormal EEG slow activity in left temporal areas in senile dementia of the Alzheimer type. *J Gerontol Med Sci* 1990;45:M145-151.

Ritchie K, Lovestone S. The dementias. *Lancet* 2002;360:1759-1766.

Robinson DJ, Merskey H, Blume WT, Fry R, Williamson PC, Hachinski VC. Electroencephalography as an aid in the exclusion of Alzheimer's disease. *Arch Neurol* 1994;51:280-284.

Rodriguez G, Vitali P, De Leo C, De Carli F, Girtler N, Nobili F. Quantitative EEG changes in Alzheimer patients during long-term donepezil therapy. *Neuropsychobiology* 2002;46:49-56.

Rogers J, Morrison JH. Quantitative morphology and regional and laminar distributions of senile plaques in Alzheimer's disease. *J Neurosci* 1985;5:2801-2808.

Rombouts SARB, Keunen RWM, Stam CJ Investigation of nonlinear structure in multichannel EEG. *Phys Lett A* 202;352-358.

Röschke J, Aldenhoff J. The dimensionality of the human's electroencephalogram during sleep. *Biol Cybern* 1991;64:307-313.

Rosen I. Electroencephalography as a diagnostic tool in dementia; a review. *Acta Neurol Scand Suppl* 1996;168:63-70.

Rosen I, Gustafson L, Risberg J. Multichannel EEG frequency analysis and somatosensory-evoked potentials in patients with different types of organic dementia. *Dementia* 1993;4:43-49.

Saletu B, Anderer P, Paulus E, Grunberger J, Wicke L, Neuhold A, Fischhof PK, Litschauer G. EEG brain mapping in diagnostic and therapeutic assessment of dementia. *Alzheimer Dis Assoc Disord* 1991;5 Suppl 1:S57-75.

Sannita WG, Maggi L, Rosadini G. Effects of scopolamine (0.25-0.75 mg i.m.) on the quantitative EEG and the neuropsychological status of healthy volunteers. *Neuropsychobiology* 1987;17:199-205.

Sarbadhikari SN, Chakrabarty K. Chaos in the brain: a short review alluding to epilepsy, depression, exercise and lateralization. *Med Eng Phys* 2001;23:445-455.

Sarter M, Bruno JP. Abnormal regulation of corticopetal cholinergic neurons and impaired information processing in neuropsychiatric disorders. *Trends Neurosci* 1999;22:67-74.

Sarter M, Bruno JP. Mild cognitive impairment and the cholinergic hypothesis: a very different take on recent data. *Ann Neurol* 2002;52:384-385.

Sarter M, Turchi J. Age- and dementia-associated impairments in divided attention: psychological constructs, animal models, and underlying neuronal mechanisms. *Dement Geriatr Cogn Disord* 2002;13:46-58.

Scheltens P, Leys D, Barkhof F, Huglo D, Weinstein HC, Vermersch P, Kuiper M, Steinling M, Wolters EC, Valk J. Atrophy of medial temporal lobes on MRI in probable Alzheimer's disease and normal ageing: diagnostic value and neuropsychological correlates. *J Neurol Neurosurg Psychiatry* 1992;55:967-972.

Scheltens P. Early diagnosis of dementia: neuroimaging. *J Neurol* 1999;246:16-20.

Scheltens P, Korf ES. Contribution of neuroimaging in the diagnosis of Alzheimer's disease and other dementias. *Curr Opin Neurol* 2000;13:391-396.

Schreiber T. Interdisciplinary application of nonlinear time series methods. *Phys Rep* 1999;308:2-64.

Schreiber T, Schmitz A. Surrogate time series. *Physica D* 2000;142:346-382.

Schreiter-Gasser U, Gasser T, Ziegler P. Quantitative EEG analysis in early onset Alzheimer's disease: a controlled study. *Electroencephalogr Clin Neurophysiol* 1993;86:15-22.

Schreiter-Gasser U, Gasser T, Ziegler P. Quantitative EEG analysis in early onset Alzheimer's disease: correlations with severity, clinical characteristics, visual EEG and CCT. *Electroencephalogr Clin Neurophysiol* 1994;90:267-272.

Selkoe DJ. Cell biology of the amyloid beta-protein precursor and the mechanism of Alzheimer's disease. *Annu Rev Cell Biol* 1994;10:373-403.

Sloan EP, Fenton GW. Serial visual evoked potential recordings in geriatric psychiatry. *Electroencephalogr Clin Neurophysiol* 84:325-331, 1992.

Sloan EP, Fenton GW. EEG power spectra and cognitive change in geriatric psychiatry: a longitudinal study. *Electroencephalogr Clin Neurophysiol* 1993;86:361-367.

Sloan EP, Fenton GW, Kennedy NS, MacLennan JM. Neurophysiology and SPECT cerebral blood flow patterns in dementia. *Electroencephalogr Clin Neurophysiol* 1994;91:163-170.

Smith MA, Casadesus G, Joseph JA, Perry G. Amyloid-beta and tau serve antioxidant functions in the aging and Alzheimer brain. *Free Radic Biol Med* 2002;33:1194-1199.

Soininen H, Partanen VJ, Helkala EL, Riekkinen PJ. EEG findings in senile dementia and normal aging. *Acta Neurol Scand* 1982;65:59-70.

Soininen H, Reinikainen KJ, Partanen J, Helkala EL, Paljarvi L, Riekkinen PJ. Slowing of electroencephalogram and choline acetyltransferase activity in post mortem frontal cortex in definite Alzheimer's disease. *Neuroscience* 1992;49:529-535.

Soong ACK, Stuart CIJM. Evidence of chaotic dynamics underlying the human alpha-rhythm electroencephalogram. *Biol Cybern* 1989;62:55-62.

Spehlmann R, Norcross K. Cholinergic mechanisms in the production of focal cortical slow waves. *Experientia* 1982;38:109-111.

Sramek JJ, Zarotsky V, Cutler NR. Review of drug development and therapeutic role of cholinesterase inhibitors in Alzheimer's disease. *Drug Dev Res* 2002;56:347-353.

Stam CJ, Tavy DL, Jelles B, Achtereekte HA, Slaets JP, Keunen RW. Non-linear dynamical analysis of multichannel EEG: clinical applications in dementia and Parkinson's disease. *Brain Topogr* 1994;7:141-150.

Stam CJ, Jelles B, Achtereekte HA, Rombouts SA, Slaets JP, Keunen RW. Investigation of EEG non-linearity in dementia and Parkinson's disease. *Electroencephalogr Clin Neurophysiol* 1995;95:309-317.

Stam CJ, Pijn JP, Suffczynski P, Lopes da Silva FH. Dynamics of the human alpha rhythm: evidence for non-linearity? *Clin Neurophysiol* 1999;110:1801-1813.

Stam CJ, van der Made Y, Pijnenburg YA, Scheltens P. EEG synchronization in mild cognitive impairment and Alzheimer's disease. *Acta Neurol Scand* 2003;108:90-96.

Stigsby B, Johannesson G, Ingvar DH. Regional EEG analysis and regional cerebral blood flow in Alzheimer's and Pick's diseases. *Electroencephalogr Clin Neurophysiol* 1981;51:537-547.

Storey E, Slavin MJ, Kinsella GJ. Patterns of cognitive impairment in Alzheimer's disease: assessment and differential diagnosis. *Front Biosci* 2002;7:e155-184.

Strijers RLM, Scheltens P, Jonkman EJ, de Rijke W, Hooijer C, Jonker C. Diagnosing Alzheimer's disease in community-dewelling elderly: a comparison of EEG and MRI. *Dementia* 1997;8:198-202.

Sutula TP. Experimental models of temporal lobe epilepsy: new insights from the study of kindling and synaptic reorganization. *Epilepsia* 1990;31 Suppl 3:S45-54.

Szelies B, Grond M, Herholz K, Kessler J, Wullen T, Heiss WD. Quantitative EEG mapping and PET in Alzheimer's disease. *J Neurol Sci* 1992;110:46-56.

Takens F. Detecting strange attractors in turbulence in dynamical systems and turbulence. *Lecture Notes in Mathematics* 1981;898:366-381.

Theiler J, Eubank S, Longtin A, Galdrikian B, Farmer JD. Testing for nonlinearity in times series: the method of surrogate data. *Physica D* 1992;58:77-94.

Theiler J, Rapp PE. Re-examination of the evidence for low-dimensional, nonlinear structure in the human electroencephalogram. *Electroencephalogr Clin Neurophysiol* 1996;98:213-222.

Toussaint O, Schneider ED. The thermodynamics and evolution of complexity in biological systems. *Comp Biochem Physiol A Mol Integr Physiol* 1998;120:3-9.

Verma NP, Greiffenstein MF, Verma N, King SD, Caldwell DL. Electrophysiologic validation of two categories of dementias--cortical and subcortical. *Clin Electroencephalogr* 1987;18:26-33.

Vicioso BA. Dementia: when is it not Alzheimer disease? *Am J Med Sci* 2002;324:84-95.

Villa AE, Tetko IV, Dutoit P, Vantini G. Non-linear cortico-cortical interactions modulated by cholinergic afferences from the rat basal forebrain. *Biosystems* 2000;58:219-228.

Visser SL, Van Tilburg W, Hooijer C, Jonker C, De Rijke W. Visual evoked potentials (VEPs) in senile dementia (Alzheimer type) and in non-organic behavioural disorders in the elderly; comparison with EEG parameters. *Electroencephalogr Clin Neurophysiol* 1985;60:115-121.

Visser SL. The electroencephalogram and evoked potentials in normal aging and dementia. *Electroencephalogr Clin Neurophysiol* 1991;Suppl 42:289-303.

Wackermann J. Towards a quantitative characterisation of functional states of the brain: from the non-linear methodology to the global linear description. *Int J Psychophysiol* 1999;34:65-80.

Wolf A, Swift JB, Swinney HL, Vastano JA. Deterministic Lyapunov exponents from a time series. *Physica D* 1985;16:285-317.

Wolf H, Jelic V, Gertz HJ, Nordberg A, Julin P, Wahlund LO. A critical discussion of the role of neuroimaging in mild cognitive impairment. *Acta Neurol Scand Suppl.* 2003;179:52-76.

Woyshville MJ, Calabrese JR. Quantification of occipital EEG changes in Alzheimer's disease utilizing a new metric: the fractal dimension. *Biol Psychiatry* 1994;35:381-387.

Yagyu T, Wackermann J, Shigeta M, Jelic V, Kinoshita T, Kochi K, Julin P, Almkvist O, Wahlund LO, Kondakor I, Lehmann D. Global dimensional complexity of multichannel EEG in mild Alzheimer's disease and age-matched cohorts. *Dement Geriatr Cogn Disord* 1997;8:343-347.

Yates FE. Complexity of a human being: changes with age. *Neurobiol Aging*. 2002;23:17-19.

Zappoli R, Versari A, Paganini M, Arnetoli G, Muscas GC, Gangemi PF, Arneodo MG, Poggiolini D, Zappoli F, Battaglia A. Brain electrical activity (quantitative EEG and bit-mapping neurocognitive CNV components), psychometrics and clinical findings in presenile subjects with initial mild cognitive decline or probable Alzheimer-type dementia. *Ital J Neurol Sci* 1995;16:341-376.

In: Depression and Dementia
Editor: Suptendra Nath Sarbadhikari, p. 245-304
ISBN 1-59454-114-0

Chapter 9

EEG in Dementia Review of the Past, View into the Future

Vesna Jelic[*]
Karolinska Institutet
Department of NEUROTEC
Sweden

Abstract

This paper briefly introduces dementia syndromes with current concept of classification, discusses a rationale for the use of EEG, and quantitative EEG in particular, as a research and potential diagnostic technique in dementia, puts a special emphasis on its most prevalent form Alzheimer's disease, and reviews selected studies that have contributed to the understanding of this topic. There is an abundance of literature on various electrophysiological indexes of cognitive impairment in dementia and this review is limited to the studies related to analysis of spontaneous EEG recordings during wakefulness in normal aging, Alzheimer's disease and related dementing disorders. It is written from a perspective of a clinician with a critical stance towards existing knowledge and prevailing theories and suggests what should be further explored in order to use the full potential of this method in clinical practice.

Key words: Electroencephalography, Dementia, Alzheimer's disease, Mild Cognitive Impairment, Diagnosis

[*] Address of the corresponding author is: Vesna Jelic, Karolinska Institutet, Dept. NEUROTEC, Karolinska University Hospital-Huddinge, 141 86 Stockholm, Sweden Email: Vesna.Jelic@neurotec.ki.se

BACKGROUND

Worldwide demographic statistics are estimating that number of demented people will increase from 25.5 million in 2000 to 63 million in 2030 (Wimo et al, 2003). Dramatic dimension of this problem has triggered efforts towards an early and accurate diagnosis of the disease where an emphasis is on a development of a reliable procedure that could detect as early as possible a disease process with its structural and functional changes and be sensitive to the progression of disease (Klunk, 1998). Such a procedure should be able to either detect a specific pathological feature of disease or be sensitive to the key symptoms of disease. Even the most advanced neuroimaging techniques are reflecting only the indirect correlates of the specific pathology of neurodegenerative disorders like dementia. Magnetic resonance imaging (MRI), positron emission tomography (PET), single photon emission tomography (SPECT) or functional MRI (fMRI) describe with more or less high spatial accuracy disturbed neuronal structure and function. However, decreased glucose metabolism and cerebral blood flow are epiphenomena of the pathology at the synapse level, Fig 1. Electroencephalography (EEG) measures electrical activity of the cortex which is reflecting summated electrical activity at the level of functional units of the cerebral cortex - synapses in a real time with a millisecond time resolution. Therefore, by its nature EEG should be a method of choice to study disturbances of cognitive functioning. With the advances in computational engineering new ways of data analysis are emerging which are of interest from both, theoretical aspects and rethinking basic mechanisms behind the mental processes, and practical aspects which reflect current need for an accurate, reliable and non-invasive diagnostic tool in dementia assessments. This paper briefly introduces dementia syndromes with current concept of classification, discusses a rationale for the use of EEG, and quantitative EEG in particular, as a research and potential diagnostic technique in dementia, puts a special emphasis on its most prevalent form Alzheimer's disease, and reviews selected studies that have contributed to the understanding of this topic. There is an abundance of literature on various electrophysiological indexes of cognitive impairment in dementia and this review is limited to the studies related to analysis of spontaneous EEG recordings during wakefulness in normal aging, Alzheimer's disease and related dementing disorders. It is written from a perspective of a clinician with a critical stance towards existing knowledge and prevailing theories and suggests what should be further explored in order to use the full potential of this method in clinical practice.

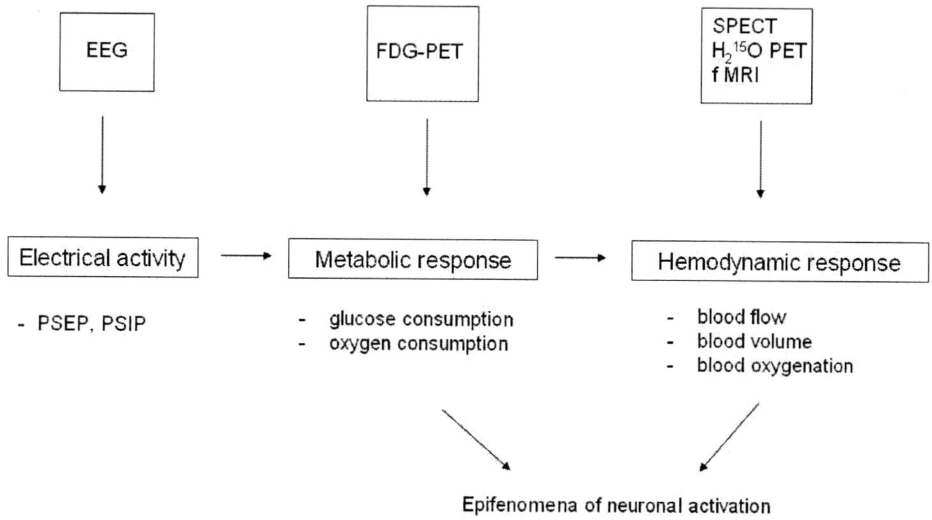

Figure 1. Diagnostic methods of different modalities are measuring various aspects of brain function. PSEP – postsynaptic excitatory potential; PSIP – postsynaptic inhibitory potential.

BRIEF OVERVIEW OF DEMENTING DISORDERS

Dementia is a clinical syndrome of cognitive decline severe enough to interfere with social and occupational functioning. It is caused by a wide spectrum of disorders that are currently classified according to the distinct clinico-pathological features into major categories: primary degenerative dementias, vascular dementias, dementia-plus syndromes, infectious or transmissible diseases and reversible or treatable causes. Category of primary degenerative dementia applies to all cases of neuronal degeneration without established cause and is the primary interest of this review. The majority of the cases, over 50% (Lobo et al, 2000) are due to Alzheimer's disease (AD). While typical clinical profile of AD is a progressive amnestic disorder which evolves into a loss in other cognitive domains, frontotemporal dementia (FTD) is characterized clinically by personality and behavioral changes, disinhibition and apathy that result from the typical topography of pathological changes primarily involving the frontal and temporal lobes. The concept of FTD has been refined recently and a syndrome of progressive aphasia (PA) has been recognized as a clinical correlate of pathological features that are predominantly involving the frontotemporal lobes of the left hemisphere. When the pathological features are predominantly characterized by bilateral atrophy of the temporal neocortex, with a multimodal loss of conceptual knowledge and consequent failure to understand meaning of words and recognize objects a syndrome of semantic dementia (SD) emerges (Neary, 1995). What in the literature appears as the Pick's disease is a frontotemporal lobe degeneration characterized by specific histopathological changes, and is not a distinguishable clinical syndrome per se.

Lewy Body Dementia (LBD) has emerged recently as a distinct subcategory of primary degenerative dementias, responsible for as much as 20% of all dementia cases (Heidebrink, 2002). Histopathologically, LBD is characterized with diffuse appearance of Lewy bodies throughout the cerebral cortex and a typical clinical presentation includes dementia, fluctuating alertness, visual hallucinations and other psychotic symptoms, mild Parkinsonism and troublesome sensitivity to neuroleptic therapy.

Vascular dementia is generally used diagnostic term when dementia is presumed to be caused by vascular disease through three major mechanisms: strategically localized single brain lesion in one of the major cerebral arteries' territories, multi-infarct dementia (MID) and subcortical arteriosclerotic encephalopathy also known as Binswanger´s disease.

In dementia-plus syndromes cognitive impairment appears in the context of more widespread neurological dysfunction with pyramidal, extrapyramidal or cerebellar signs as in Parkinson's disease, progressive supranuclear palsy, Huntington disease, amyotrophic lateral sclerosis, and corticobasal degeneration. Among the infectious or transmissible diseases Creutzfeldt-Jakob disease and AIDS dementia complex are of special interest when EEG is considered as an aid in differential diagnosis of dementia.

Early identification and differentiation of various forms of dementia is important for therapeutical interventions and prognosis of the individual patient. However, according to the clinicopathological correlative studies there are rarely "pure" forms of distinct dementia subtypes (Gearing et al, 1995; Kosunen et al, 1996). Prevalence of vascular dementia (VaD) is estimated to 20% of all dementias, 15% of which has mixed vascular and AD pathology. Similarly, LBD has estimated prevalence of 15-20 % of all dementias, where 12% has mixed LBD and AD pathology. Since these "mixed" types could differ in terms of prognosis and therapeutical approach, it is of interest to review EEG characteristics in major subtypes of dementing disorders. Hypothetically, if a patient with a clinical presentation of AD has some EEG characteristics of VaD that could imply possible silent comorbidity and consequent worse prognosis.

ALZHEIMER'S DISEASE: NEUROBIOLOGICAL SUBSTRATES AND THEIR RELEVANCE TO EEG GENERATION

This review is biased to the most prevalent form of dementia, Alzheimer's disease (AD). The definite diagnosis of AD is based on the examination of the brain tissue. The main neuropathological hallmarks of the disease are intracellular presence of neurofibrillary tangles (NFT) and the extracellular appearance of senile plaques (SP) with its main component β-amyloid, accompanied by other structural changes like granulovacuolar degeneration, dendritic atrophy and neuron and synapse loss (Terry, 1994). Within cerebral cortex all NFT-bearing neurons are large pyramidal projection cells. The prevailing theory of the evolution of AD pathology recognizes a specific hierarchical pattern of neuronal changes where the limbic cortex is particularly vulnerable to the disease process, projection neurons in the transentorhinal cortex being first affected by neurofibrillary changes, while isocortex is being affected last with preferential involvement of associative neocortical areas (Braak & Braak, 1991). This stepwise progression of degenerative changes along the cortico-cortical connections forms a basis for the disconnection hypothesis of Alzheimer's disease (de Lacoste & White III, 1993). Interestingly, the pattern of appearance of the neurofibrillary changes resembles the inverse sequence of cortical myelination (Braak H & Braak E, 1996). Neurobiological parameters that best correlate with the degree of dementia in AD are increased density of NFT and decreased density of synapses (Arriagada et al, 1992). It has been hypothesized that particular vulnerability of certain brain areas is based on their high degree of structural plasticity which allows modification of the synaptic connections as the basic mechanism behind the higher brain functions (Arendt, 2001).

Disturbance of projection neurons in the entorhinal cortex leads to functional changes in association areas long before the pathology is present there. It has been hypothesized that early metabolic deficits in AD arise from synaptic failure in association cortical areas and not neuronal loss. This is mirrored in findings obtained by neuroimaging methods of different modalities early during the course of disease, when MRI visualizes atrophy and site of neuronal loss in medial temporal lobe structures and functional imaging methods like PET and SPECT visualize and quantify remote effects of neuronal loss and deficient synaptic activity like decreased glucose metabolism and cerebral blood flow in temporo-parietal association cortex (Grady et al, 1988; Jobst et al, 1992).

What relevance has this characteristic pathogenesis of AD for the generation of the electrical activity of the brain and choice of analyzing method?

Although alpha activity is controversial in its origin and that is still a subject of debate, a prevailing theory assumes that pyramidal neurons with its somata and basal dendrites in cortical layers IV/V form biological dipoles that generate EEG activity, more specifically alpha rhythms of visual cortex (Lopes da Silva and Storm van Leeuwen, 1977). Via cortico-cortical connections of pyramidal neurons spread the alpha rhythms in different directions across the cortex. As it has been discussed above, Alzheimer's disease is primarily a disorder of cerebral cortex, a highest organizational level of the human brain. The major principle of organization is cortico-cortical connectivity via streams of feedforward axonal projections reciprocated by feedback axons and sending also lateral projections (Van Hoesen, 1997). It is logical to believe that pathology that affects origins and end stations of this system, in particular cortical layers should have consequences on the generation of the EEG activity and its propagation across the cortex. Recent studies employing analysis of event-related cortical responses- EEG reactivity (event related desynchronisation, ERD and event related synchronisation, ERS) in combination with topographic mapping have shown abnormal coupling of cortical response and movement timing in AD patients, suggesting that AD is a global brain network disease including even sensorimotor processing in the absence of an overt movement disorder (Babiloni et al, 2000b; Babiloni et al, 2004b).

EEG rhythmic activity has a wide range of frequencies, which cluster in bands that have functional significance: slow frequency range like delta and theta, and high frequency range like alpha and beta. Delta activity has been related, among other causes like i.e. ischemic vascular changes in the brain and cytotoxic processes, to the cholinergic deafferentation of the cortex (Detari and Vanderwolf, 1987; Buszaki et al, 1988). Relationship between the cortical choline acetyltransferase content and EEG delta-power has been demonstrated in the animal study after lesion of nucleus basalis (Riekkinen et al, 1990). In Alzheimer's disease cholinergic deafferentation of the cerebral cortex results as a selective loss of the cholinergic neurons in the basal forebrain (Davies et al, 1976; Whitehouse et al, 1981). Cholinergic deficits have been shown to be the best neurochemical correlates of dementia severity in AD (Bierer et al, 1995). Consequently, currently prevailing treatment strategies in AD are based on cholinergic substitution (Francis et al, 1999) and quantitative EEG has demonstrated reduced slow activity as the effect of treatment with acetylcholinesterase inhibitors (Jelic et al, 1998).

Theta activity or the rhythmic slow activity (RSA) has been shown in experimental studies to generate in the limbic cortex and is related to the transmission of signals through the entorhino-hippocampal pathway (Lopes da Silva et al, 1990). Rae-Grant et al (1987) found a high correlation between excessive theta activity as rated by visual analysis and neuronal loss in the hippocampus. However, it is questionable whether theta activity recorded at the scalp corresponds to this hippocampal theta rhythm that could be propagated to the cortex via hippocampo-cortical feed-back loops. This relationship has been demonstrated by showing that both hippocampal theta and EEG theta recorded at the scalp synchronize with increasing task demands (Klimesch, 1996). The remaining question is how could be the appearance of theta activity explained in a resting EEG of a demented subject in the absence of any activation paradigm? Does the disease process induce stress and increased demands on healthy neuronal populations and related neuronal networks with a consequent increase of theta activity? Is it just a shift from another frequency, for example, increased frequency of delta activity? Or, does the scalp recorded theta activity reflect just a slowing of the main background alpha activity i.e. increased synchronization? Von Stein and Sarnthein (2000) have proposed that behind the resting state there is an active cortex with internal mental activity, i.e. top-down processing, where long-range interactions in the alpha and theta range seem specifically involved to subserve functional integration of multiple simultaneous brain activities. It remains to be shown whether the disease process modifies this dynamics of the resting state by increasing synchronization with consequent shift towards slow activities.

Brief Overview of Methods of Quantitative EEG Analysis

Conventional and Widely Used Methods

While visual analysis of EEG recordings still prevails in a routine clinical practice, the most commonly used methods in research are a frequency analysis of single EEG channels or by using bipolar recording montage, topographic mapping or more complex but spatially non-ambiguous source computations. The most commonly used is a frequency analysis by means of Fast Fourier Transform (FFT) that quantifies the power at each discrete frequency point of the EEG averaged across the entire sample, which leads to the loss of temporal resolution.

Digital EEG has enabled statistical approach to the data analysis like "brain electrical activity mapping" (BEAM) (Duffy et al, 1979) and the "neurometrics" (John et al, 1977). These methods have being criticized as tools for clinical decision-making, since statistical concept of abnormality in terms of 2 to 3 standard deviations below the norms does not necessarily imply medical abnormality and could lead to false-positive findings (Oken & Chiappa, 1986; Fisch & Pedley, 1989).

Coherence analysis of EEG, which is a correlation between a pair of signals expressed as a function of frequency, has been very much exploited in dementia research and given means to study functional cortico-cortical connections and possibly underlying structural connectivity (Shaw et al, 1978; Thatcher et al, 1986). Coherence is independent of the amplitude of two recorded EEG signals because it is normalized by the power of a chosen frequency band and therefore should be a complementary measure to the EEG power. In other words, while EEG amplitude predominantly reflects amount of synchronized activity recorded by one channel, coherence measures the degree of interactions between two signals.

The concept of EEG coherence has been very much exploited in the field of dementia and AD research in particular with an interest in finding an index for a neocortical disconnection (Thatcher et al, 1986; Cook & Leuchter, 1996). Most of the studies analyzed coherence by means of FFT transformation and averaged multiple bipolar recordings (Leuchter et al, 1992; Dunkin et al, 1994; Jelic et al, 1996) or between one electrode and all surrounding electrodes (Besthorn et al, 1994; 1997). However, this type of analysis suffers from methodological problems like the influence of the reference electrode or volume conduction which could induce false high coherence values (Fein et al, 1988; Nunez et al, 1997; Nunez et al, 1999). Another problem is impossibility to differentiate contribution of the single brain regions from the bipolar recordings that reflect signal differences between two channels commonly recorded more or less over the same cerebral regions that consequently gives low coherence values. It is still a highly controversial issue whether there is a straight forward correspondence between scalp electrodes and underlying brain structures and it has been generally accepted that interpretation of surface scalp measurements in terms of "brain regions" and source localizations is not possible without performing inverse calculation of the data. Therefore, conclusions based on findings from most of published empirical studies employing coherence method in differentiating AD from healthy aging are remaining speculative.

Novel Advanced Methods of Analysis

Novel approaches to EEG analysis such as EEG source localizations (Lehmann & Michel, 1989), EEG-microstates (Dierks et al, 1997) and non-linear dynamics (Stam et al, 1996; Yagyu et la, 1997) have been applied in dementia research in order to evaluate whether these new parameters could provide additional classification accuracy between demented and healthy subjects.

The method of FFT Dipole Approximation uses Fourier coefficients (sine- and cosine values) of a given frequency point to approximate a potential field generated by intracerebral electrical dipoles (Lehman & Michel, 1989). Resulting FFT Dipole Approximation values constitute a potential distribution map which can be used for conventional three-dimensional dipole source estimation. The variance of the amplitude of all channels could be detected for a certain frequency point and corresponds to the Global Field Power (GFP). Therefore GFP corresponds to the generalized EEG amplitude in a dipole model of brain function. This method has an advantage that it is reference free and allows data reduction in a multichannel recording resulting in only 6 parameters per frequency band: magnitude in μV, antero-posterior, left-right localisation and depth of equivalent dipole in mm and direction of a dipole.

Among the recent techniques emerging in the field of source localization techniques is a low resolution electromagnetic tomography (LORETA) (Pascual-Marqui et al, 1994; 1999), which computes estimates of the 3-dimensional distribution of electrical neuronal activity through the full brain volume which are then displayed in a human head model. This method enables visualization and relative unambiguous localization of sources of electrical brain activity, as well as analysis of individual data sets.

Conventional spectral analysis by means of FFT is based on time epochs of 2 seconds which are averaged over longer time duration of the recording; therefore the high temporal resolution of the EEG is lost. The spontaneous brain activity is highly discontinuous and is characterized by rapid transition between microstates in the sub-second range with stable spatial configuration which constitute momentary field maps (landscapes) (Lehman, 1971; Lehman & Koenig, 1997). It has been hypothesized that different spatial configurations correspond to the activity of the different neuronal generators of the electrical activity.

Recently, there have been attempts to develop another methods to measure synchronized brain activity, like Global Field Synchronization (GFS) where in contrast to coherence, synchronization is measured on a spatially global level within given frequency band with an assumption that EEG signals are stationary only within single short EEG epochs (Koenig et al, 2001). In the resting EEG in the absence of stimulation there is ongoing brain activity that is spontaneously changing and stimulus induced changes reflect largely the dynamics of the ongoing activity (Tononi et al, 1998).

Another method to track rapid changes in interdependencies between two EEG signals is derived from the theory of non-linear dynamic systems and takes into account non-linear couplings between EEG signals as well as their non-stationary nature (Stam & van Dijk, 2002). This synchronization likelihood (SL) is a measure of the statistical interdependencies between 2 time series and can be computed with a high time resolution, but using information from single channels suffer from the same methodological disadvantages as coherence data.

Methods of non-linear dynamics are more appropriate to study the non-stationary EEG data and irregular aperiodic time series, which could not only be the result of noise but could also bring biologically relevant information and be related to i.e. degree of desynchronization in EEG. From a practical point of view methods of nonlinear quantitative EEG analysis are attractive because they reduce information from multichannel recordings to the single measure like Global Dimensional Complexity (GDC) or the correlation dimension (D2) (Pritchard & Duke, 1992).

However, one should keep in mind that most of these analyzing techniques are based on a signal analysis driven by a theoretical model and may not reflect the physiological properties of brain function.

EEG Findings in Normal Aging

The main confounding variable in AD is that of age. Several studies on EEG changes in dementia have reported abnormal EEG for the healthy control population, their rates being 29 % in study of Soinen et al (1982a), 27% in study of Rae-Grant et al (1987), 36,7 % in study of Robinson et al (1994), the later two used visual interpretation of the recordings. Therefore the crucial question is whether human EEG does change in normal aging and whether these changes follow the same directions as in dementia. If the later is true are differences in neurophysiological variables between physiological and pathological aging only quantitative? Several studies have reported a decrease of dominant alpha frequency, an increase of slow activity in the delta and theta range, a decrease of beta activity and focal temporal slowing with aging (Roubicek 1977; Soininen et al, 1982a; Torres et al, 1983; Giaquinto & Nolfe, 1986; Visser et al, 1987). Elmståhl et al (1994) subdivided according to age their control sample of 56 elderly women and found that there was a significant tendency for theta power to increase with age from 75 to 90 years, whereas the oldest group above 90 years showed a relative decrease in theta power. However, 13 subjects from this study had borderline results in both spatial and vocabulary tests, or a pathological result in one test. Longitudinal study of Coben et al (1985) followed for 2, 5 years quantitatively the EEGs of normal elderly subjects aged 65-82 years and reported decrease in delta activity, decrease in beta activity and average frequency, and stable alpha and theta frequency. A 9 year follow-up study of Nakano et al (1992) found that slowing of EEG, increase of theta and decrease of alpha activity, became obvious in late senescence in late seventies or beyond eighties and was correlated with the decline of mental functions. Both, EEG slowing and the lower scores on psychometrics were inversely corelated to the longevity of life in this study.

However, most of these studies used simple neuropsychological tests and did not apply extensive clinical or radiological evaluations to search for subclinical brain disorders. Indeed, slight left-sided antero-temporal focal abnormalities were related to deterioration of language function (Visser et al, 1987) and poor performance on memory tests (Rice et al, 1991) in normal aged subjects. The presence of white matter hyperintensities on MRI was also reported to be related to intermittent temporal slowing in healthy elderly subjects over age 84 (Oken & Kaye, 1992). In 46 % of healthy volunteers with cerebrovascular risk factors, aged 45 to 74 years, focal slowing was present on brain mapping (Logar et al, 1993).

Hartikainen et al (1992) showed an inverse correlation between delta amplitude and AChE activity in the CSF of old subjects with errors on the list learning test. In addition, quite a few studies did not find increases in slow wave activity with age (Breslau et al, 1989; Duffy et al, 1984; Williamson et al, 1990). There are several well-documented reports on age-related increase in EEG desynchronization with age and increased beta power in elderly subjects when compared to the younger ones (Koyama et al, 1997; Duffy et al, 1984b; Duffy et al, 1993; Pollock et al, 1990a). Potential explanation of this finding is that there is a decreased coherence or cortical coupling between brain regions, possibly related to age-related reduction of cortical connectivity (Duffy et al, 1996). The later hypothesis stems from the study of Duffy et al (1996) where 371 healthy subjects aged 20-30 were studied with 2-years follow-up to ensure that they remain medically healthy.

Interestingly, Knott et al (2001) compared spectral EEG values of 30 healthy control subjects with a mean age of 74 years with adult age-regressed EEG population norms according to "neurometrics" by John et al (1977), derived from 278 adults in age range from 18-82 years and found that "optimally healthy" controls from the study sample had significantly reduced theta absolute power compared to population norms and a tendency to reduced relative delta power.

There is a growing evidence that in the context of a good health status no significant EEG slowing should be expected in elderly. Therefore, when evaluating the effect of aging on physiologic measures of CNS function, it is important to control for factors that are associated with increasing age and which may produce subclinical functional and structural CNS changes: i.e. hypertension, diabetes, and use of different medications.

METHODOLOGICAL CRITERIA FOR A DIAGNOSTIC TEST

Overview of methodological challenges for a validity of a diagnostic test, as well as quality of evidence ratings of scientific studies are given in Table 1 and Table 2. There are some formal requirements for the acceptance of a diagnostic technique in clinical routine, which include: increasing certainty of the presence or absence of disease, supporting clinical management, assessing prognosis and monitoring clinical course (Knottnerus et al, 2002). The later objective could be extended to the assessment of treatment efficacy.

Table 1. Methodological challenges and validity of a diagnostic test

1. Well accepted standards to define the disese – "gold standard".
2. Spectrum and selection bias.
3. Observer variability and bias.
4. Test-retest reliability
5. Sample size.
6. Impact on clinical decision making, yield over already available methods.

Modified from Knottnerus et al (2002) and Hughes & John (1999).

In determining the accuracy of a diagnostic test, there should be a suitable reference standard, or the "gold standard". In the absence of reliable biomarkers, the role of a "gold standard" in the diagnosis of AD have standardized operational clinical criteria such as those proposed by the NINCDS-ADRDA Work Group (McKhann et al, 1984), the DSM-III-R (American Psychiatric Association, 1987), ICD-10 (World Health Organization, 1992) and DSM-IV (American Psychiatric Association, 1994) criteria. Several studies based on clinicopathological series have reported good validity for NINCDS-ADRDA criteria and diagnostic accuracy rates 80-90% (Galasko et al, 1994; Klatka et al, 1996). The accuracy of a potential diagnostic test for AD should not fall bellow that of standardized clinical criteria.

Table 2. Published studies - Quality of evidence ratings

Class of evidence	**Provided by:**	
I	one or more well-designed, prospective, blinded, controlled clinical studies	
II	one or more well-designed clinical studies such as case control, cohort studies, etc.	
III	expert oppinion, nonrandomized historical controls or case reports	
Strenght of reccomendation		
Type	**Recommendation**	**Based on**
A	Strong positive	class I evidence, or overhelming class II evidence
B	Positive	clas II evidence
C	Positive	strong consensus of class II evidence
D	Negative	inconclusive or conflicting class II evidence
E	Negative	evidence of ineffectiveness or lack of efficacy

Modified from Nuwer (1998) and Hughes & John (1999).

Therefore, to increase the certainty of the presence or absence of disease the test should have sufficient discriminatory power. The most common measures of discriminatory power, or in other words indexes of accuracy, are sensitivity (proportion of diseased patients with positive test results) and specificity (proportion of nondiseased patients with negative test results) or likelihood ratios (odds of finding a particular test result in diseased versus nondiseased patients) (Carrington Reid et al, 1995). While sensitivity and specificity are not sufficient to establish clinical usefulness, the likelihood ratio is critical for the assessment of clinical utility. However, the later is strongly dependent on the disease prevalence which is very high in preselected clinical samples.

Although review of the table 3 indicates that there is a consistency among the findings from different studies, results from most of the studies could not be generalized because they suffer from a methodological weaknesses like too small sample size, spectrum bias (limited range of disease severity), they are mainly taking retrospective samples and not consecutively referred patients which reflect reality of clinical practice. Furthermore, selection strategies for the controls are not based on population-based reference groups, there is often bias of selection procedures towards healthier individuals and, therefore, contrast between patients and a reference group are increased.

Comparison of the diagnostic abilities of two or more diagnostic tests is usually based on comparison of their respective sensitivities and specificities, as in Table 5. However, it has been shown that using likelihood ratios one can show that a test can be superior to its competitor in terms of predictive values, while having either sensitivity or specificity smaller (Biggerstaff, 2000).

Another problem in the interpretation of the accuracy indexes arises from the statistical procedure used for the group classification. There are several approaches reviewed and criticized by Besthorn et al (1997) like: 1) classification by group means which is a method that lacks optimization; 2) discriminant analysis which gives the best linear combination of the input variables but with too many predictors entered it can give very high classification rates by chance; combined with a stepwise selection of predictors by their relative predictive power it reduces the number of predictors but discards many variables; 3) principal component analysis (PCA) which precedes discriminant analysis and uses factor loadings or actual data related to the factors with highest loadings; 4) neuronal networks approach using back propagation which due to its non-linearity could be superior to other methods.

Very few studies have used area under receiver operating characteristic (ROC) curves in order to determine optimal cutoffs of different parameters and to quantify the accuracy of discrimination at multiple cutoff points. This method is superior to the traditional one which defines indexes of accuracy in terms of a single 2 times 2 table and consequently confound discrimination capacity and decision criterion (Swets, 1986).

Another important aspect of validity of diagnostic tests is reliability of a given index. Few studies, have addressed intrasubjects short- and long-term EEG variability (Gasser et al, 1985; Salinsky et al, 1991; Pollock et al, 1991) and to our knowledge only one (Hooijer et al, 1990) has addressed this problem in a study sample of demented subjects. So far, only reliability measures for indexes of conventional frequency analysis are available and continued efforts should be directed towards the novel methods of analysis. This is also of importance if we want to establish these measures as state markers of the disease and markers of treatment efficacy in the future.

EEG Findings in Alzheimer's Disease Versus Normal Aging

Brief Overview of EEG Changes in AD

Slowing of EEG background activity, i.e. alpha frequency, either assessed visually or by means of computer analysis is a consistent finding in dementia and AD, in particular. It was already observed and first published by Hans Berger, the inventor of EEG, in 1932 (Berger, 1932). It has generally been accepted that there is a temporal dynamics of EEG changes during the disease process. Early changes are detected as an increase in theta and decrease in beta, followed by a decrease in alpha, and later in the moderate and severe stages, an increase in delta band power (Coben et al, 1985; Pentillä et al, 1985; Dierks et al, 1991). Slowing of EEG is typically diffuse, but some studies which focused on topographic measures found it particularly pronounced in temporal and parietal areas (Duffy et al, 1984; Breslau et al, 1989; Rice et al, 1990; Dierks et al, 1991; Duffy et al, 1995). Another consistent finding in AD patients is a reduced alpha blocking upon eyes opening (Pritchard et al, 1994; Signorino et al, 1995; Duffy et al, 1995). Worse qEEG findings, in terms of increased theta and decreased alpha power were reported in patients with an earlier onset (Schreiter-Gasser et al, 1994). Similarly, Miyauchi et al (1994) reported a more severe slowing in the range of delta and theta activity in patients with presenile AD. Studies describing equivalent EEG sources in AD subjects found that they have higher amplitudes in a slow frequency range and a shift of alpha and beta activity towards frontal brain regions (Dierks et al, 1993; Huang et al, 2000). It is, however, disputable whether there is a shift of the sources of alpha activity from their physiological location in posterior brain regions, or some other sources of alpha activity are becoming more dominant during the disease process.

EEG pattern during tonic REM sleep in AD patients show similar changes in the power spectra as during wakefulness although these changes are more augmented during sleep probably because the role of cholinergic input from the basal forebrain in cortical activation is more central for EEG desynchronization during REM sleep than in wakefulness when several other neurotransmitter systems are engaged in cortical activation (Petit et al, 1992).

In contrast to observed changes in spectral power, studies on EEG coherence in AD reported decreased coherence in high frequency bands (O'Connor et al, 1979; Leuchter et al, 1987; 1992; Besthorn et al, 1994; Dunkin et al, 1994; Locatelli et al, 1998) and unchanged or even increased coherence in slow frequency bands (Besthorn et al, 1994; Locatelli et al, 1998; Comi et al, 1998). While most of the studies found specific regional pattern with decreased coherence in temporo-occipito-parietal areas, Besthorn et al, (1994) reported more pronounced decrease in frontal and central areas, probably due to methodological differences among studies.

EEG coherence, calculated between pairs of bipolar channels representing origins and terminations of long cortico-cortical association fibers, has been reported to be decreased in alpha band in temporo-parietal scalp regions in subjects with only mild cognitive impairment implying that functional disconnection could be the earliest change appearing in preclinical stages of the disease (Jelic et al, 1996). Similarly, Stam et al (2003) demonstrated recently that the synchronization likelihood (SL), a novel type of coherence measure that combines sensitivity to linear and non-linear information with a high time resolution, was significantly decreased in fast frequency bands in the beta range in AD patients as compared to those with MCI and healthy subjects. In a subsequent multicentre study Babiloni et al (2004a) reported reduction of SL in fronto-parietal and inter-hemispherical electrode pairs in mild AD, especially in alpha 1 sub-band, 8-10.5 Hz. The authors proposed, based on functional relation of slow alpha rhytm to attentional processing (Klimesch, 1999), that reduced coupling of the low alpha rhytm could reflect an abnormal increase in cortical excitation or disinhibition in patients with AD.

Table 3. Selected studies reporting accuracy of EEG method in dementia diagnosis

Author, year	Study sample	Age (years) Mean+SD, (range)	Disease severity	Diagnostic criteria	Method of analysis	Main findings	Indexes of accuracy* (%)
AD vs controls (C)							
Soininen et al, 1982a	56 AD 84 C	78±6 74±7	moderate to severe	not specified	visual analysis, 4 grades of severity	dominant occipital rhytm highest coefficient in DA	SS (82) SP (89) OA (86)
Brenner et al, 1986	35 AD 61 C	67±9 67±7	MMSE 9-29	NINCDS-ADRDA	frequency analysis	increased theta & alpha1 power	AD (MMSE ≤ 22) vs C: SS (79) SP (93) OA (89) AD (MMSE ≥ 23) vs C: SS (36) SP (93) OA (85)
John et al, 1988	125 demented: (93 AD, 32 MID) 76 MCI 120 C	70 (mean) 17-90	demented: GDS>3 MCI: GDS 2	DSM-III	neurometric evaluation DA, split-half replication	central theta, fronto- -temporal alpha, composite variables theta all regions, anterior power, total slow-wave asymmetry, total delta coherence accounted for most of the variance	Initial discriminant: SS (77) SP (79) Independent replication: SS (75) SP (77)
Coben et al, 1990	Sample 1 38 AD, 41 C Sample 2: 21 AD, 22 C	72±5 (63-83)	mild, CDR 1	CDR	frequency analysis, right occipital-vertex derivation	higher % theta: lower mean frequency: (cut-off score set before)	SS (24) SP (100) PPV (100) SS (19) SP (100) PPV (100)

Table 3. Selected studies reporting accuracy of EEG method in dementia diagnosis (Continued)

Author, year	Study sample	Age (years) Mean+SD, (range)	Disease severity	Diagnostic criteria	Method of analysis	Main findings	Indexes of accuracy* (%)
Hooijer et al, 1990	43 AD 41 psychiatric patients 51 C	76±5 74±7 73±5	not specified	DSM-III	visual analysis + frequency analysis	visual analysis variable (amount of alpha substracted from theta/delta amount); quantitative EEG variable (percentage of fast divided by a percentage of slow frequencies)	DA visual analysis AD vs C: SS (71) SP (79) OA (74); DA frequency analysis AD vs C: SS (86) SP (76) OA (83).
Robinson et al, 1994	86 AD 17 mixed, AD +MID 56 C	73±9 76±8 72±11	ESD 57±63 ESD 98±51 (dementia threshold ESD score 221)	autopsy confirmed diagnoses	visual analysis, 5 increasing grades of severity	grade 2-5 abnormality in 78% AD and 77% mixed AD	grades 2-5: SS (87) SP (63) PPV (81) NPV (74) grades 3&4: SS (50) SP (96) PPV (83) NPV (83) LR+ (2.5)
Elmståhl et al, 1994	23 AD (females) 56 C (females)	85±5 84±4	Severe MMSE 5-14 in 10 patients (rest scored 0) disease duration 8±4 years	NINCDS-ADRDA	frequency analysis, absolute & relative power from 4 head quadrants	absolute delta power from posterior quadrant best predictor	predictive value 0.94 via logistic regression analysis (no data available for SS,SP)
Printz et al, 1992	39 AD 43 C	70±7 68±8	MMSE 22±3 DRS 116 ±13	NINCDS ADRDA DSM-III	tonic REM sleep, variance-normalised power spectra	increased delta & theta, reduced beta power	SS (92) SP (95) OA (94)

Table 3. Selected studies reporting accuracy of EEG method in dementia diagnosis (Continued)

Author, year	Study sample	Age (years) Mean+SD, (range)	Disease severity	Diagnostic criteria	Method of analysis	Main findings	Indexes of accuracy* (%)
Pritchard et al, 1994	14 AD 25 C	72±10 69±6	mild to moderate MMSE 19±3 (14-23)	DSM-III-R (?)	linear (frequency analysis) & non-linear (dimensional complexity, DCx) measures	AD: increased frontal delta & diffuse theta reduced parieto-occipital alpha and beta 1 activity lower DCx over frontal & central midline loci, higher over occipital loci.	linear prediction (DA): SS (72) SP (80) OA (77) neural-net (NN) prediction: SS (86) SP (96) OA (92)
Duffy et al, 1995	60 AD 129 C	69 (53-89) 64 (51-80)	mild to moderate DRS 116	INCDS-ADRDA	frequency analysis, topographic mapping, split-half replication study	increased theta, decreased beta activity, 19 ROIs predominantly temporo- parietal distinguished AD & C	DA training set: SS (77) SP (98) OA (91) DA test set: SS (77) SP (91) OA (86)
Stam et al, 1996	15 AD 15 C	80±6 70±5	ADS-6 < 5	NINCDS-ADRDA	frequency analysis relative power & D2 cutt-offs from ROC curves.	AD: increased theta relative power and lower reactivity of D2 (correlation dimension) during eyes open in AD	At SP 100%: relative theta SS (47); D2 reactivity SS (33); Relative theta + D2 SS (60).

Table 3. Selected studies reporting accuracy of EEG method in dementia diagnosis (Continued)

Author, year	Study sample	Age (years) Mean+SD, (range)	Disease severity	Diagnostic criteria	Method of analysis	Main findings	Indexes of accuracy* (%)
Jelic et al, 1996	18 AD 19 MCI 17 SMC 16 C	61±5 62±7 60±6 64±11	mild to moderate, MMSE in AD 21+4; MMSE in MCI 27+2	NINCDS-ADRDA MCI diagnosis: 1-2 SD below average on standardized NP tests	frequency analysis + coherence analysis according to Newton et al (1993)	increased theta relative power and decreased alpha relative power and temporo-parietal coherence distinguished AD & C	DA AD vs C: SS (78) SP (100) OA (89) DA AD vs MCI: SS (89) SP (84) OA (86) DA AD vs SMC: SS (72) SP (94) OA (83)
Besthorn et al, 1997	32 probable AD 18 possible AD 42 controls	68±9 (all AD) 66±7	moderate to severe, MMSE 12±8 CDR 2±0.8 illness duration 66±41 months	NINCDS-ADRDA	frequency analysis + coherence analysis according to Besthorn et al, 1994	alpha blocking index lower in alpha 1 & 2, increased delta & theta power in AD	classification, group means: OA (83) classification, stepwise DA: OA (86%) classification, NN: OA (84) combined DA + PCA, all: SS (82) SP (93) OA (87) probable AD: SS (94) SP (98) OA (96)
Claus et al, 1999	86 AD 49 C (population-based)	79±6 78±5	AD: MMSE 18+6 CAMCOG 62+16 C: MMSE 25+4 CAMCOG 79+14	NINCDS-ADRDA	visual assessment, 2 raters, the grand total of EEG (GTE) score according to Jonkman, 1989 & de Werd et al, 1990	reduced frequency of rhytmic background activity & its reactivity, diffuse slow activity in AD	GTE cut-off 3: SS (45) SP (89) PPV (88) at pre-test probability 63 %, at SP 100% SS 13%

Table 3. Selected studies reporting accuracy of EEG method in dementia diagnosis (Continued)

Author, year	Study sample	Age (years) Mean+SD, (range)	Disease severity	Diagnostic criteria	Method of analysis	Main findings	Indexes of accuracy* (%)
Knott et al, 2000	35 AD 30 C	72±8 74±6	MMSE 19±8	NINCDS-ADRDA & DSM-IV	raw & Z-transformed (Prichep & John, 1992) coherence for 8 inter- & intrahemispheric site pairs	reduced interhemispheric coherence in all bands & reduced intrahemispheric in delta & theta band in AD	raw values/5 predictors: SS (77) SP (73) OA (75) Z-scores/5 predictors: SS (74) SP (73) OA (74)
Ihl et al, 2000	36 AD 44 C	73±9 69±10	MMSE 14±6 BCRS 4±0.9 SKT 20±5	NINCDS-ADRDA	frequency analysis, comparison with discriminative power of ADAS	topography of beta and delta and amplitude of delta activity best discriminators of AD vs C	DA, 4 EEG variables: SS (94) SP 93 OA (94) DA, 6 ADAS variables: SS (100) SP (100)
Stevens et al, 2001	37 AD 28 C	70±10 68±8	MMSE 21±6 illness duration 21 months	NINCDS-ADRDA	frequency & coherence analysis for 3 states: rest, EC, EO & watching a pendulum	group differences in power spectra and coherence largest during rest EO	DA 3 coherence variables during rest, EO: SS (80) SP (75) OA (77)

Table 3. Selected studies reporting accuracy of EEG method in dementia diagnosis (Continued)

Author, year	Study sample	Age (years) Mean+SD, (range)	Disease severity	Diagnostic criteria	Method of analysis	Main findings	Indexes of accuracy* (%)
Knott et al, 2001	35 AD 30 C	72±8 74±6	MMSE 19±8	NINCDS-ADRDA & DSM-IV	raw & Z-transformed (Prichep & John, 1992) values for absolute & relative power	increased absolute raw &. Z-transf. delta, theta, decreased absoloute and Z-transf. relative alpha power & mean frequency in AD	raw averaged values/9 predictors: SS (69) SP (80) OA (74) Z-scores averaged/7 predictors: SS (69) SP (83) OA (75)
Bennys et al, 2001	35 AD 35 C	70±7 62±9	MMSE 19±5 range (10-27) ilnesses duration 3±2 years	NINCDS-ADRDA & DSM-IV	frequency analysis absolute power + spectral ratios	theta/alpha+beta ratio (parieto-occipital) strongly differentiate groups	optimal cut-off from ROC curves: SS (70) SP (90); at SP 100% SS is 40%
AD vs Multi-infarct dementia (MID) vs controls (C)							
Erkinjunti et al, 1988	AD 67 MID 77 PVD 45	70±1 73±1 75±2	mild to severe	DSM-III + Hachinski score + CT (autopsy validation on a subsample)	visual + frequency analysis	focal slowing: 18% AD, 36% MID, 13% PVD paroxysmal activity: 45% AD, 64% MID; 58% PVD	Focal slowing MID vs AD: RR 21; SS (50); SP(96); paroxysmal activity, MID vs AD: RR 2.1
Leuchter et al, 1987	AD 12 MID 6 C 6	75 (SD?) 75 (SD?) 73 (SD?)	MMSE 22 (14-30) 16 (14-26)	DSM-III	frequency & coherence analysis	spectral ratio high/slow frequency decreased in AD & MID; multiple elevated coherence values in MID vs AD&C	combination of spectral ratio and 3 antero-post. coherence variables in DA gave OA 92%

Table 3. Selected studies reporting accuracy of EEG method in dementia diagnosis (Continued)

Author, year	Study sample	Age (years) Mean+SD, (range)	Disease severity	Diagnostic criteria	Method of analysis	Main findings	Indexes of accuracy* (%)
Leuchter et al, 1992	AD 49 MID 29 C 38	72±8 78±7 72±8	MMSE 17±7 16±9	DSM-III-R NINCDS-ADRDA	frequency & coherence analysis	"trans-Rolandic" coherence lowered in AD, "pre- & post-Rolandic" in MID	coherence measures in DA gave 76% correct classification of AD & MID
Leuchter et al, 1993	AD 49 MID 29 C 38	72±8 78±7 72±8	MMSE 17±7 16±9	DSM-III-R NINCDS-ADRDA	frequency analysis (absolute, relative power & spectral ratios)	no significant difference between AD and MID	highest classification by absolute power measures AD 77%, MID 81%; AD vs MID 66%
Anderer et al, 1994	sample 1: AD 54, MID 57 sample 2: AD 45, MID 51 C 56	82 (58-98) 82 (61-96) 68 (60-87)	MMSE, sample 1+2: 10-25 SCAG 1, 70 (40-90) SCAG 2, 68 (45-90)	DSM-III + Hachinski score + CT	frequency analysis (absolute, relative power & Z-transformed values); neural networks (NN), Z-statisics & DA classification		NN classification superior to Z-statistics and DA; for AD at SP 100%, SS 71%, at SP 80%, SS 87%, ROC area 0.89; for MID at SP 100%, SS 69%, at SP 80%, SS 88%, ROC area 0.90;
Robinson et al, 1994	86 AD 17 mixed (AD + MID) 56 C	73±9 76±8 72±11	ESD 57±63 ESD 98±51 (dementia threshold ESD score 221)	autopsy confirmed diagnoses	visual analysis, 5 increasing grades of severity	Grade 2-5 abnormality in 78% AD and 77% mixed AD	Mixed AD+MID vs C: SS (77) SP (65) LR+ (2.2)

Table 3. Selected studies reporting accuracy of EEG method in dementia diagnosis (Continued)

Author, year	Study sample	Age (years) Mean+SD, (range)	Disease severity	Diagnostic criteria	Method of analysis	Main findings	Indexes of accuracy* (%)
AD vs frontotemporal dementia (FTD) vs controls (C)							
Yener et al, 1996	26 AD 13 FTD 27 C	75±7 65±5 66±7	CDR 0.5-3 CDR 0.5-3	NINCDS-ADRDA FTD criteria (Brun et al, 1994)	frequency analysis	AD: generalised increase in delta and theta and decrease in posterior alpha; FTD: 63% preserved dominant posterior alpha; 69% slowing anteriorly, 31% normal EEG.	DA, FTD vs C: SS (77) SP (100); AD vs C: SS (73) SP (82); AD vs FTD: 81% AD 85% FTD correctly classified.
Förstl et al, 1996	10 AD 10 FTD 10 C	62±6 61±8 61±7	AD: CDR 2±1; AD:MMSE 9±7 FTD: CDR 2±1; FTD: MMSE: 15±11	NINCDS-ADRDA FTD criteria (Gustafson & Nilson, 1982)	frequency analysis	AD: increase of delta & theta, decrease of alpha & beta compared to C & FTD; FTD vs C no difference.	Fz delta, Pz theta & beta 1 correctly classified 70 % AD and 90% FTD; SS (?)
Lindau et al, 2003	16 AD 19 FTD 19 C	59±6 59±8 62±10	MMSE 20±3 MMSE 22±7	DSM-IV criteria & Lund & Manchester criteria (Neary et al, 1998)	frequency analysis (GFP)	FTD compared to AD had less delta and theta and less alpha and beta GFP.	FTD vs AD: theta GFP OA (69), delta GFP OA (63); combined delta and theta GFP and psychometric tests OA (93%)

Table 3. Selected studies reporting accuracy of EEG method in dementia diagnosis (Continued)

Author, year	Study sample	Age (years) Mean+SD, (range)	Disease severity	Diagnostic criteria	Method of analysis	Main findings	Indexes of accuracy* (%)
AD vs major depressive disorder							
Brenner et al, 1986	35 AD 23 Depr. 61 C	67±9 70±8 67±7	MMSE 9-29 MMSE ≥25	NINCDS-ADRDA SADS-C Hamilton rating > 14	frequency analysis	Lower delta & theta in Depr.vs AD, lower mean freq. & beta in Depr. vs C	AD (MMSE ≤ 22) vs Depr: SS (58) SP (100) OA (89); AD (MMSE ≥23) vs Depr: SS (27) SP (100) OA (76)
John et al, 1988	125 demented: (93 AD, 32 MID) 76 MCI 120 Depressed (68 unipolar, 35 bipolar) 120 C	70 (mean) 53 (mean) 17-90	demented: GDS>3 MCI: GDS 2	DSM-III	neurometric evaluation DA, split-half replication	central theta, fronto--temporal alpha, composite variables theta all regions, anterior power, total slow-wave asymmetry, total delta coherence accounted for most of the variance	Initial discriminant, AD vs Depression: SS (79) SP (72) Independent replication, AD vs Depression: SS (77) SP (85)
Prinz & Vitiello, 1989	41 AD 22 Depr. 50 C	71±8 62±5 68±7	MMSE: 23±3 29±1	NINCDS-ADRDA DSM-III SADS-C, HDRS	visual rating of dominant occipital frequency (DOF)	DOF significantly lower in AD vs C & Depr. lower DOF in Depr. vs C	DA AD vs C: SS (71) (82) OA (77); AD vs Depr: SS (66) SP (83)OA (72)
Moe et al, 1993	35 AD 24 Depr. 8 Depr+MCI 43 C	72±1 63±1 67±2 67±1	MMSE: 22±1 29±0.3 28±1	NINCDS-ADRDA DSM-III SADS-C, HDRS	frequency analysis of tonic REM sleep	Lower fast alpha power in Depr. vs C; higher beta, lower delta, theta & slow alpha in Depr. & C vs AD	DA: SS/Depr. (88) SS/AD (89), SP (100) Depr+MCI 100% correct prediction of outcome

Table 3. Selected studies reporting accuracy of EEG method in dementia diagnosis (Continued)

Author, year	Study sample	Age (years) Mean+SD, (range)	Disease severity	Diagnostic criteria	Method of analysis	Main findings	Indexes of accuracy* (%)
Dykierek et al, 1998	35 AD 39 Depr 42 C	62±9 68±10 64±8	MMSE: 20±5 28±2	NINCDS-ADRDA DSM-III-R HDRS, CAMDEX subscale	frequency analysis of tonic REM sleep	REM density & REM percentage lower in AD; REM latency shorter in Depr.	DA: SS/AD (96) SP/Depr. (76) OA (86)

* Where it has not been specifically mentioned, indexes of accuracy were obtained via discriminant analysis; DA – discriminant analysis; SS – sensitivity; SP specificity; OA – overall accuracy; PPV – positive predictive value; NPV – negative predictive value; LR+ - positive likelihood ratio; CDR - Clinical Dementia Rating scale (); DRS – Dementia Rating Scale (Mattis, 1976); ROI – region of interest; MCI – mild cognitive impairment; SMC – subjective memory complaints; NP – neuropsychology; NN – neuronal network; PCA – principal component analysis; CAMCOG – cognitive test from the CAMDEX-N (The Dutch version of the Cambridge Mental Disorders of the Elderly Examinations); BCRS – Brief Cognitive Rating Scale; SKT – Syndrom-Kurz-Test; ADAS – Alzheimer's Disease Assessment Scale; EC – eyes closed; EO – eyes open; ESD – Extended Scale for Dementia (Hersch, 1978); SADS-C – Schedule for Affective Disorders and Schizophrenia; HRS – Hamilton Depression Rating Scale; CMRglu-cerebral metabolic rate of glucose; GFP-global field power; ADS-6 – Amsterdamse Dementie Screening Test 6, a Dutch demenita screening test composed of subtests for visual and auditive memory, orientation, fluency, and constructional ability;

Few studies focused on the time domain in spontaneous EEGs in demented patients. One of them used a limited number of 10 controls and 10 healthy subjects and reported a decreased number and a longer duration of brain microstates implying that fewer brain generators were active in patients with AD (Ihl et al, 1993). Another study performed on a larger sample of 133 subjects with various degrees of cognitive decline and 21 controls found more anterior center of gravity of the microstate topography and, in contrast to the first study, reduced segment durations. The later discrepant finding authors explained as an incapability of the diseased brain to establish stable states of communicating neuronal activation patterns necessary for the attentional focusing and adequate information processing (Dierks et al, 1997).

Emerging novel non-linear methods of analysis have demonstrated decreased dimensional complexity in Alzheimer patients as measured by correlation dimension (D2) or global dimensional complexity (GDS) (Pritchard et al, 1994; Besthorn et al, 1995; Yagyu et al, 1997; Jeong et al, 1998; Jelles et al, 1999). Theoretically, neuronal and synapse loss characteristic of AD results in reduced number of functional neural networks and their dynamical interplay which influences complexity of EEG signal.

Although, there is a wealth of publications on use of EEG, and qEEG method in particular, in separating demented individuals from healthy elderly, only a selected number of articles could be assessed against the methodological criteria, Tables 3 to 5, and this review is mainly based on reports that could be classified as a class IB or class II A, II B evidence.

Cross-Sectional Studies, Classification Rates

Soinen et al (1982) published one of the first studies which applied discriminant analysis on EEG data of a representative study sample encompassing 56 patients with AD and 84 healthy elderly and resulted with a sensitivity of 82% and a specificity of 89% based on a dominant occipital rhythm. The limitations of this study are a visual analysis of the EEG data with a semiquantitative grading of severity, moderate to severe stage of the disease of the enrolled patients and lack of standardized clinical diagnostic criteria in the selection of the study population. Robinson et al (1994) also applied visual analysis to their EEG data, however the "gold standard" in their study is autopsy confirmed diagnosis. They reported that 87% of AD patients had abnormal EEG initially giving 87% sensitivity and when only moderately and severely abnormal EEGs were considered in a subgroup of AD patients with shorter duration of illness sensitivity was 50%, specificity 96% and negative predictive value 82.5%, meaning that absence of moderate to severe abnormality excludes the disease with a high certainty.

Study of Coben et al (1990) used two samples with mildly impaired AD patients and controls, 79 from the original study and 43 from a starting longitudinal study, with an aim to replicate earlier findings and asses the ability of each EEG measure to detect individual AD patients. Percentage theta power and a mean frequency were showing consistently difference across the two samples; however the most effective measure, percentage theta power, showed very modest sensitivity about 20% at 100% specificity and positive predictive value, meaning that in clinical settings test would be false negative in 4 out of 5 patients. However, this study used only one occipital-vertex derivation and did not apply current standardized clinical diagnostic criteria which limits its comparability with more recent studies.

Study of Elmståhl et al (1994) focused on qEEG differences between 23 female patients with rather advanced AD and 56 control subjects and via logistic regression analysis found predictive value of 0.94 for absolute delta power from the posterior head quadrant. This study does not provide data for measures of accuracy indexes which is hardly relevant since AD patients had a very severe form of the disease and, therefore, the study suffers from a spectrum bias. Diagnostic accuracy of topographic distributions of EEG alterations in mild to moderately impaired AD patients has been evaluated in study by Duffy et al (1995) on a large sample size of 60 patients and 129 controls by a split-half replication approach. Increased theta and decreased beta activity in 19 predominantly temporoparietal ROIs distinguished patients and controls and of these 5 variables were highly significant in discriminant function analysis which in training set correctly classified 77% of patients and 98% of controls and in the test set gave identical sensitivity with slightly lower specificity of 91%. This study primarily validated consistency of topographic patterns of spectral power distribution in AD, but given high prior probability of the disease the accuracy indexes are not so impressive to suggest optimal discriminators for clinical purposes.

Study of Jelic et al (1996) studied 54 subjects encompassing an equal number of AD patients, subjects with mild cognitive impairment (MCI) supposed to have a preclinical manifestation of the disease, those with subjective memory complaints but without objective evidence of memory decline and healthy controls. The authors found that the best discriminators between the groups were theta relative power from the fronto-central bipolar derivation and alpha relative power from parietooccipital derivation and that decreased alpha band temporo-parietal coherence appear as discriminating variable only between AD patients and controls, but not between AD and MCI which suggested that coherence should be further explored as a discriminating variable in very early stages of the disease. Besthorn et al (1997) studied 4 classification procedures in a data set of 50 probable and possible AD patients and 42 controls and found that discriminant analysis combined with PCA was superior to the classification based on group means, stepwise discriminant analysis, neuronal networks giving overall classification rate of 87% as compared to 83%, 86% and 84%, respectively. The best predictors were delta and theta power in eyes-open and eyes-closed condition and classification rates did not improve by addition of fast frequencies and coherence measures, but when introducing age and AD-subtypes overall classification accuracy increased to 90 and 96 %, respectively. Study of Knott et al (2000) reported similar lower sensitivity and specificity around 75 and 73 respectively, when both raw and Z-transformed coherence values according to population norms were used. Stevens et al (2001) reported slightly higher classification accuracy of 77% of coherence measures in fast bands during rest condition with eyes open and suggested as promising further assessment of dynamic coherence in future studies.

In their study Claus et al (1999) investigated diagnostic value of visually assessed EEG in patients with predominantly mild AD and reported quite low diagnostic accuracy with sensitivity of 45% at specificity of 89 % and positive predictive value 88% with pre-test diagnostic probability of 63%. Translated into clinical reality that would mean that among patients with positive test result 88% have AD. However, incremental ruling-in and ruling-out curves showed that maximum diagnostic gain is 38% for positive test result at pre-test probability of 30-40% and cca 10% when pre-test probability is high, 80-90 % meaning that visually assessed EEG could be clinically relevant only when there is a diagnostic doubt. These results are probably reflecting a lack of spectrum bias since AD patients were consecutively referred patients to the memory clinic and control subjects came from the general population. This study did not escape from the problem inherent to the procedures of visual analysis such as interrater reliability. The kappa statistics was 0.58, indicating only moderate agreement between two observers, so the final scoring was a result of a consensus. Knott et al (2001) tried to advance further clinical usefulness of quantitative EEG by comparing EEG data of AD patients to 2 normative groups, a normal age-matched control group and published adult age-regressed EEG population norms (Prichep & John, 1992), obtained on more than 200 adults in wide age range. Both, raw EEG data and age-regressed Z-score population normative values showed similar and very modest classification rates of only 75%.

An attempt to compare discriminative power of neuropsychometric tests like Alzheimer's disease Assessment Scale (ADAS) with EEG measures resulted in study of Ihl et al (2000) in almost optimal classification rate of both methods. ADAS gave 100% accuracy clearly because of inherent circularity in the design, since items of the test are very close to clinical symptoms. Four EEG variables in this study, topography of beta and delta activity and amplitude of delta activity, gave independent 94% correct classification rate.

Bennys et al (2001) addressed in their study another important methodological problem, a lack of a simple single reliable discriminating qEEG parameter. They demonstrated that a single theta/(alpha+beta) ratio from parieto-occipital region gave at optimal cut-off derived from the ROC curve sensitivity of 70% and specificity of 90%. Advantage of such ratios is that they are independent of the absolute power values which may largely differ among the subjects.

It has been reported that the addition of non-linear EEG measures like dimensional complexity (DCx) and neural-net (NN) modeling improve classification accuracy of AD patients and controls giving 92% overall diagnostic accuracy as compared to 77% achieved by traditional linear techniques like discriminant analysis (Pritchard et al, 1994). Potential usefulness of trained recurrent neural networks (RNN) combined with wavelet preprocessing to discriminate between AD and healthy aging has been suggested in a pilot study on a small sample of 20 patients and subjects where network achieved cca 80% sensitivity and 100% specificity (Petrosian et al, 2001).

Although sleep recordings are not user-friendly for the clinical routine, it is nevertheless worthwhile mentioning consistently reported across several studies high classification rates of frequency spectra during tonic REM sleep. (Petit et al, 1992; Prinz et al, 1992; Hassania et al, 1997; Dykierek et al, 1998). During wakefulness both cholinergic but also diffuse cortical projections of noradrenergic system are responsible for cortical activation, while during the REM sleep cholinergic activation prevails (Hobson et al, 1986) and, therefore it seems plausible that differences in EEG measures between AD patients and healthy controls observed during resting awake EEG could be augmented during sleep. In study of Petit et al (1992) ratio of slow to fast frequencies or percent power in conventional frequency bands from temporal regions resulted in no overlap among patients and controls and Hassania et al (1997) reported for ratio of slow to fast frequencies classification rate of 90% with sensitivity of 82% and specificity of 100%, while same measures in wakefulness classified correctly 81% of subjects with sensitivity 67% and specificity 96%. In subsequent study of Petit et al (1993) regional differences in EEG slowing, expressed by the ratio of slow to fast frequencies, during REM sleep were more prominent than during wakefulness, particularly in the temporal region. Prinz et al (1992) analyzed frequency spectra during tonic REM sleep and found reduced beta and increased delta and theta activity in AD patients. It is important to note that patients in this study were mildly impaired with mean MMSE scores of 22 and achieved indexes of accuracy were high, with sensitivity of 92% and specificity 95%.

Cognitive and Functional Relevance of EEG Indexes

A test that should contribute to the diagnostic process as well as have characteristics of a state marker should be related to the key symptoms of the disease – cognitive and functional impairment that are central to dementia. In what way are previously discussed quantitative EEG indexes related to the cognitive status of a demented subject and disease severity? Quite a few studies (Brenner et al, 1986; Primavera et al, 1990; Mody et al, 1991; Knott et al, 2001; Kowalski et al, 2001) reported correlations between qEEG measures and the Mini Mental Test Scores (MMSE) (Folstein et al, 1975). In general, positive correlation with a mean frequency and negative correlation with slow activity has been found by a conventional frequency analysis.

Dierks et al (1995) correlated peak frequency of equivalent dipoles generating brain electrical activity in different frequency bands, and found that neither MMSE or other psychometric scales used correlated with delta and theta activity, while there was positive correlation with alpha intensity. A method of MMSE is a simple measure of a global cognitive function used in most of the studies to stratify the severity of dementia and follow its progression, see Table 3, but cannot describe more precisely focal deficits in certain cognitive domains characteristic for AD. More detailed neuropsychological assessment is needed to describe neuropsychological profile of AD which is characterized by a specific sequence and pattern of cognitive decline during the course of AD, related to the topographical evolution of the disease pathology. Early changes are observed in the domain of secondary memory, particularly episodic memory, visuospatial function and attention (Almkvist & Bäckman, 1993; Storey et al, 2002). This is followed by impairment of verbal functions, and in fully developed disease short-term or primary memory. Several studies have reported that increased slowing in EEG and decreased fast activity were associated with poor test performance (Duffy et al, 1984; 1995; Pozzi et al, 1995; Jelic et al, 1996). Duffy et al (1995) used qEEG with topographic mapping and reported in their study that relative theta power during eyes open condition, predominantly from posterior and parietal temporal regions, was significantly correlated with the delayed verbal recall score, a measure of episodic memory which is impaired in early stages of the disease. The absolute beta power correlated significantly with neuropsychological measures representing memory, executive function and language. In another study lower alpha relative power was significantly associated with a worse performance on tests of attention, memory and language (Pozzi et al, 1995). This is not surprising, since alpha power has been traditionally associated with attentional processes and attention is also an important prerequisite for a memory performance.

Quantitative EEG has been also proposed as a confirmatory test of localization following a syndrome analysis approach to neurological assessment (Shenal et al, 2001). It has been demonstrated via this approach that EEG slow wave activity in dementia, represented by the low frequency of posterior dominant rhythm and increased percentage of delta and theta activity, reflects parietal lobe dysfunction (Edman et al, 1995).

An important aspect is the evidence of heterogeneity of cognitive profiles among AD patients which implies existence of clinical subtypes of the disease and could have importance for a prognosis and treatment (Petersen, 1998). Neuropsychological assessment is crucial in distinguishing these subgroups, however there is a possibility of a false-positive rate and in this context qEEG measures could add independent confirmatory information. Albert et al (1990) used brain electrical activity mapping in 16 patients subdivided into 2 groups according to their cognitive profile. It has been found that a patient group with a pronounced decline in spatial abilities, as compared to the group with a profound memory deficit, had less beta activity in 14 EEG and EP regions, 11 of which belonged to the parietal area and were mostly bilateral. Topography of beta activity was also reported to distinguish two subgroups of AD patients, with severely affected patients having the lowest activity and a map with flat distribution without centro-parieto-occipito-temporal maxima observed in controls (Ihl et al, 1989).

Some authors argue that integrity of widespread cortical networks linking specific regions is equally or even more crucial for complex cognitive functions than specific topography. In that context EEG coherence or similar measurements of statistical interrelationships between time series recorded at different sites, could be a more precise way to localize brain function than the conventional spectral analysis (Leuchter et al, 1992; Dunkin et al, 1995; Gevins et al, 1998).

Several studies have done an attempt to relate index of EEG dimensional complexity to cognitive performance and found that it was related to the intelligence quotient in healthy subjects (Lutzenberger et al, 1992). In a couple of studies on AD patients it showed weak correlations with scores on neuropsychological tests representing frontal dysfunctions (Jelles et al, 1999), general intellectual function and tests from verbal memory domain (Ikawa et al, 2000).

For research and clinical settings staging of the severity of the disease is often performed by clinical rating scales such as the Global Deterioration Scale (GDS) (Reisberg et al, 1982). Several studies have found significant correlations between GDS stages and EEG measures, implying that the later could be used independently for functional staging of the disease and eventually become established as state markers of the disease (Prichep et al, 1993; Chiaramonti et al, 1997; Rodriguez et al, 1999). Using the Neurometric method in a large sample of 319 elderly with a broad spectrum of cognitive decline Prichep et al (1994) found that increased theta activity shows the greatest and earliest deviations from the population norms, starting already in GDS phase 2 and growing significant differences across stages 3-6, while absolute alpha power remains largely within normal limits throughout the range of clinical deterioration.

To summarize, resting state qEEG variables correlate with specific cognitive and functional deficits in AD, although straight forward interpretation of their direct link to specific cognitive processes remains speculative without validation in activation studies and correlative studies with functional neuroimaging methods.

Longitudinal Studies, Prognosis and Prediction

A prospective longitudinal study design is the best way to validate cross-sectional findings and to determine their prognostic significance in terms of wide range of outcomes.

Several longitudinal studies have examined prevalence of EEG abnormalities in AD patients, their evolution during disease progress and predictive power of future cognitive or functional decline in subjects at risk of developing AD. Review of selected longitudinal studies is given in table 4.

Prognosis

One of the largest cohorts reported in the literature consisted of 139 patients with AD and mixed dementia and 148 age-matched healthy controls, who were followed with sequential EEG recordings during the variable period of time up to 4 years (Rae-Grant *et al*, 1987). Using visual ratings authors demonstrated that progression and pattern of EEG changes varied with time, but was stable in individual patients showing good correlation between successive recordings, most probably due to the initial severe stage of illness. Interestingly 12% of AD patients improved and in 21% of subjects who came to autopsy there was correlation with psychometric scores, neuronal loss and EEG grade. Coben *et al* (1985) followed 43 patients with mild AD and 43 healthy control subjects for a 2.5 years period and reported linear changes in EEG power for all 4 frequency bands with time: increase of delta and theta and decrease of alpha and beta power, where for theta there was also an exponential component in addition to the linear one since change occurred between entry and 1 year follow up, not afterwards. Theta relative power also distinguished between all four stages of AD at 1 year after entry, however no significant differences at entry were found for two AD subgroups who had after the 1 year follow-up either progressed to the moderate dementia or remained stable. Possible explanation for a lack of prognostic significance of EEG variables could be already advanced disease process at entry and ceiling effect of some EEG variables. In study of Soininen et al (1991) data from only one temporo-occipital bipolar derivation were analyzed and it was found that absolute theta power was the best discriminating variable between the patients who progressed more rapidly during the first year of the follow up, as well as between those who after 3 years remained at home and those who were institutionalized or died, giving 87, 5 % correct classification of cases. An important source of bias is high drop-out rate with only 54% of patients being left after the 3 years follow-up, which in addition decreases final number of subjects, reduces statistical significance and limits interpretation. Another study demonstrated on the same data set that patients with deteriorating EEG showed also a decline of praxic functions, confrontation naming, automatic speech functions and a tendency towards a higher frequency of extrapyramidal symptoms (Helkala *et al*, 1991). In contrast to previous two studies Kuskowski *et al* (1993) found that absolute alpha power analyzed over all electrode sites correlated with computed rate of MMSE decline in 15 AD patients with mild to moderate disease followed for up to 4 years, meaning that alpha power could be an index of cognitive deterioration or in another words a state marker of the disease. Slowing of the posterior dominant EEG rhythm was reported in a multicenter study to be a predictor of disease progression (Richards *et al*, 1993). In line with these findings lower fast activities in alpha and/or beta range were reported to predict survival in a prospective cohort study of more than 100 patients with early Alzheimer's disease as well as more decline in global cognitive function and activities in daily living (Claus *et al*, 1998a; Claus *et al*, 1998b; Claus *et al*, 1998c). Loss of activities of daily living (ADL) and onset of incontinence are among the final clinical milestones in the progression of the disease and delta and theta power respectively predicted their occurrence in 31 AD patients followed for a mean time of 26 months (Rodriguez *et al*, 1996).

Table 4. Selected longitudinal studies on EEG changes in demented and high- risk subjects: EEG as a prognostic marker and a predictor of differential outcome.

Source (year)	Sample	Age in yrs (SD)	Follow up	Outcome measures and end-points	Results
Coben et al, 1985	43 mild AD (CDR 1) 43 controls	72 (4) 71 (5)	2.5 years, annual recordings	CDR	Theta relative power distinguished all 4 stages of AD after 1 year; no EEG variables at baseline distingusihed AD subgroup which progressed after 1 year (2 channel montage)
Rae-Grant et al, 1987	139 AD and mix-AD 148 controls	73 (8.9)	1 – 4 yrs with annual evaluations	ESD, London Psycho- geriatric Rating Scale	EEG (visual ratings) varied in progression and pattern, 12% AD improved; correlation between EEG grade, psychometric scores and neuron loss (21% came to autopsy)
Soininen et al, 1991	24 AD patients mild to moderate stage (1 severe); 54% remained after 3 years	66 (6)	3 years	CDR, BCRS institutionalisation death	Absolute theta amplitude best discriminating variable of poor outcome; 87.5% correct classification home care vs institutionalisation vs death (data from T6-O2)
Helkala et al, 1991	24 AD patients	66 (6)	3 yrs with annual evaluations	CDR, BCRS, PDRS	abnormal (composite index criteria) qEEG predicts more severe cog. decline higher frequency of extrapyramid symptoms and institutionalization
Leuchter 1994	Group 1: 50 AD, 24 MID Group 2:AD 23, MID 17	74 (mean) 75 (mean)	2 years (15-37 months)	IADL, ADL institutionalisation (via structured telephone questionnaire)	decreased coherence across the Rolandic fissure in the left hemisphere was significantly associated with poorer functional status as measured by ADL
Rodriguez et al, 1996	31 AD patients (baseline GDS 3-6)	69 (8.4)	26.4 months	ADL, urinary incontinence, death	delta power predicted loss of ADL and death, theta power incontinence
Elmståhl et al, 1997	33 healthy old females (population registry)	75-95	5 years	MMSE (<27), NP assesment	low beta activity + orthostatic blood pressure reaction predicted cog. decline

Table 4. Continued.

Source (year)	Sample	Age in yrs (SD)	Follow up	Outcome measures and end-points	Results
Strijers et al, 1997	58 MCI subjects (community-based)	65-75	5 years	CAMDEX, AD (NINCDS-ADRDA)	classification accuracy (stable vs converters) of qEEG 84% compared to 72% of MRI (cut-offs derived from ROC curves)
Lopez et al, 1997	95 AD patients	72.7 (7)	3.6	MMSE, BDRS, ADL	abnormal EEG and psychosis independent predictors of cognitive and functional impairment
Claus et al, 1998	82 AD patients	79.1 (6)	6 months	CAMCOG, ADL, RMBPC	lower parieto-occipital beta and higher theta power predictive variables for decline in both cognition and function
Claus et al, 1998	101 AD patients	79.2 (6.3)	4.4 yrs (survivors) 2.6 yrs (non-survivors)	Mortality	beta and alpha activity independent predictors of survival
Jelic et al, 2000	27 MCI subjects	58 (6)	21 months (12-39)	MMSE, transition to AD (NINCDS-ADRDA)	baseline MMSE and alpha and theta relative power predicted transition to AD in 85% of cases (only MMSE in 70%)
Huang et al, 2000	31 MCI subjects	61 (8)	26 months (12-48)	MMSE, transition to AD (NINCDS-ADRDA)	in linear DA "anteriozation" of alpha activity gave 77% classification accuracy between MCI subjects who remained stable and those who developed AD

ADL – Activities of Daily Living; BDRS – Blessed Dementia Rating Scale; BCRS – Brief Cognitive Rating Scale; ESD – Extended Scale of Dementia; PDRS – Parkinson's Disease Rating Scale; RMBPC-Revised Memory and Behavioral Problems Checklist (Dutch version); DA – discriminant analysis.

Prediction

It is of a great research interest as well as a potential practical utility at the clinical level to be able to predict with diagnostic instruments development of the disease in subjects who are at greater risk to develop dementia than a general population or have a preclinical phase of the disease. A new operational definition of mild cognitive impairment (MCI) has been proposed for the subjects who have subjective and objective memory deficits which do not cause functional impairment necessary for the clinical diagnosis of dementia (Petersen et al, 1999). Studies with structural imaging methods such as MRI have shown cca 80-85%

prediction accuracy of reduced volumes of medial temporal lobe structures in MCI subjects who later develop AD (Visser et al, 2002; Wolf et al, 2003). Similarly, reduced temporoparietal blood flow and glucose metabolism, measured by SPECT and PET, demonstrated 80 to 90%, correct classification rate of those individuals who progressed to AD (Johnson et al, 1998; Arnaiz et al, 2001). Could EEG variables with a similar precision predict transition from MCI to AD? In their longitudinal study Jelic et al (2000) followed 27 MCI individuals for 2 years, after which 54% developed AD. Combined alpha and theta relative power and the mean frequency from the left temporo-occipital derivation, controlled for the baseline MMSE in a logistic regression model, were the best predictors of MCI outcome, giving 85% classification accuracy.

Authors from the same group have applied the method of FFT approximation on the slightly enlarged sample in a similar study design and demonstrated in a linear discriminant analysis that the best predictor of future development of AD in MCI subjects was "anteriorization" of alpha frequency, giving 71% sensitivity and 82% specificity (Huang et al, 2000). Compared to the MCI subjects who remained stable, those MCI individuals who progressed to AD had decreased alpha GFP and a more anterior localization of sources of theta, alpha and beta frequency, Fig 3.

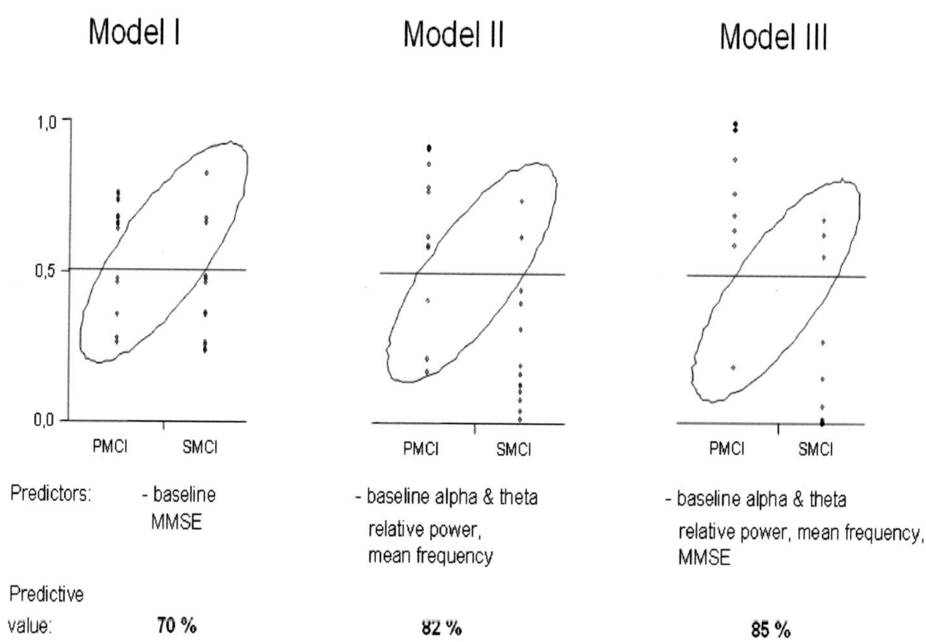

Figure 2. Plots of predictive probabilities obrtained from the logistic regression models using baseline MMSE scores (Model I), baseline qEEG variables (Model II), baseline MMSE scores + baseline EEG variables (Model III) as predictors of clinical outcome in subjects with MCI at baseline, after on average 2 years follow-up period. Misclassified subjects are marked by elipses. SMCI- stable MCI; PMCI – progressive MCI; for the misclassified PMCI subject from Model III an alternative diagnosis of corticobasal degeneration was considered after repeated clinical evaluation, performed blind of the results from this analysis. (figure from Jelic, 1999)

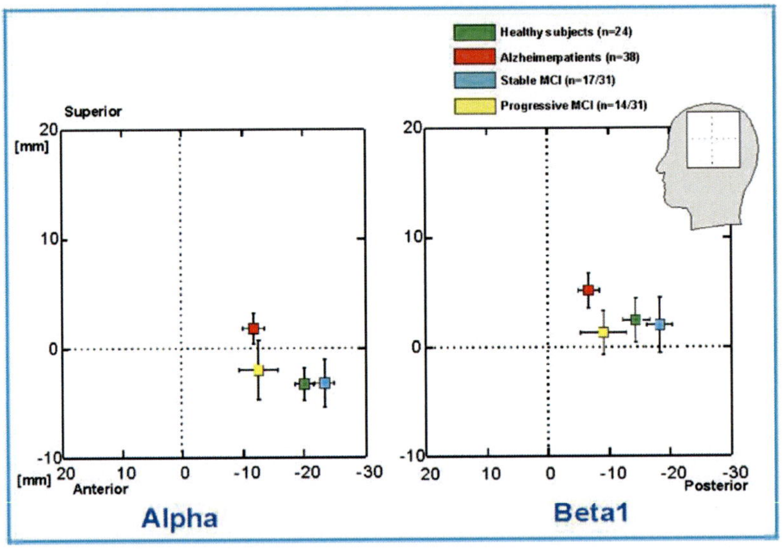

Figure 3. Spatial characteristics of EEG activity in patients with AD, MCI subjects and healthy individuals. Figure demonstrates that there is anteriorization of alpha and beta 1 GFP in MCI subjects who deteriorated clinically and were diagnosed with AD after a mean follow up of 26 months. (based on data from Huang et al, 2000).

Recent cross sectional studies have also addressed various measures of EEG synchronization in MCI subjects as compared to AD patients and healthy controls (Stam et al, 2003; Koenig et al, in press). It would be of interest to explore their predictive power of differential outcome in a prospective longitudinal study design. Furthermore, it should be explored whether there is a gain in classification accuracy by adding activation paradigms to the conventional resting EEG, as the recent cross-sectional study demonstrated better separation between MCI and healthy subjects by means of increased theta power in MCI during a haptic tasks (Grunwald et al, 2002).

Correlative Studies with Neuroimaging Methods

Interest in correlative studies of EEG and neuroimaging methods of other modalities, structural as well as functional is twofold. Firstly, these studies could provide information on relation between brain structure and various aspects of brain function on one side and electrical brain activity on the other. Secondly, they could demonstrate comparative advantage or disadvantage or complementary diagnostic value of EEG method in classifying correctly demented subjects and healthy individuals in clinical settings.

EEG findings in AD, in particular the regional power of delta and theta bands and the resulting changes in mean frequency, have been shown in earlier studies to correlate with other measures of cerebral functions such as cerebral blood flow (Johanesson et al, 1977; Ingvar et al, 1979; Stigsby et al, 1981; Passero et al, 1995; Siennicki-Lantz, 1998; Rodriguez et al, 1998). A large study of Claus et al (2000) on 163 consecutive patients with probable and possible AD found significant correlation between lower temporo-parietal rCBF and lower parieto-occipital alpha activity, and this association remained unchanged when leukoaraiosis or indices of cortical atrophy were added to the regression model. Kwa et al (1993) et al found that patients with normal EEG peak frequency and a normal SPECT scan had a tendency towards a shorter duration of illness when compared to patients with normal EEG peak frequency but abnormal SPECT scan, suggesting that typical hypoperfusion of temporoparietal area precedes slowing in the EEG. However, a small number of subjects in these subgroups, 5 and 3 respectively, make this hypothesis speculative without confirmation on a larger sample.

The most recent study using a new imaging method of dynamic susceptibility contrast MRI averaged temporoparietal and sensorimotor regional cerebral blood volume into a total perfusion index and demonstrated negative correlation with antero-central theta relative power and positive correlation with alpha relative power over central regions (Mattia et al, 2003). EEG slowing showed also regional correlations with lower oxygen metabolism in AD patients (Buchan et al, 1997).

Sheridan et al (1988) described a higher cerebral glucose metabolism, as measured by PET, in patients with preserved alpha background activity and correlated these findings with psychometric tests for parietal lobe function. In another study AD patients and healthy controls performed a verbal memory task during the uptake of FDG and authors found that AD patients had significantly greater left temporal delta amplitude which showed higher correlations with hippocampal metabolic rate than metabolic rate measured in the brain area under the electrode (Valladeras-Neto et al, 1995).

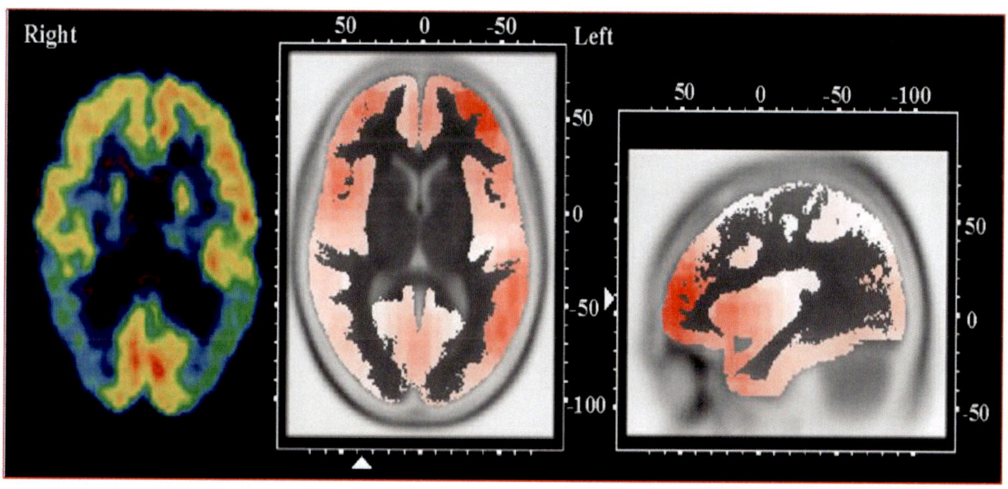

Figure. 4 Correlation between spatial pattern of glucose metabolism and localisation of intracerebral EEG generators. Left. PET image of cerebral glucose metabolism of a patient with Alzheimer's disease with MMSE score 23; Right: EEG LORETA-KEY©® (Pasqual-Marqui, 1999) image of the estimated source distribution of the same patient displayed in Talaraich space; images were scaled to the maximum activity, darlker yellow and red reflecting higher glucose metabolism, and more intense red indicating higher activity of EEG. (modified from Dierks et al, 2000)

Recent study aimed to show similarity between regional cerebral metabolic rate of glucose (rCMRglu) and EEG spatial patterns in a population with varying degrees of cognitive dysfunction (Dierks et al, 2000). Authors demonstrated that localization of EEG generator in antero-posterior direction correlated with CMRglu in the frequency bands between 7 and 15 Hz, while superior-inferior ratio of CMRglu in the brain correlated positively with the localization of the EEG generator in superior-inferior direction in the frequency band between 21 and 26 Hz. Furthermore, asymmetry index of the metabolic ratio showed a positive correlation with the localization of the generator of the brain electrical activity in the left-right direction. In this study PET images were contrasted to the LORETA images of the same subjects, ilustrating similarity between metabolic and neurophysiological spatial patterns, Fig 4.

A few studies compared EEG and structural imaging methods on clinical samples. An early study by Kaszniak et al (1979) examined 78 hospital patients with memory impairment and found in multiple regression analysis that EEG slowing rated visually, and cerebral atrophy as assessed by CT scans had independent negative correlations with several cognitive variables, indicating that EEG slowing and cerebral atrophy might reflect independent pathological processes. Interestingly, EEG slowing had much stronger influence on cognition than atrophy. Structural imaging methods have also revealed that presence of leukoaraiosis and white matter hyperintensities (WMH) is a common finding in AD patients and could, probably due to subtle cerebrovascular changes, additionally influence severity of a clinical presentation of the disease and its progression. Correlation between presence of leukoaraiosis and increased absolute delta and theta activity (Claus *et al*, 2000), as well as, a relation between visually graded EEG abnormality and periventricular WMH (Lopez *et al*, 1995) have been reported. These findings further support hypothesis that cortical deafferentation via white matter lesions could induce increase in delta activity in EEG. It is intriguing that the correlation dimension (D2) was correlated with periventricular white matter hyperintensities as visualized by CT and not with cortical atrophy (Jelles *et al*, 1999). It seems that pathology in deeper brain structures has a global effect on brain electrical activity and complexity of cortical dynamics.

Another point of interest in correlative studies is comparison of diagnostic accuracies of structural and various functional imaging methods. Several studies addressing this topic are listed in Table 5. One of the earliest comparative studies with CT found that in discriminant function analysis the best discriminator was dominant occipital rhythm, classifying correctly 86% of patients and healthy controls. Adding an index of cortical atrophy, width of the third ventricle, increased classification accuracy till 90% (Soininen et al, 1982b). Another study focused on differential diagnosis of dementia and included in analysis 50 patients with AD, multiinfarct dementia (MID) or mixed type, 32 of them got final diagnosis at the autopsy (Ettlin et al, 1989). In the group with autopsy proven diagnoses of 3 clinical subgroups, CT measures of cortical atrophy and ventricular size and EEG criteria based on the visual analysis gave comparable sensitivity in differentiating subgroups. However, although each method classified AD patients with 80% sensitivity they were very poor in classifying MID patients giving only 18% sensitivity, while EEG failed in classifying correctly mixed cases. Both AD and MID patients in this study were moderately to severely impaired, which implies that once the dementing process is clinically advanced, irrespective of underlying pathology there is also increased cortical atrophy and consequences on brain function and its neurophysiological parameters are similar in, from pathological perspective, different dementing diseases.

Table 5. Selected review of clinical studies comparing diagnostic accuracies of EEG and neuroimaging methods of various modalities.

Author, year	Study sample	Age Mean +SD, (range)	Disease severity	Diagnostic criteria	Methods of analysis	Main findings & Indexes of accuracy (%)
Etlin et al, 1989	15 AD 11 MID 6 MIX	83±15 82±6 86±8	MMSE 8±7 9±7 17±6	autopsy-based study	EEG: visual rating (overall disturbance asymmetry, bifrontal delta waves) CT: cortical atrophy ventricular size rating, presence of infarcts	CT or EEG: AD vs other forms SS (80 each) SP (35,29); MID vs other forms SS (18 each) SP (100, 90); MIX vs other forms SS (17,0) SP (81,92); combined methods: AD vs other SS (47), SP (65); MID vs others SS (9), SP (100); MIX vs others SS (16) SP (35).
Szelies et al, 1992	42 AD 15 C	67±8 56±7	mean GDS 4±1 (3-6)	NINCDS-ADRDA	FDG-PET: quantitative regional analysis ($rCMR_{Glu}$) EEG: frequency analysis; comparison by ROC curves area.	Temporoparietal $rCMR_{Glu}$ SS(87) vs global & temporoparietal relative theta power SS (86); at SP (100) $rCMR_{Glu}$ SS(72), global theta power SS (43); at SP (93) global theta power SS (79); for mild AD patients global theta power SS (71) at SP (93).
Szelies et al, 1994	24 AD 19 VaD 15 C	66±8 69±10 60±7	GDS 3.4±0.5 3.4±0.5	NINCDS-ADRDA NINCDS-AIREN	FDG-PET: quantitative regional analysis ($rCMR_{Glu}$) and metabolic ratio; EEG: frequency analysis.	DA correct classification by metabolic ratio: AD (75) VaD (53) C (7) OA (66); DA correct classification by relative theta power and occipital/frontal alpha ratio: AD (58) VaD (47) C (53) OA (53) DA combined PET & EEG variables: AD (79) VaD (53) C (80) OA (71).
Vallada res-Neto et al, 1995	36 AD 17 C	73±9 70±7	MMSE 19±5	NINCDS-ADRDA	FDG-PET: quantitative regional analysis ($rCMR_{Glu}$) and metabolic ratio; EEG: frequency analysis. Discriminant analysis (DA).	Absolute left temporal delta amplitude and lateral rCMRGlu best discriminators. DA with EEG variables only: SS (71) SP (88) DA with rCMRGlu only: SS (77) SP (94).

Table 5. Selected review of clinical studies comparing diagnostic accuracies of EEG and neuroimaging methods of various modalities. (Continued)

Author, year	Study sample	Age Mean +SD, (range)	Disease severity	Diagnostic criteria	Methods of analysis	Main findings & Indexes of accuracy (%)
Strijers et al, 1997	58 community dwelling elderly: 9 AD, 49 Non-AD (31 MCI 18 normal)	81±5 78±5	MMSE: 18±7 25±4	NINCDS-ADRDA CAMDEX criteria	MRI: visual rating of MTA; EEG: visual rating & frequency analysis. ROC analysis	EEG visual rating, : SS (67) SP (84) OA (81) EEG delta & theta power, centroparieto occipital derivations: SS (44-67) SP (90) OA (81-84). MRI (MTA): SS (71) SP (72) OA (72).
Rodriguez et al, 1998	42 AD 18 C	72±9 65±6	MMSE 15±7 GDS 4±1	NINCDS-ADRDA	rCBF by Xe-inhalation technique; EEG: frequency analysis. Discriminant analysis.	EEG variables, right hemisphere: SS (71; 47 for GDS 3 only) SP (89) OA (77) rCBF variables, right hemisphere: SS (74; 65 for GDS 3 only) SP (78) OA (75) EEG+rCBF variables: SS (88; 77 for GDS 3) SP (89) OA (88).
Jelic et al, 1999	40 AD 14 C	61±7 57±9	MMSE 24±3 FSIQ 82±12	NINCDS-ADRDA	FDG-PET: quantitative regional analysis ($rCMR_{Glu}$) and metabolic ratio; EEG: frequency analysis. Discriminant analysis.	EEG relative theta power: SS (83) SP (71) OA (80) PET metabolic ratio: SS (80) SP (100) OA (85) EEG+PET variables: SS (88) SP (100) OA (91).

AD-Alzheimer's disease; SS- sensitivity; SP- specificity; OA- overall accuracy; MID-Multiinfarct dementia; MIX-mixed dementia; C-healthy controls; ROC-Receiver Operator Characteristic; VaD-vascular dementia; MTA-medial temporal lobe atrophy; rCBF-regional cerebral blood flow; FSIQ-full scale intelligence quotient;

A couple of studies compared diagnostic accuracies of regional glucose metabolism as measured by PET and qEEG parameters. Szelies et al (1992) and Jelic et al (1999) both reported that relative temporo-parietal theta power showed an accuracy close to that of glucose metabolic values from PET in differentiating between mildly to moderately impaired AD patients and healthy elderly. In the first study receiver operator characteristic (ROC) curves were applied and showed very similar areas under the curve for either PET or EEG, 86% versus 87% respectively. In the later study by Jelic et al (1999) in the discriminant analysis EEG and PET combined gave an almost optimal classification accuracy of 91%. It is interesting that healthy controls that were misclassified as diseased by means of EEG parameter performed significantly worse than correctly classified controls on tests representing visuospatial functions and attention. This observation suggests that EEG could provide sensitive state markers but should be combined with another method with higher specificity to achieve the optimal diagnostic accuracy. This line of thinking is supported by the results from the study which correlated rCBF as measured by ^{133}Xe-inhalation technique and qEEG parameters (Rodriguez et al, 1998). Authors reported that while sensitivity of a relative power in slow frequency bands alone was reaching 89%, adding rCBF measures of right hemisphere increased specificity from 71% to 88%. However, this study included patients with a wide range of disease severity (MMSE 1-24), which makes the reported figures on diagnostic accuracy less impressive.

Surprisingly very few studies compared diagnostic accuracy of qEEG with a method that is most often discussed in the literature as the potential neuroimaging marker of the AD: MRI. The study of Strijers et al (1997) is unique because the population studied encompassed a community-dwelling population enriched with subjects with minimal dementia, which reflects more realistically daily practice in a memory clinic. Furthermore, the authors compared with MRI measures of medial temporal lobe atrophy both, visually analyzed EEG as well as qEEG and found that MRI measure showed a total classification accuracy of 72%, while visually assessed EEG and qEEG measures (delta and theta power in centro-parieto-occipital derivations) 81% and 84% respectively. It is important to note that there was an overlap in subjects showing EEG or MRI abnormalities, which imply that two methods are complementary to each other in the diagnostic, process probably because they have different sensitivity to various aspects of the disease or stages during the disease progression.

EEG in Differential Diagnosis of Dementia

EEG in Major Depression, Comparison with AD

An important challenge to the clinician is to differentiate subjects with depression as a behavioral manifestation of AD and those with depression-related cognitive impairment, so called pseudodementia. Converging evidence from the literature suggests that EEG variables could be successful in this discrimination, since EEG is in general normal in depression. Most of the studies using quantitative EEG, as reviewed by Pollock and Schneider (1990b), reported increases in both alpha and beta power and no increase in slow activities. Increased alpha activity was present in elderly subjects even after recovery from depression (Pollock and Schneider, 1989).

Brenner et al (1986) studied a sample of 35 AD patients, 23 patients with major depression and 61 healthy elderly controls and found that depressed patients had significantly less delta and theta activity when compared to AD patients and decreased parasagittal mean frequency and beta power when compared to controls. Although specificity in this study was optimal, sensitivity was only 58% and 27% when AD patients were divided into subgroups with MMSE ≤22 and ≥23, respectively. In study of Prinz and Vitiello (1989) a simple visual rating of dominant occipital frequency in a sample of 41 AD patients in early stage of the disease, 22 subjects with major depressive disorder and 50 healthy control subjects, achieved an overall correct classification rate of 77% for AD versus controls (criterion level 8.88 Hz) and 72% for AD versus depressed subjects (criterion level 8.98 Hz).

An early study of O'Connor et al (1979) differentiated by EEG coherence measures at 10 Hz between right parietal and temporal derivation 3 relatively small groups of healthy subjects, patients with depression and arteriosclerotic dementia. No replication of these results on a larger sample appeared later in the literature.

Ihl and Brinkmeyer (1999) compared in their study GFP and EEG segmentation in 11 young and 10 aged controls, 12 patients with mild AD, 10 young and 12 aged patients with endogenous monopolar depression in order to investigate possible alterations due to aging, AD and depression. The main findings of this study were increased number of different EEG segments in the beta frequency band in aged controls and aged patients with depression as compared to AD patients which supports the hypothesis of unchanged EEG parameters in depression and suggests increased variability in brain function and increased complexity of the EEG in elderly subjects. In contrast to these findings, Strik et al (1995) did not find differences in the topography of the microstates, while there was only a trend to shorter microstates when all segments were considered in a sample of 22 depressive patients compared to 22 controls with a wide age range. Authors speculated that a deficit in sustained attention during spontaneous cognition could explain a finding of shorter microstates in depression.

Several studies have suggested that sleep EEG, especially REM sleep physiology, could add additional sensitivity to the differentiation between AD and depressive illness in elderly (Reynolds III et al, 1985; Bahro et al, 1993; Moe et al, 1993; Dykierek et al, 1998). Theoretical background for this empirical data are results from animal experiments showing that cholinergic cell groups in the brain stem trigger and maintain REM sleep, in complex interaction with noradrenergic and serotonergic nuclei in the brainstem (Hobson et al, 1986).

Due to cholinergic hyperactivity REM latency is assumed to be shortened in depression and prolonged in AD patients. Reynolds et al (1985) used visual analysis of REM sleep EEG and found in a prospective study on a 25 healthy aged subjects, 25 elderly depressives and 25 elderly demented patients with mild to moderate dementia, that the sleep of the depressed subjects was characterized by a reduced REM sleep latency, increased REM percent and altered temporal distribution of REM, REM density when compared to the AD patients. In addition AD patients had less severe sleep maintenance difficulties than depressives. Combination of REM latency cut-off score of <30 minutes, REM density and sleep maintenance percent correctly classified 68% of depressives and 60% of demented patients. It has to be mentioned that demented patients in this study were not classified on the basis of possible etiological background. Results from the study of Bahro et al (1993), which also applied visual scoring of sleep variables, confirmed lower REM percentage, total REM density in AD patients but did not find increased REM sleep latency. Possible explanation could be more advanced disease process in AD patients in this sample, where also noradrenergic pathways originating in the locus coeruleus which inhibit REM sleep are affected. However, this is just a speculation due to the methodological problem of this paper: lack of the control group.

In their methodologically more advanced study which used qEEG analysis of tonic REM data, Moe et al (1993) found that a complex diagnostic score based on a correspondence of depressed subject's spectra with frequency microbins of known AD and control populations, correctly classified 88% of patients with a major unipolar depressive disorder, 89% of mild

AD patients and 100% of the controls. In addition, clinical outcome after 4 years follow-up of 8 subjects with depression and initially cognitive impairment was correctly predicted with baseline diagnostic score. The strengths of this study were recruitment of the depressed patients from the community at large and 4-years follow-up of cognitive and health status of the study sample. Similar high classification rates were obtained in study by Dykierek et al (1998) where stepwise discriminant analysis using REM density, REM latency, and REM percentage correctly classified 96% of AD patients and 76% of patients with old age depression. Interestingly, discriminative power of REM density was higher than that of REM latency.

Studies addressing qEEG changes in depressed subjects without dementia and depressed AD patients are still very rare. Pozzi et al (1995) examined 18 non-depressed AD patients, 13 non-demented patients with major depression or dysthymia, 17 AD patients who also met criteria for either dysthymia or major depression and 10 healthy control subjects. When compared to non-depressed AD patients, depressed AD patients showed significant increases in both delta and theta relative power and significant reduction of alpha relative power in posterior brain regions, mainly bilaterally. Depressed non-AD patients had decreased alpha power unilaterally, over the right hemisphere. Depressed non-AD patients had also a significant global decrease of delta power, while depressed patients with AD had significant increase of delta power in posterior brain areas. It would be of clinical interest to examine whether these qEEG differences between AD patients with and without depression predict faster progression of the disease. Another important issue is whether qEEG variables could predict in subjects with depression future development of AD, since depressive symptoms have been observed before the diagnosis of AD and depression has been recognized as a risk factor for Alzheimer's disease (Berger et al, 1999; Green et al, 2003).

One has to be aware of the limitation of the studies with depressed subjects which are in general not drug naive and even with temporary withdrawals some influence of centrally active drugs can still remain and could influence functional diagnostic test, such as EEG.

EEG in other Dementing Disorders, Comparisons with AD and Controls

Vascular Dementia

The concept of vascular and mixed dementia is still controversial with several unresolved issues like lack of specificity of the diagnostic criteria which should play a "gold standard" in clinical studies, various pathogenetic processes behind the single nosological term, synergistic effects of vascular and degenerative lesions in producing cognitive deficit, influence of white matter changes, etc (Leys et al, 1999). Vascular dementia is a diagnostic challenge because its progression could be modified by preventive strategies. Could EEG have a role in this process?

Early studies employing visual analysis found similar EEG abnormalities in AD and MID in terms of over-all disturbance, lower average frequency of dominant occipital rhythm, accentuation of theta and delta rhythms, fluctuations in alertness, paroxysmal activity and driving response (Soininen et al, 1982a). The EEG findings of the MID patients differed significantly from those of AD patients and controls only in asymmetric findings which were more common in MID. Interestingly, mild asymmetric findings in a form of focal abnormalities, mostly theta activity in the left temporal region, were even present in 33% of the controls which might be due to the presence of silent vascular pathology. This speculation could be supported by study of Logar et al (1993) who investigated a sample of 72 healthy individuals with age range 45-74 years and found focal changes on EEG mapping in 46% of the subjects who had cerebrovascular risk factors, while this applied to only 11% of those without presence of risk factors, giving sensitivity of 46% and specificity of 89%. By taking into account a number of risk factors present, sensitivity increased to 59%.

Erkinjuti et al (1988) applied both, visual and frequency analysis on EEG data from a large sample of 67 AD, 77 MID and 45 probable vascular dementia (PVD) patients and found that patients with different types of dementia did not differ significantly in regard to diffuse abnormality, occurrence of driving response, mean background frequency or other parameters of quantitative EEG. However, all these measures were related to the degree of dementia in this study. In agreement with other studies, authors also reported increased focal slowing which was present in 18% of AD, 36% of MID and 13% of PVD patients resulting in relative risk (RR) of 2.1 for MID compared to AD, which gave sensitivity of 50% and specificity of 96%. Paroxysmal activity was seen in 45% of AD, 64% pf MID and 58% of PVD, giving RR of 2 for MID compared to AD. Since the criteria for vascular dementia also include cases with a combination of degenerative and vascular changes, lack of more pronounced focal findings in PVD could be explained by more prevalent mixed cases in this group. The clinical accuracy of diagnoses authors confirmed on a smaller subsample who came to autopsy which was for AD 100%, for MID 89% and for PVD only 60%.

John et al (1988) compared percentages of abnormal findings in two subgroups of patients with cerebrovascular disease: symptomatic patients with completed stroke and asymptomatic patients with reversible ischemic neurologic deficits and transient ischemic attacks, using ^{133}Xe measures of regional cerebral blood flow (rCBF) and neurometric evaluation of EEGs using overall frequency abnormality. Authors reported that abnormal rCBF was present in 69% of symptomatic and 53% of asymptomatic subjects, while neurometric abnormality was present in 91% of symptomatic and 90% of asymptomatic individuals.

Robinson et al (1994) found by means of visual analysis of initial EEG data of 86 AD patients and 17 patients with mixed AD and MID, autopsy confirmed, abnormal EEGs in 77% of mixed group, resulting in sensitivity of 77%, specificity 65% and positive likelihood ratio of 2.2 when compared to the pure AD group. Interestingly, only 6% of mixed cases had pronounced focal abnormality classified as grade 5, while 41 % had moderate excessive theta activity and/or bursts of bisynchronous diffuse rhythmic 2-3 Hz waves classified as a grade 3 of 5.

In order to increase sensitivity of the EEG method in distinguishing vascular dementia and AD, Signorino et al (1995) performed spectral analysis in two conditions, eyes closed (EC) and eyes open (EO) on a sample of 50 AD, 37 VaD patients and 46 controls with a wide range of disease severity (MMSE 0-26; GDS 3-6). 97% of VaD as compared to 44% of AD patients had in EC condition a spectrum with a dominant activity in the 6.5-12 Hz band with a slow frequency peak between 6.5 7.5 as compared to 9-11 Hz peak in normal controls. Majority of remaining AD patients had high power in 1-6.5 Hz band. No data were available for calculation of indexes of accuracy for these measures and it is also worth mentioning that this study did not report increased prevalence of left-right asymmetry in slow frequency bands, an index of focal slowing. On the other hand, Martin-Loeches et al (1991) using brain electrical activity mapping suggested that topography of theta band could be considered as an important discriminator between AD and MID, since in their study 10 AD patients showed a higher power over right posterior regions when compared to 10 MID patients during 3 behavioral conditions: resting with eyes open, memorizing a list of words and recalling the same list of words. Sloan et al. (1993) reported similar observations on a larger number of initially 135 patients and healthy subjects. In their longitudinal study AD patients had more delta and theta power and less alpha power than MID patients and these changes were relatively stable during the 2 years follow-up period, although high drop-out rate could have biased the results. Anderer et al (1994) tried to optimize classification accuracy of MID patients versus healthy elderly by means of artificial neural networks and receiver operating characteristics and reported 69% sensitivity at specificity of 100%, figure similar to those obtained for AD versus controls. The two dementia subgroups differed in power asymmetry scores. Study of Partanen et al (1997) also explored in addition to conventional background EEG analysis EEG measures of brain reactivity like EC/EO ratio. In their study they compared 17 VaD patients with moderate or severe stage of the disease with 11 healthy controls, reference AD group was not included, and found that VaD patients did not have less activity in the alpha band when compared to the controls, but the alpha amplitude ratio EC/EO condition was decreased in VaD and showed significant correlations with several neuropsychological variables like visuo-spatial and speech function and learning. Authors speculated that diminution of alpha activation during visual stimulation as well as impaired cortical functions reflect dysfunctional cortical networks. As it has been mentioned before, coherence has been proposed as a neurophysiological index of cortical connectivity, sensitive to differential anatomical disconnection occurring in AD and VaD. While in AD specific pathology is distributed in the neocortex and interferes with the origins and termination of long cortico-cortical association fibers, in VaD or more specifically MID, a diffuse deep-white matter ischemia causes a wide-spread demyelination which involves a broad complex networks of cortico-cortical and corticosubcortical fibers (Rogers & Morrison, 1985; Pantoni et al, 1999). A most recent study using conventional and magnetization transfer magnetic resonance images has found evidence of subtle gray-matter pathologic changes in healthy individuals with nonspecific white matter hyperintensities (WMH), which further supports speculated mechanism of disconnection in VaD (Mezzapesa et al, 2003). Group of AF Leuchter has tried in several studies to test this hypothesis by examining coherence averaged according to Thatcher et al (1986) over groups of bipolar channels representing "trans-Rolandic" projections and structural integrity of superior longitudinal fasciculus and "pre- and post-Rolandic" projections involving complex networks of frontal and visual cortex vulnerable to the presence of periventricular white matter hyperintensities (Leuchter et al, 1987; 1992; 1993; 1994; Cook & Leuchter, 1996). Trans-Rolandic coherence at 14-18 Hz band was reduced in AD patients and post-Rolandic coherence at 10-14 Hz in MID patients and based on these measures authors were able to classify correctly 76% of demented subjects into two clinical subgroups (Leuchter et al, 1992). In the subsequent study the same group confirmed previous results and validated them by showing relation between lower pre- and post-Rolandic coherence measures and periventricular white matter hyperintensities as visualized by MRI. Interestingly, in patients with AD and WMH these coherence measures did not differ from MID patients (Leuchter et al, 1994). This could explain the results of Jelic et al (1997) who found an association between reduced temporo-parieto-occipital alpha band coherence and APOE e4 allele, a risk factor associated with Alzheimer's disease pathology but also with cerebrovascular disease (Frisoni et al, 1994).

In summary, although AD and VaD are statistically distinguishable on a group level based on linear spectral EEG and coherence measures, the distinction is not sufficiently reliable to be used in daily clinical practice for diagnosing individual patients.

Frontotemporal Dementia

EEG is has been proposed as a suitable test to differentiate AD and frontotemporal dementia (FTD), since EEGs of FTD patients were not significantly different from controls at least in early stages of the disease as compared to those of AD patients with similar disease severity (Johanesson et al, 1979; Julin et al, 1995; Gustafson et al, 1992). In a correlative study which examined the presence of specific qEEG changes in dementia patients with relatively lower frontal or parietal blood perfusion as demonstrated by SPECT, qEEG changes typical of dementia were not related to perfusion deficits in frontal brain areas (Pozzi et al, 1996). Quantitative EEG changes have been reported in two studies on relatively small samples of FTD patients which limits the power of a study. In study of Rosen et al (1993) 7 FTD patients had a well preserved alpha power, no significant change of absolute power for any of the conventional frequency bands studied and a rather weak EEG power over a wide frequency range except for relative theta power which was moderately increased anteriorly as well as posteriorly. In study of Förstl et al. (1996) 10 patients with a clinical diagnosis of frontal lobe degeneration were compared to 10 AD patients with, according to MMSE scores, severe to moderate stages of the disease and to 10 healthy elderly. FTD patients did not differ from the controls in absolute band power across the wide range of frequency spectrum as well as in coherence measurements. However, authors presented data from only two derivations, Fz and Pz, and even performed a discriminant analysis with resulting 15 variables on a total sample of 20 demented subjects which resulted in 3 misclassified AD patients and 1 misclassified FTD patient on a basis of 3 variables: Fz delta and Pz theta and beta 1. Yener et al (1996) compared 3 clinical groups: 27 healthy subjects, 26 patients with AD and 13 patients with FTD and found that preservation of posterior dominant alpha rhythm was frequent in FTD and that overall degree of slowing in FTD was less severe than in AD. Five most informative quantitative EEG parameters between 2 dementia groups were right parietal alpha and beta 2 bands, left parietal theta and beta 2 bands, and left temporal beta 2 bands, resulting in 81% correctly classified AD and 85% FTD patients. The most recent study by Lindau et al (2003) was performed on a sample of 19 healthy subjects, 19 FTD and 16 AD patients and reported lack of significant increase in slow, delta and theta GFP in FTD patients when compared to AD patients and a strong tendency towards decrease in fast, alpha and beta 1-3 GFP when compared to the controls. Using a logistic regression analysis the authors showed that the best predictors of AD and FTD diagnosis were combined delta and theta GFP and scores from neuropsychological tests from visuospatial and episodic memory domain, giving classification accuracy of 93 %.

Extended study from the same group, performed on the so far largest reported sample which included 26 FTD and 24 AD patients and 17 controls confirmed previous findings and in addition showed that FTD patients had decreased EEG synchronization as expressed by GFS in all frequency bands when compared to AD patients and controls (Jelic et al, 2002). In this study combined GFP in delta and theta frequency bands together with GFS in fast frequency bands, alpha and beta 2 correctly classified 90% of AD and controls, while combined GFP in delta, theta and beta 1-3 bands with GFS in all bands correctly classified 94% of AD and FTD patients in a discriminant function analysis. Combined GFP in fast frequency bands, alpha and beta 1-3 and GFS in all frequency bands correctly classified 93% of FTD cases and controls. Authors conclude that lower amplitudes and anteriorization of alpha activity in AD, but not in FTD and lower alpha GFS in both diseases could imply that alpha activity in AD disintegrates both in time and space, while in FTD disintegration occurs in time. Finding is possibly related to the selective occurrence of AD pathology in parietooccipital regions, postulated site of main generators of alpha activity.

Other Dementing Diseases

Classical subdivision of dementing diseases to cortical dementias such as AD and FLD and subcortical dementias including Parkinson's disease (PD), Huntington's disease and progressive supranuclear palsy (PSP) has become debatable lately. Increasing knowledge on neurodegenerative diseases as processes which have many pathological mechanisms in common (Hardy & Gwinn-Hardy, 1998) could explain autopsy findings of mixed pathologies in distinct clinical entities of different dementing disorders. Patients with Parkinson disease could also have cortical involvement and majority of patients with Lewy body dementia (LBD) have also AD pathology (Lopez et al, 2002). Therefore it is not surprising that PD patients with dementia show in general similar EEG features as AD patients, the degree of abnormality depending on the degree of motor disability and severity of dementia (Neufeldt et al, 1994). In patients with progressive supranuclear palsy, frontal EEG slowing in wakefulness, mainly increase in theta relative power, and a reduction in sleep spindles of stage 2 sleep have been described (Montplaisir et al, 1997). The greater slowing of EEG in LBD as compared to the AD has been reported in autopsy-based studies (Byrne et al, 1989; Crystal et al, 1990; Hely et al, 1996; Briel et al, 1999). In addition patients with LBD had loss of alpha activity as the dominant rhythm and half of them had also slow wave transient activity in areas corresponding to the temporal lobes (Briel et al, 1999) as well as bilateral frontal intermittent rhythmic delta activity (FIRDA) (Calzetti et al, 2002). More pronounced slowing in LBD is probably related to a greater loss of acetylcholinetransferase in LBD than in AD. Slow-wave transients defined as episodes of delta or theta with duration less than 1 second that occurred in the temporal lobe regions are probably related to the clinical history of the episodic loss of consciousness typical for LBD. Although fluctuating cognition (FC) is common in all major dementias, it is particularly present in LBD. Walker et al (2000) evaluated mean EEG frequency across 90 seconds and reported that FC occurs on second to second basis in patients with LBD and have greater prevalence and severity than in AD or VaD patients.

Finally, the appearance of periodic sharp wave complexes occurring on a diffusely slow background in a patient with a recent onset of dementia is highly suggestive of Creutzfeldt-Jacob disease (Brown et al, 1986). However, it may be necessary to perform repeated EEG recordings before these changes appear or to do recording during the REM sleep phase and still there will be a subgroup of patients in which these periodic discharges do not occur. This EEG pattern is not pathognomonic of the disease and has been described also in toxic-metabolic causes of dementia and severe AD (reviewed by Rosén, 1996).

Perspectives

Advances in EEG methodology should be introduced into empirical studies in dementia research. There are some main areas of interest that could be relevant to the studies of cognition: increased spatial resolution of EEG recordings, computation of better dipole models and estimates of neuronal disconnection (Gevins et al, 1995; Gevins, 1998; Koles, 1998). Better spatial sampling could be achieved by introducing more electrode sites and by using a realistic model of individual's head constructed from his/her MRI (Merlet et al, 1999; Babiloni et al, 2000). In this way fine structural details like localization of gray matter could be provided. Localization of sources of generators of electrical activity should be achieved by better dipole modeling which is more realistic from the anatomical and neurophysiological point of view. A single dipole model is an oversimplification of complex neuronal activity and co-registration of different paradigms of evoked/event-related potentials with three-dimensional functional imaging methods such as fMRI and PET (Heinze *et al*, 1994) would give more valid spatiotemporal information on cognitive processes, both in health and disease. Functional disconnection of widely distributed neuronal networks could be tested and visualized in the future by computing coherence of spatially unambiguous dipole data, i.e. between LORETA voxels or by using similar methods that are calculating and displaying regional sources.

As the main interest in dementia research is shifting towards an early recognition of cognitive deficits and neuronal dysfunction, even before clinically manifest dementia, applications of above mentioned methods in analysis of EEG recordings during various cognitive activation paradigms will become more suitable to study brain function than a resting spontaneous EEG.

Concluding Remarks

In order to look into the future and evaluate progress, one has to be aware what has been done in the past. In contrast to other articles that are introducing new ways of EEG analysis, this article aimed to show that the methodology of diagnostic, clinical research does not follow in the same pace development of new diagnostic techniques. Recent evidence-based review by The Diagnosis of Dementia Committee addressed major issues in the diagnosis of dementia and in the resulting practice parameter on dementia diagnosis did not consider qEEG among the laboratory tests that could improve diagnostic accuracy of dementing illness or be used in the presymptomatic detection of the disease (Knopman et al, 2001). What should be done in the future towards a different consensus with regard to the qEEG technique? Although there is a lot of converging evidence and consistency in reported findings from the studies performed so far, one has to address their methodological limitations with a constructive criticism in order to give guidelines for future research. One of the problems that qEEG brings as a potential useful investigation in clinical reality is a multitude of parameters it produces, their relation to neurobiological substrates and cognitive and behavioral symptoms of the disease and still remaining question which of qEEG parameters could be the best candidates for potential discrimination of patients. Table 3 illustrates that various authors did not use exactly same inclusion criteria (spectrum of tested patients not specified in detail), analyzing technique (reference electrode choice, arbitrary montage selections, etc) or EEG parameters. Therefore, so far it has been impossible to make a metaanalysis for validation purposes.

More prospective, preferably multicentre, studies on unselected and larger samples are needed for the validation of respective techniques. Implications of this evidence-based approach are twofold: optimal clinical practice based on the best available evidence and selection of the most promising areas of the future research. We still need qEEG parameters proven to be sufficiently reliable to be used for diagnosing individual patients.

In addition, multivariate approach should be used to evaluate the added value of qEEG in combination with another diagnostic techniques. Comparative studies which apply different imaging modalities together with EEG on the same patient population are still very rare. Of interest is not only comparative advantage or disadvantage of EEG in comparison with other diagnostic techniques, but also a supplementary information that it could give on brain function. The characteristic of a disease process is a tension between the pathophysiological cascade of events on one side and neuronal reparation and compensation mechanisms on the other side, the later being highly individual trait under influence of genetic and environmental factors. In other words, natural history of the disease is determined not only by what has been lost, but also by what has been left during the disease process. Therefore, beside the development of the tests which show accurately and with a precision how much the brain has been affected structurally and functionally during the disease process, attempts should be made towards a procedure that reflects how much of brain function has been left and towards understanding a mechanism of cognitive brain reserve (Stern, 2002) which delays clinical manifestation of dementia. Could varying figures on sensitivities derived from EEG studies in dementia be discussed and explained in this way? Obviously, a larger number of prospective studies is needed not only aiming to confirm the dementia diagnosis from a longitudinal perspective, but also to reveal a heterogeneous nature of disease progression.

It seems that we are facing a new era where neurodegenerative diseases, including dementia, will not be defined as clinicopathological entities but as a processes with overlapping pathogenetic mechanisms (Hardy, 2003). Could we, therefore, in differential diagnosis expect optimal specificity with respect to patients groups classified clinically into different dementia syndromes?

Clinically important question with respect to new emerging methods of qEEG analysis is whether these new methods have significant diagnostic value comparable to the conventional parameters. So far, diagnostic accuracies of non-linear parameters did not show convincing additional advantage over the conventional parameters. However, it should be further explored what is their functional significance and if they could add complementary information to the diagnostic process and prognosis.

Finally, if any of qEEG variables is going to be validated and established as a biomarker of disease with sufficiently high sensitivity and specificity, it could be incorporated in the algorithmic approach used in presymptomatic/preclinical detection of disease. This approach is a major avenue of future research.

REFERENCES

Albert MS, Duffy FH, McAnulty Gloria. Electrophysiologic comparisons between two groups of patients with Alzheimer's disease. Arch Neurol 1990; 47: 857-863

Almkvist O, Bäckman L. Detection and staging of early clinical dementia. Acta Neurol Scand 1993; 88: 10-15

Anderer P, Saletu B, Klöppel B, Semlitsch HV, Werner H. Discrimination between demented patients and normals based on topographic EEG slow wave activity; comparison between z statistics, discriminant analysis and artificial neuronal network classifiers. Electroencephalogr Clin Neurophysiol 1994; 91: 108-117

Arendt T. Disturbance of neuronal plasticity is a critical pathogenetic event in Alzheimer's disease. Int J Devl Neuroscience 2001;19:231-245

Arriagada PV, Growdon JH, Hedley-Whyte ET, Hyman BT. Neurofibrillary tangles but not senile plaques parallel duration and severity of Alzheimer's disease. Neurology 1992; 42:631-639

Arnaiz E, Jelic V, Almkvist O, et al. Impaired cerebral glucose metabolism and cognitive functioning predict deterioration in mild cognitive impairment. Neuroreport 2001; 12:851-855

Babiloni F, Babiloni C, Locche L, Cincotti F, Rossini PM, Carducci F. High-resolution electroencephalogram: source estimates of Laplacian-transformed somatosensory-evoked potentials using a realistic subject head model constructed from magnetic resonance images. Med Biol Eng Comput 2000a; 38:512-9

Babiloni C, Babiloni F, Carducci F, et al. Movement-related electroencephalographic reactivity in Alzheimer disease. Neuroimage 2000b; 12:139-146

Babiloni C, Ferri R, Moretti DV, et al. Abnormal fronto-parietal coupling of brain rhytms in mild Alzhemier's disease: a multicentric EEG study. Eur J Neurosci 2004; 19:2583-2590

Babiloni C, Babiloni F, Carducci F, et al. Human cortical rhytms during visual delayed choice reaction time tasks. A high-resolution EEG study on normal aging. Behavioural Brain Res 2004b; 153:261-271

Bahro M, Riemann D, Stadtmüller G, Berger M, Gattaz WF. REM sleep parameters in the discrimination of probable Alzheimer's disease from old-age depression. Biol Psychiatry 1993; 34:482-486

Bennys K, Rondouin G, Vergnes C, Touchon J. Diagnostic value of quantitative EEG in Alzheimer's disease. Neurophysiol Clin 2001; 31: 153-60

Berger A-K, Fratiglioni F, Forsell Y, Winblad B, Bäckman L. The occurrence of depressive symptoms in the preclinical phase of AD. A population-based study. Neurology 1999; 53:1998-2002

Berger H. Über das Elektroenkephalogramm des Menschen: Fünfte Mitteilung. Arch Psychiatr Nervenkr 1932; 98:231-254

Besthorn C, Forstl H, Geiger-Kabish C, Sattel H, Gasser T, Schreiter-Gasser U. EEG coherences in Alzheimer disease. Electroenceph Clin Neurophysiol 1994; 90: 242-245

Besthorn C, Sattel H, Geiger-Kabisch C, Zerfass R, Förstl H. Parameters of EEG dimensional complexity in Alzhemier's disease. Electroenceph Clin Neurophysiol 1995; 95:84-89

Besthorn C, Zerfass R, Geiger-Kabisch C, Sattel H, Daniel S, Schreiter-Gasser U, Förstl H. Discrimination of Alzheimer's disease and normal aging by EEG data. Electroenceph Clin Neurophysiol 1997; 103: 241-248

Bierer LM, Haroutunian V, Gabriel S, et al. Neurochemical correlates of dementia severity in Alzhemier's disease: relative importance of cholinergic deficits., J Neurochem 1995; 64:740-760

Biggerstaff BJ. Comparing diagnostic tests: a simple graphic using likelihood ratios. Statist Med 2000; 19:649-663

Braak H, Braak E. Neuropathological staging of Alzheimer-related changes. Acta Neuropathol 1991; 82: 239-259

Braak H, Braak E. Development of Alzheimer-related neurofibrillary changes in the neocortex inversely recapitulates cortical myelogenesis. Acta Neuropathol 1996, 92. 197-201

Brenner RP, Ulrich RF, Spiker DG, et al. Computerized EEG spectral analysis in elderly normal, demented and depressed subjects. Electroenceph Clin Neurophysiol 1986; 64: 483-492

Breslau J, Starr A, Sicotte N, Higa J, Buchsbaum MS. Topographic EEG changes with normal aging and SDAT. Electroencephalogr Clin Neurophysiol 1989;72(4):281-289.

Briel RCG, McKeith IG, Barker WA, et al. EEG findings in dementia with Lewy bodies and Alzheimer's disease. J Neurol Neurosurg Psychiatry 1999; 66:401-403

Brown P, Cathala F, Castaigne P, Gajdusek D. Creutzfeldt-Jakob disease: clinical analysis of a consecutive series of 230 neuropathologically verified cases. Ann Neurol 1986; 20:597-602

Brun A, Englund B, Gustafson L, et al. Clinical and neuropathological criteria for frontotemporal dementia. J Neurol Neurosurg Psychiatry 1994; 57:416-418

Buchan RJ, Nagata K, Yakoyama E, et al. Regional correlations between the EEG and oxygen metabolism in dementia of Alzhemier's type. Electroenceph Clin Neurophysiol 1997; 103:409-417

Buszaki G, Bickford RG, Ponomareff G, Thal LJ, Mandel R, Gage FH. Nucleus basalis and thalamic control of neocortical activity in the freely moving rat. J Neurosci 1988; 8:4007-4026

Byrne EJ, Lennox G, Lowe J, et al. Diffuse Lewy body disease: clinical features in 15 cases. J Neurol Neurosurg Psychiatry 1989; 52: 709-717

Calzetti S, Bortone E, Negrotti A, Zinno L, Mancia D. Frontal intermittent shytmic delta activity (FIRDA) with dementia with Lewy bodies: A diagnostic tool? Neurol Sci 2002; 23 [Suppl 2]: S65-6

Chiaramonti R, Muscas GC, Paganini M, et al. Correlations of topographical EEG features with clinical severity in mild to moderate dementia of Alzheimer type. Neuropsychobiology 1997; 36:153-158

Claus JJ, Ongerboer de Visser BW, Walstra GJM, Hijdra A, Verbeeten B, van Gool WA. Quantitative spectral electroencephalography in predicting survival in patients with early Alzhemier's disease. Arch Neurol 1998a; 55: 1105-1111

Claus JJ, van Gool WA, Teunisse S, et al. Predicting survival in patients witrh early Alzhemier's disease. Dement Geriatr Cogn Disord 1998b; 9:284-293

Claus JJ, Kwa VIH, Teunisse S, et al. Slowing on quantitative spectral EEG is a marker for rate of subsequent cognitive and functional decline in early Alzheimer disease. Alzhemier Dis Assoc Disorder 1998; 12:167-174

Claus JJ, Strijers RLM, Johkman EJ, et al. The diagnostic value of electroencephalography in mild senile Alzheimer's disease. Clin Neurophysiology 1999; 110: 825-832

Claus JJ, Ongerboer de Visser BW, Bour LJ, et al. Determinants of quantitative spectral electroencephalography in early Alzheimer's disease: Cognitive functioning, regional cerebral blood flow, and computed tomography. Dement Geriatr Cogn Disord 2000; 11:81-89

Coben LA, Danziger W, Storandt M. A longitudinal EEG study of mild senile dementia of Alzheimer type: changes at 1 year and at 2.5 years. Electroencephalogr Clin Neurophysiol 1985;61(2):101-112.

Coben LA, Chi D, Snyder AZ, Storandt M. Replication of a study of a frequency analysis of the resting awake EEG in mild probable Alzheimer's disease. Electroencephalogr Clin Neurophysiol 1990; 75:148-154

Comi GC, Fornara C, Locatelli T, et al. EEG coherence in Alzheimer and multiinfarct dementia. Arch Gerontol Geriatr 1998; [suppl 6]:91-8

Cook IA & Leuchter AF. Synaptic dysfunction in Alzheimer's disease: clinical assessment using quantitative EEG. Behavvioural Brain Res 1996; 78:15-23

Crystal HA, Dickson DW, Lizardi JE, et al. Antemortem diagnosis of diffuse Lewy body disease. Neurology 1990; 40:1523-1528

Davies P, Maloney AJ. Selective loss of central cholinergic neurons in Alzheimer's disease. Lancet 1976; 2: 1403.

Detari L. and Vanderwolf CH. Activity of cotically projecting and other basal forebrain neurons during large slow waves and cortical activation in anesthetized cat. Brain Res 1987; 437: 1-8

De LaCoste M-C & White III CL. The role of cortical connectivity in Alzheimer's disease pathogenesis: A review and model system. Neurobiology of Aging 1993; 14; 1-16

de Weerd AW, Perquin WVM, Jonkman EJ. Role of the EEG in the prediction of dementia in Parkinson's disease. Dementia 1990; 1: 115-118

Dierks T, Perisic I, Frölich L, Ihl R, Maurer K. Topography of the quantitative electroencephalogram in dementia of the Alzheimer type: Relation to severity of dementia. Psychiatry Res Neuroimaging 1991; 40: 181-194

Dierks T, Ihl R, Frolich L, Maurer K. Dementia of the Alzheimer type: effects on the spontaneous EEG described by dipole sources Psychiatry Res 1993; 50: 151-162

Dierks T, Frölich L, Ihl R, Maurer K. Correlation between cognitive brain function and electrical brain activity in dementia of Alzheimer type. J Neural Transm [GenSect] 1995; 99:55-62

Dierks T, Jelic V, Julin P, Maurer K, Wahlund L-O, Almkvist O, Strik WK, Winblad B. EEG-microstates in mild memory impairment and Alzheimer's disease: possible association with disturbed information processing. J Neural Transm 1997; 104:483-495

Dierks T, Jelic V, Pascual-Marqui RD, et al. Spatial pattern of cerebral glucose metabolism (PET) correlates with localization of intracerebral EEG-generators in Alzhemier's disease. Clin Neurophysiology 2000; 11:1817-1824

Duffy FH, Burchfiel JL, Lombroso CT. Brain electrical activity mapping (BEAM): a method for extending the clinical utility of EEG and evoked potential data. Ann Neurol 1979; 5 (4): 309-21

Duffy FH, Albert MS, McAnulty G. Brain electrical activity in patients with presenile and senile dementia of the Alzheimer's type. Ann Neurol 1984a; 16: 439-448

Duffy FH, Albert MS, McAnulty G, Garvey AJ. Age-related differences in brain electrical activity of healthy subjects. Ann Neurol 1984b; 16 (4): 430-8

Duffy FH, McAnulty GB, Albert MS. The pattern of age-related differences in electrophysiological activity of healthy males and females. Neurobiol Aging 1993; 14: 73-84

Duffy FH, McAnulty GB, Albert MS. Temporoparietal electrophysiological differences characterize patients with Alzheimer's disease: a split-half replication study. Cereb Cortex 1995; 5(3): 215-21

Duffy FH, McAnulty GB, Albert MS. Effects of age upon interhemispheric EEG coherence in normal adults. Neurobiol Aging 1996; 17(4):587-99

Dunkin JJ, Leuchter AF, Newton TF, Cook IA. Reduced EEG coherence in dementia: state or trait marker? Biol Psychiatry 1994; 35:870-879

Dunkin JJ, Osato S, Leuchter AF. Relationship between EEG coherence and neuropsychological tests in dementia. Clin Electroencephalography 1995; 26: 47-59

Dykierek P, Stadtmüller G, Schramm P, et al. The value of REM sleep parameters in differentiating Alzheimer's disease from old-age depression and normal aging. J Psychiatric Research 1998; 32: 1-9

Edman Å, Matousek M, Wallin A. EEG findings in dementia are related to the parietal lobe syndrome. Dementia 1995; 6:323-329

Elmståhl S, Rosén I, Gullberg B. Quantitative EEG in elderly patients with Alzheimer's disease and healthy controls. Dementia 1994; 5:119-124

Elmståhl S, Rosén I. Postural hypotension and EEG variables predict cognitive decline: Results from a 5-year follow-up of healthy elderly women. Dement Geriatr Cogn Disord 1997; 8: 180-187

Erkinjuti T, Larsen T, Sulkava R, Ketonen L, Laaksonen R, Palo J. EEG in the differential diagnosis between Alzheimer's disease and vascular dementia. Acta Neurol Scand 1988; 77:36-43

Ettlin TM, Staehelin HB, Kischka U, et al. Computed tomography, electroencephalography, and clinical features in the differential diagnosis of senile dementia. Arch Neurol 1989; 46: 1217-1220

Fein G, Raz J, Brown FF, Merrin EL. Common reference coherence data are confounded by power and phase effects. Electroencephalogr Clin Neurophysiol 1988; 69:581-4

Fisch BJ, Pedley TA. The role of quantitative topographic mapping or "neurometrics" in the diagnosis of psychiatric and neurological disorders: the cons. Electroencephalogr Clin Neurophysiol 1989; 73:5-9

Folstein MF, Folstein SE, McHugh PR. "Mini-Mental State": A practical method for grading the cognitive state of patients for the clinician. J Psychiatr Res 1975; 12: 189-198

Francis PT, Palmer AM, Snape M, Wilcock GK. The cholinergic hypothesis of Alzheimer's disease: a review of progress. J Neurol Neurosurg Psychiatry 1999; 66:137-147

Frisoni GB, Calabresi L, Geroldi C, et al. Apolipoprotein E epsilon 4 allele in Alzheimer's disease and vascular dementia. Dementia 1994; 5:240-2

Förstl H, Besthorn C, Hentschel F, Geiger-Kabisch C, Sattel H, Schreiter-Gasser U. Frontal lobe degeneration and Alzheimer's disease: A control study on clinical findings, volumetric brain changes and quantitative electroencephalography data. Dementia 1996; 7:27-34

Galasko D, Hansen LA, Katzman R, et al. Clinical-neuropathological correlations in Alzhemier's disease and related dementias. Arch Neurol 1994; 51: 888-895

Gasser T, Bacher P, Steinberg H. Test-retest reliability of spectral parameters of the EEG. Electroencephalogr Clin Neurophysiol 1985; 60:312-319

Gevins A. The future of electroencephalography in assessing neurocognitive functioning. Electroencephalogr Clin Neurophysiol 1998,106: 165-172

Gearing M, Schneider JA, Rebeck GW, Hyman BT, Mirra SS. Alzheimer's disease with and without coexisting Parkinson's disease: apolipoprotein E genotype and neuropathologic correlates. Neurology 1995; 45: 1985-1990

Gevins A, Leong H, Smith ME, Le J, Du R. Mapping cognitive brain function with modern high resolution electroencelophalography. Trends Neurosci 1995; 18:429-436

Giaquinto S, Nolfe G. The EEG in normal elderly: a contribution to the interpretation of aging and dementia. Electroencephalogr Clin Neurophysiol 1986; 63: 540-546

Grady CL, Haxby JV, Horwitz B, et al. Longitudinal study of the early neuropsychological and cerebral metabolic changes in dementia of Alzheimer type. J Clin Exp Neuropsychol 1988; 10:576-596

Green RC, Cupples LA, Kurz A, et al. Depression as a risk factor for Alzheimer disease. A MIRAGE study. Arch Neurol 2003; 753-759

Grunwald M, Busse F, Hensel A, et al. Theta power differences in patients with mild cognitive impairment under rest condition and during haptic tasks. Alzheimer Dis Assoc Disord 2002; 16:40-48

Gustafson L, Nilsson L. Differential diagnosis of presenile dementia on clinical grounds. Acta Psychiatr Scand 1982; 65:194-209

Gustafson L, Brun A, Passant U. Frontal lobe degeneration of non-Alzheimer type. Baillieres Clin Neurol 1992; 1: 559-582

Hardy J, Gwinn-Hardy K. Genetic classification of primary neurodegenerative disease. Science 1998; 282: 1075-1079

Hassainia F, Petit D, Nielsen T, Gauthier S, Montplaisir J. Quantitative EEG and statistical mapping of wakefulness and REM sleep in the evaluation of mild to moderate Alzhemier's disease. European Neurology 1997; 37: 219-224

Hardy D. The relationship between Lewy Body disease, Parkinson's disease, and Alzheimer's disease. Ann N Y Acad Sci 2003; 991:167-170

Hartikainen P, Soininen H, Partanen J, Helkala EL, Riekkinen P. Aging and spectral analysis of EEG in normal subjects: a link to memory and CSF AchE. Acta Neurol Scand 1992; 86:148-155

Heidebrink JL. Is dementia with Lewy bodies the second most common cause of dementia. J Geriatr Psychiatry Neurol 2002; 15: 182-7

Heinze HJ, Mangun GR, Burchert W, et al. Combined spatial and temporal imaging of brain activity during visual selective attention in humans. Nature 1994; 372: 543-546

Helkala E-L, Laulumaa V, Soininen H, Partanen J, Riekkinen P. Different patterns of cognitive decline related to normal or deteriorating EEG in a 3-year follow-up study of patients with Alzhemier's disease. Neurology 1991; 41:528-532

Hely MA, Reid WGJ, Halliday GM, et al. Diffuse Lewy body disease: clinical features in nine cases without coexistent AD. J Neurol Neurosurg Psychiatry 1996; 60: 531-538

Hobson JA, Lydic R, Baghdoyan HA. Evolving concepts of sleep cycle generation: from brain centers to neuronal populations. Behavioural Brain Science 1986; 9:371-448

Hooijer C, Jonker C, Posthuma J, Visser SL. Reliability, validity and follow-up of the EEG in senile dementia: sequelae of sequential measurement. Electroenceph Clin Neurophysiol 1990; 76: 400-412

Huang C, Wahlund L-O, Dierks T, Julin P, Winblad B, Jelic V. Discrimination of Alzheimer's disease and mild cognitive impairment by equivalent EEG sources: a cross-sectional and longitudinal study. Clin Neurophysiology 2000; 111: 1961-1967

Hughes JR, John ER. Conventional and quantitative electroencephalography in psychiatry. J Neuropsychiatry Clin Neurosci 1999; 11: 190-208

Ihl R, Maurer K, Dierks T, Frölich L, Perisic I. Staging in dementia of the Alzheimer type: Topography of electrical brain activity reflects the severity of the disease. Psychiatry Research 1989; 29: 399-401

Ihl R, Dierks T, Froelich L, Martin E-M, Maurer K. Segmentation of the spontaneous EEG in dementia of the Alzheimer type. Neuropsychobiology 1993; 27:231-236

Ihl R, Brinkmeyer J. Differential diagnosis of aging, dementia of Alzheimer type and depression with EEG-segmentation. Dement Geriatr Cogn Disord 1999; 10:64-69

Ihl R, Brinkmeyer J, Janner M, Kerdar MS. A comparison of ADAS and EEG in the discrimination of patients with dementia of the Alzheimer type from healthy controls. Neuropsychobiology 2000; 41:102-7

Ikawa M, Nakanishi M, Furukawa T, Nakaaki S, Hori S, Yoshida S. Relationship between EEG dimensional complexity and neuropsychological findings in Alzhemier's disease. Psychiatry and Clinical Neurosciences 2000; 54:537-541

Ingvar DH, Rosén I, Johanesson G. EEG is related to cerebral metabolism and blood flow. Pharmacopsychiatry 1979; 12:200-209

Jelic V, Shigeta M, Julin P, Almkvist O, Winblad B, Wahlund L-O. Quantitative electroencephalography power and coherence in Alzheimer's disease and mild cognitive impairment. Dementia 1996; 7:314-323

Jelic V, Julin P, Shigeta M, et al. Apolipoprotein E ε4 allele decreases functional connectivity as measured by EEG coherence. J Neurol Neurosurg Psychiatry 1997; 63:59-65

Jelic V, Dierks T, Amberla K, Almkvist O, Winblad B, Nordberg A. Longitudinal changes in quantitative EEG during long-term tacrine treatment of patients with Alzheimer's disease. Neurosci Lett 1998; 254: 85-88

Jelic V. Early diagnosis of Alzheimer's disease. Focus on quantitative EEG in relation to genetic, biochemical and neuroimaging markers. Doctoral Thesis. Stockholm, Karolinska Institutet, 1999a.

Jelic V, Wahlund L-O, Almkvist O, et al. Diagnostic accuracies of quantitative EEG and PET in mild Alzheimer's disease. Alzheimer's Reports 1999b; 2:291-298

Jelic V, Johansson S-E, Almkvist O, et al. Quantitative EEG in mild cognitive impairment: longitudinal changes and possible prediction of Alzheimer's disease. Neurobiol Aging 2000; 21:533-540

Jelic V, Koenig T, Lindau M, Dierks T, Wahlund L-O. EEG amplitude and synchronisation distinguish Alzheimer's disease, frontotemporal dementia and normal aging. Neurobiol Aging 2002; 23 [1Suppl]: S355

Jelles B, van Birgeln JH, Slaets JPJ, Hekster REM, Jonkman EJ, Stam CJ. Decrease of non-linear structure in the EEG of Alzheimer patients compared to healthy controls. Clin Neurophysiology 1999; 110:1159-1167

Jeong J, Kim SJ, Han S-H. Non-linear dynamical analysis of the EEG in Alzhemier's disease with optimal embedding dimension. Electroenceph Clin Neurophysiol 1998; 106: 220-228

Jobst KA, Smith AD, Barker CS, et al. Association of atrophy of the medial temporal lobe with reduced blood flow in the posterior parietotemporal cortex in patients with a clinical and patjological diagnosis of Alzheimer's disease. J Neurol Neurosurg Psychiatry 1992;55:190-194

Johanesson G, Brun A, Gustafson I, Ingvar DH. EEG in presenile dementia related to cerebral blood flow and autopsy findings. Acta Neurol Scand 1977; 56:89-103

Johanesson G, Hagberg B, Gustafsson L, Ingvar DH. EEG and cognitive impairment in presenile dementia. Acta Neurol Scand 1979; 59: 225-240

John ER, Karmel BZ, Corning WC, et al. Neurometrics: numerical taxonomy identifies different profiles of brain functions within groups of behaviourally similar people. Science 1977; 196:1393-1410

John ER, Prichep LS, Fridman J, Easton P. Neurometrics: Computer-assisted differential diagnosis of brain dysfunctions. Science 1988; 239: 162-169

Jonkman EJ. A simple EEG scoring method for senile dementia of the Alzheimer type. Electroenceph Clin Neurophysiol 1989; 72: 44P

Johnson KA, Jones K, Holman BL, et al. Preclinical prediction of Alzheimer's disease using SPECT. Neurology 1998; 50: 1563-1571

Julin P, Wahlund L-O, Basun H, Persson A, Måre K, Rudberg U. Clinical diagnosis of frontal lobe dementia and Alzheimer's disease: Relation to cerebral perfusion, brain atrophy and electroencephalography. Dementia 1995; 6:142-147

Kaszniak AW, Garron DC, Fox JH, Bergen D, Huckman M. Cerebral atrophy, EEG slowing, age, education, and cognitive functioning in suspected dementia. Neurology 1979; 29:1273-1279

Klatka LA, Schiffer RB, Powers JM, Kazee AM. Incorrect diagnosis of Alzheimer's disease. Arch Neurol 1996; 53:35-42

Klimesch W. Memory processes, brain oscillations and EEG synchronization. Int Journal fo Psychophysiology 1996; 24:61-100

Klimesch W. EEG alpha and theta oscillations reflect cognitive and memory performance: a review and analysis. Brain Res Rev 1999; 29:169-195

Klunk WE. Biological markers of Alzheimer's disease. Neurobiol Aging 1998; 19:145-147

Knopman DS, DeKosky ST, Cummings JL, *et al.*, Practice parameter: Diagnosis of dementia (an evidence-based review). Report of the quality standards subcommittee of the American Academy of Neurology, *Neurology,* 2001; **56**:1143-1153

Knott V, Phil D, Mohr E, Mahoney C, Ilivitsky V. Electroencephalographic coherence in Alzhemier's disease: Comparisons with a control group and population norms. J Ger Psychiatry and Neurology 2000; 13: 1-8

Knott V, Mohr E, Mahoney C, Ilivitsky V. Quantitative electroencephalography in Alzhemier's disease: comparison with a control group, population norms and mental status. J Psychiatry Neurosci 2001; 26:106-16

Knottnerus JA, van Weel C, Muris JWM. Evaluation of diagnostic procedures. BMJ 2002; 324:477-80

Koenig T, Lehmann D, Saito N, Kuginuki T, Kinoshita T, Koukkou M. Decreased functional connectivity of EEG theta-frequency activity in first-episode, neuroleptic-naive patients with schizophrenia: preliminary results. Schizophr Res 2001; 1-2: 55-60

Koenig T, Prichep L, Dierks T, Hubl D, Wahlund L-O, John ER, Jelic V. Decreased EEG synchronisation in Alzheimer's disease and mild cognitive impairment. Neurobiol Aging, in press

Koles ZJ. Trends in EEG source localization. Electroencephalogr Clin Neurophysiol 1998; 106: 127-37

Kosunen O, Soininen H, Paljarvi L, Heinonen O, Talasniemi S, Riekkinen PJ Sr. Diagnostic accuracy of Alzhemier's disease: a neuropathologic study. Acta Neuropathol 1996; 91: 185-193

Kowalski JW, Gawel M, Pfeffer A, Barcikowska M. The diagnostic value of EEG in Alzheimer disease. Correlation with the severity of mental impairment. J Clin Neurophysiol 2001; 18: 570-575

Koyama K, Hirasawa H, Okubo Y, Karasawa A. Quantitative EEG correlates of normal aging in elderly. Clinical Electroencephalography 1997; 28: 160-165

Kuskowski MA, Mortimer JA, Morley GK, Malone SM, Okaya AJ. Rate ofr cognitive decline in Alzhemier's disease is associated with EEG alpha power. Biol Psychiatry 1993; 33: 659-662

Kwa VIH, Weinstein HC, Meyjes Posthumus EG, et al. Spectral analysis of EEG and 99m-Tc-Hmpao SPECT-Scan in Alzheimer's disease. Biol Psychiatry 1993; 33:100-107

Lehman D. Multichannel topography of human alpha EEG fields. Electroencephalogr Clin Neurophysiol 1971; 31: 439-449

Lehman D, Michel CM. Intracerebral dipole sources of EEG FFT power maps. Brain Topogr 1989;2:155-164

Lehmann D, Koenig T. Spatio-temporal dynamics of alpha brain electrical fields and cognitive modes. Int J Psychophysiology 1997; 26: 99-112

Leuchter AF, Spar JE, Walter DO, Weiner H. Electroencephalographic spectra and coherence in the diagnosis of Alzheimer's type and multi-infarct dementia: a pilot study. Arch Gen Psychiatry 1987; 44:993-998

Leuchter AF, Newton TF, Cook IA, Walter DO, Rosenberg-Thompson S, Lachenbruch PA. Changes in brain functional connectivity in Alzheimer-type and multiinfarct dementia. Brain 1992; 115:1543-1561

Leuchter AF, Cook IA, Newton NF, et al. Regional differences in brain electrical activity in dementia: use of spectral power and spectral ratio measures. Electroenceph Clin Neurophysiology 1993; 87: 385-393

Leuchter AF, Dunkin JJ, Luftkin RB, Anzai Y, Cook IA, Newton TF. Effect of white matter disease on functional connections in the aging brain. J Neurol Neurosurg Psychiatry 1994; 57:1347-1354

Leys D, Erkinjuntti T, Desmond DW, et al. Vascular dementia: The role of infarcts. Alzheimer Dis Assoc Disorders 1999; 13[Supppl 3]:S38-S48

Lindau M, Jelic V, Johansson S-E, Andersen C, Wahlund L-O, Almkvist O. Quantitative EEG abnormalities and cognitive dysfunctions in frontotemporal dementia and Alzheimer's disease. Dement Geriatr Cogn Disord 2003; 15: 106-114

Lobo A, Launer LJ, Fratiglioni L, et al. Prevalence of dementia and major subtypes in Europe: A collaborative study of population-based cohorts. Neurology 2000; 54[Suppl5]:S4-S9

Locatelli T, Cursi M, Liberati D, Franceschi M, Comi G. EEG coherence in Alzheimer's disease. Electroenceph Clin Neurophysiology 1998; 106: 229-237

Logar Ch, Schmidt R, Freidl W, Reinhart B, Scala M, Lechner H. EEG mapping in middle aged normal volunteers: The impact of cerebrovascular risk factors. Brain Topography 1993; 6:111-115

Lopes da Silva FH and Storm van Leeuwen W. The cortical source of the alpha rhytm. Neurosci Lett 1977; 6:237-241

Lopes da Silva FH, Witter MP, Boeijinga PH, Lohman AHM. Anatomic organization and physiology of the limbic cortex. Physiol Rev 1990; 70:453-511

Lopez OL, Brenner RP, Becker JT, Jungreis CA, Rezek D, DeKosky ST. Electroencephalographic correlates of periventricular white matter lesions in probable Alzheimer's disease. Dementia 1995; 6:343-347

Lopez OL, Becker JT, Kaufer DI, Hamilton RL, Sweet RA, Klunk W, DeKosky ST. Research evaluation and prospective diagnosis of dementia with Lewy bodies. Arch Neurol 2002; 59:43-6.

Lutzenberger W, Birbaumer N, Flor H, Rockstroh B, Elbert T. Dimensional analysis of the human EEG and intelligence. Neurosci Lett 1992; 143: 10-14

Martin-Loeches M, Gil P, Jimenez F, et al. Topographic maps of brain electrical activity in primary degenerative dementia of the Alzheimer type and multiinfarct dementia. Biol Psychiatry 1991; 29:211-233

Mattia D, Babiloni F, Romigi A, et al. Quantitative EEG and dynamic susceptibility contrast MRI in Alzhemier's disease: a correlative study. Clin Neurophysiology 2003; 114:1210-1216

McKhann G, Drachman D, Folstein M, Katzman R, Price D, Stadlan M. Clinical diagnosis of Alzheimer's disease: report of the NINCDS-ADRDA Work Group under the auspices of Department of Health and Human Services Task Force on Alzheimer Disease. Neurology 1984; 34: 939-944

Merlet I, García-Larrea L, Froment JC, Maguière F. Simplified projection of EEG dipole sources onto human brain anatomy. Neurophysiol Clin 1999; 29: 39-52

Mezzapesa DM, Rocca MA, Pagani E, Comi G, Filippi M. Evidence of subtle gray-matter pathologic changes in healthy elderly individuals with nonspecific white-matter hyperintensities. Arch Neurol 2003; 60:1109-1112

Miyauchi T, Haginoto H, Ishii M, et al. Quantitative EEG in patients with presenile and senile dementia of the Alzhemier type. Acta Neurol Scand 1994; 89:56-64

Mody CK, McIntyre HB, Miller BL, Altman K, Read S. Computerized EEG frequency analysis and topographic brain mapping in Alzheimer's disease. Ann New York Acad Sci 1991; 620:45-56

Moe KE, Larsen LH, Prinz PN, Vitiello MV. Major unipolar depression and mild Alzheimer's disease: differentiation by quantitative tonic REM EEG. Electroencephalogr Clin Neurophysiol 1993;86:238-246

Montplaisir J, Petit D, Décary A, et al. Sleep and quantitative EEG in patients with progressive supranuclear palsy. Neurology 1997; 49:999-1003

Nakano T, Miyasaka M, Ohtaka T, Ohmori K. Longitudinal changes in computerized EEG and mental function of the aged: A nine-year follow-up study. Int Psychogeriatrics 1992; 4: 9-23

Neary D. Frontotemporal degeneration, Pick disease, and corticobasal degeneration. Arch Neurol 1997; 54: 1425-1426

Neary D, Snowden JS, Gustafson L, et al. Frontotemporal lobar degeneration. A consensus on clinical diagnostic criteria. Neurology 1998; 51:1546-1554

Neufeldt M, Blumen S, Aitkin I, Parmet I, Korczyn A. EEG frequency analysis in demented and nondemented parkinsonian patients. Dementia 1994; 5:23-28

Newton TF, Leuchter AF, Walter DO, et al. EEG coherence in man with AIDS: association with subcortical metabolic activity. J Neuropsychiatry Clin Neurosci 1993; 5:316-321

Nunez PL, Srinivasan R, Westdorp AF, et al. EEG coherency I: statistics, reference electrode, volume conduction, Laplacians, cortica imaging, and interpretation at multiple scales. Electroencephalogr Clin Neurophysiol 1997; 103:499-515

Nunez PL, Silberstein RB, Shi Z, et al. EEG coherency II: experimental comparisons of multiple measures. Clin Neurophysiology 1999; 110:469-486

Nuwer MR. Assessing digital and quantitative EEG in clinical settings. J Clin Neurophysiol 1998; 15: 458-463

O'Connor KP, Shaw JC, Ongley CO. The EEG and differential diagnosis in psychogeriatrics. Br J Psychiatry 1979; 135:156-162

Oken BS, Chiappa KH. Statistical issues concerning computerized analysis of brainwave topography. Ann Neurol. 1986;19:493-7.

Oken BS, Kaye JA. Electrophysiologic function in the healthy, extremely old. Neurology 1992; 42:519-526

Pantoni L, Didier L, Fazekas F, et al. Role of white matter lesions in cognitive impairment of vascular origin. Alzheimer Dis Assoc Disord 1999; 13[Suppl3]:S49-S54

Partanen J, Soininen H, Helkala E-L, Könönen M, Kilpeläinen R, Riekkinen P. Relationship between EEG reactivity and neuropsychological tests in vascular dementia. J Neural Transm 1997; 104:905-912

Pascual-Marqui RD, Michel CM, Lehman D. Low resolution electromagnetic tomography: a new method for localizing electrical activity in the brain. Int J Psychophysiol 1994; 18:49-65

Pascual-Marqui RD, Lehman D, Koenig T, et al. Low resolution brain electromagnetic tomography (LORETA) functional imaging in acute, neuroleptic-naïve, first episode, productive schizophrenics. Psychiat Res-Neuroimaging 1999;

Passero S, Rocchi R, Vatti G, Burgalassi L, Battistini N. Quantitative EEG mapping, regional cerebral blood flow, and neuropsychological function in Alzhemier's disease. Dementia 1995; 6:148-156

Pentillä M, Partanen JV, Soininen H, Riekkinen PJ. Quantitative analysis of occipital EEG in different stages of Alzheimer's disease. Electroencephalogr Clin Neurophysiol 1985; 60:1-6

Petersen RC. Clinical subtypes of Alzheiemer's disease. Dement Geriatr Cogn Disord 1998; 9 [Suppl 3]:16-24

Petersen R, Smith G, Waring S, Ivnik R, Tangalos E, Kokmen E. Mild cognitive impairment:clinical characterization and outcome. Arch Neurol 1999; 56:303-308

Petersen RC, Doody R, Kurz A, et al. Current concepts in mild cognitive impairment. Arch Neurol 2001; 58: 1985-92

Petit D, Montplaisir J, Lorrain D, Gauthier S. Spectral analysis of the rapid eye movement sleep electroencephalogram in fight and left temporal regions: A biological marker of Alzheimer's disease. Ann Neurol 1992; 32:172-176

Petrosian AA, Prokhorov DV, Lajara-Nanson W, Schiffer RB. Recurrent neural network-based approach for early recognitivon of Alzheimer's disease in EEG. Clin Neurophysiol 2001; 112:1378-1387

Pollock VE, Schneider LS. Topographic electroencephalographic apha in recovered depressed elderly. J Abnorm Psychol 1989; 98:268-273

Pollock VE, Schneider LS, Lyness SA. EEG amplitudes in healthy, late-middle-aged and elderly adults: Normality of the distributions and correlations with age. Electroencephalogr Clin Neurophysiol 1990a; 75: 276-288

Pollock VE, Schneider LS. Quantitative, waking EEG research on depression. Biol Psychiatry 1990b; 27: 757-780

Pollock VE, Schneider LS, Lyness SA. Reliability of topographic quantitative EEG amplitude in healthy late-middle aged and elderly subjects. Electroencephalogr Clin Neurophysiol 1991; 79: 20-26

Pozzi D, Petracchi M, Sabe Liliana, Golimstock A, Garcia H, Starkstein S. Quantified electroencephalographic correlates of neuropsychological deficits in Alzheimer's disease. J Neuropsychiatry Clinical Neurosciences 1995a; 7:61-67

Pozzi D, Golimstock A, Petracchi M, Garcia H, Starkstein S. Quantified electroencephalographic changes in depressed patients with and without dementia. Biol Psychiatry 1995b; 38:677-683

Pozzi D, Vazquez S, Petracchi M, Dancygier G, Garcia H, Starkstein S. Quantified electroencephalographic correlates of relative frontal or parietal hypoperfusion in dementia. J Neuropsychiatry Clin Neurosci 1996; 8:26-32

Prichep L, John E. QEEG profiles of psychiatric disorders. Brain Topogr 1992; 4:249-57

Prichep LS, John ER, Ferris H, et al. Quantitative EEG correlates of cognitive deterioration in the elderly. Neurobiol Aging 1994; 15:85-90

Primavera A, Novello P, Finocchi C, Canevari E, Corsello L. Correlation beteen Mini-Mental State Examination and quantitative electroencephalography in senile dementia of Alzheimer type. Neuropsychobiology 1990; 23: 74-78

Prinz PN, Vitiello MV. Dominant occipital (alpha) rhytm frequency in early stage Alzheimer's disease and depression. Electroencephalogr Clin Neurophysiol 1989; 73: 427-432

Prinz PN, Larsen LH, Moe KE, Vitiello MV. EEG markers of early Alzheimer's disease in computer selected tonic REM sleep. Electroencephalogr Clin Neurophysiol 1992; 83: 36-43

Pritchard WS, Duke W. Measuring chaos in the brain: a tutorial review of non-linear dynamical EEG analysis. Intern J Neuroscience 1992; 67:31-80

Pritchard WS, Duke DW, Coburn KL, et al. EEG-based, neural-net predictive classification of Alzhemeir's disease versus control subjects is augmented by non-linear EEG measures. Electroencephalogr Clin Neurophysiol 1994; 91:118-130

Rae-Grant A, Blume W, Lau C, Hachinski VC, Fisman M, Merskey H. The electroencephalogram in Alzheimer-type dementia. A sequential study correlating the electroencephalogram with psychometric and quantitative pathologic data. Arch Neurol 1987;44(1):50-54.

Reisberg B, Ferris SH, de Leon MJ, Crook T. The global deterioration scale for assessment of primary degenerative dementia. Am J Psychiatry 1982; 139: 1136-1139

Reynolds III CF, Kupfer DJ, Taska LS, et al. EEG sleep in elderly depressed, demented, and healthy subjects. Biol Psychiatry 1985; 20:431-442

Rice DM, Buchsbaum MS, Starr A, Auslander L, Hagman J, Evans WJ. Abnormal EEG slow activity in left temporal areas in senile dementia of the Alzheimer type. J Gerontol 1990;45(4):M145-151.

Rice DM, Buchsbaum MS, Hardy D, Burgwald L. Focal left temporal slow EEG activity is related to a verbal recent memory deficdit in a non-demented elderly population. J Gerontol 1991; 46:144-151

Richards M, Folstein M, Albert M, et al. Multicenter study of predictors of disease in Alzheimer disease (the "Predictors study"). II Neurological, psychiatric, and demographic influences on baseline measuresof disease severity. Alzheimer Dis Assoc Disorders 1993; 7:22-23

Riekkinen P. Jr, Sirviö J, Riekkinen P. Relationship between the cortical choline acetyltransferase content and EEG delta-power. Neuroscience Ressearch 1990; 8:12-20

Robinson DJ, Merskey H, Blume WT, Fry R, Williamson PC, Hachinski VC. Electroencephalography as an aid in the exclusion of Alzheimer's disease. Arch Neurol 1994;51(3):280-284.

Rodriguez G, Nobili F, Arrigo A, et al. Prognostic significance of quantitative electroencephalography in Alzheimer patients: preliminary observations. Electroencephalogr Clin Neurophysiol 1996; 99: 123-128

Rodriguez G, Nobili F, Rocca G, de Carli F, Gianelli MV, Rosadini G. Quantitative electroencephalography and regional cerebral blood flow: discriminant analysis between Alzheimer's patients and healthy controls. Dementia 1998; 9:274-283

Rodriguez G, Copello F, Vitali P, Perego G, Nobili F. EEG spectral profile to stage Alzheimer's disease 1999; 110:1831-1837

Rogers J, Morrison JH. Quantitative morphology and regional laminar distributions of senile plaques in Alzheimer's disease. J Neurosci 1985; 5:2801-2808

Rosen I, Gustafson L, Risberg J. Multichannel EEG frequency analysis and somatosensory-evoked potentials in patients with different types of organic dementia. Dementia 1993; 4: 43-49

Rosén I. Electroencephalography as a diagnostic tool in dementia: a review. Acta Neurol Scand 1996; Suppl 168:63-70

Roubicek J. The electroencephalogram in the middle-aged and elderly. J Am Ger Soc 1977;25:145-152

Salinsky MC, Oken BS, Morehead L. Test-retest reliability in EEG frequency analysis. Electroencephalogr Clin Neurophysiol 1991; 79:382-.392

Schreiter-Gasser U, Gasser T, Ziegler P. Quantitative EEG analysis in early onset Alzheimer's diseae: correlations with severity, clinical characteristics, visual EEG and CCT. Electroencephalogr Clin Neurophysiol 1994; 90:267-262

Shaw JC, O'Connor K, Ongley C. EEG coherence as a measure of cerebral functional organisation. In: Brazier MAB & Petsche H (Eds) "Arhitectonics of the cerebral cortex", Raven Press, New York 1978; pp 245-255

Shenal BV, Rhodes RD, Moore TM, Higgins DA, Harrison DW. Quantitative electroencephalography (QEEG) and neuropsychological syndrome analysis. Neuropsychology review 2001; 11:31-44

Sheridan PH, Sato S, Foster N, et al. Relation of EEG alpha background to parietal lobe function in Alzheiemr's disease as measured by positron emission tomography and psychometry. Neurology 1988; 38:747-750

Siennicki-Lantz A, Lilja B, Rosén I, Elmståhl S. Cerebral blood flow in white matter is correlated with systolic blood pressure and EEG in senile dementia of Alzhemier type. Dement Geriatr Cogn Disord 1998; 9:29-38

Signorino M, Pucci E, Belardinelli N, Nolfe G, Angeleri F. EEG spectral analysis in vascular and Alzheimer dementia. Electroencephalogr Clin Neurophysiol 1995; 94: 313-325

Soininen H, Partanen VJ, Helkala EL, Riekkinen PJ. EEG findings in senile dementia and normal aging. Acta Neurol Scand 1982a;65(1):59-70.

Soininen H, Partanen JV, Puranen M, Riekkinen PJ. EEG and computed tomography in the investigation of patients with senile dementia. J Neurol Neurosurg Psychiatry 1982b; 45:711-714

Soininen H, Partanen J, Laulumaa V, Pääkkönen A, Helkala E-L, Riekkinen P. Serial EEG in Alzheimer's disease:3 year follow-up and clinical outcome. Electroencephalogr Clin Neurophysiol 1991; 79: 342-348

Stam CJ, Jelles B, Achtereekte HAM, van Birgeln JH, Slaets PJ. Diagnostic usefulness of linear and nonlinear quantiative EEG analysis in Alzheimer's disease. Clin Electroencephalography 1996; 27:69-77

Stam CJ, van Dijk BW. Synchronisation likelihood: an un-biased measure of generalised synchronisation in multivariate data sets. Physica D 2002; 163:236-51

Stam CJ, van der Made Y, Pijnenburg YAL, Scheltens Ph. EEG synchronisation in mild cognitive impairment and Alzheimer's disease. Acta Neurol Scand 2003; 108:90-96

Steriade M, Gloor P, Llinás R, Lopes da Silva F, Mesulam M. Basic mechanisms of cerebral rhytmic activities. Electroencephalogr Clin Neurophysiol 1990; 76: 481-508

Stern Y. What is cognitive reserve? Theory and research application of the reserve concept. J Int Neuropsychol Soc 2002; 8: 448-60

Stevens A, Kircher T, Nickola M, Bartels M, Rosellen N, Wormstall H. Dynamic regulation of EEG power and coherence is lost early and globally in probable DAT. Eur Arch Psychiatry Clin Neurosci 2001; 251:199-204

Stigsby B, Johanesson G, Ingvar D. Regional EEG analysis and regional cerebral blood flow in Alzhemier's and Pick's disease. Electroencephalogr Clin Neurophysiol 1981; 51:537-547

Storey E, Slavin MJ, Kinsella GJ. Patterns of cognitive impairment in Alzheimer's disease: assessment of differential diagnosis. Frontiers in Bioscience 2002; 7: 155-184

Strijers RLM, Scheltens Ph, Jonkman EJ, de Rijke W, Hooijer Ch, Jonker C. Diagnosing Alzheimers' disease in community-dwelling elderly: A comparison of EEG and MRI. Dement Geriatr Cogn Disord 1997; 8:198-202

Strik WK, Dierks T, Becker T, Lehman D. Larger topographical variance and decreased duration of brain electric microstates in depression. J Neural Transm [GenSect] 1995; 99:213-222

Szelies B, Grond M, Herholz K, Kessler J, Wullen T, Heiss W-D. Quantitative EEG mapping and PET in Alzheimer's disease. J neurological Sciences 1992; 110:46-56

Szelies B, Mielke R, Herholz K, Heiss W-D. Quantitative topographical EEG compared to FDG PET for classification of vascular and degenerative dementia. Electroencephalogr Clin Neurophysiol 1994; 91: 131-139

Swets JA. Indices of discrimination of diagnostic accuracy: Their ROCs and implied models. Psychological Bulletin 1986; 99:100-117

Terry RD. Chapter 29. Neuropathological changes in Alzhemier's disease. In: L. Svennerholm, AK Asbury, RA Reisfeld, K Sandhoff, K Suzuki, G Tettamanti and G Toffano (Eds.) Elsevier Science BV, Progress in Brain Research, vol 101, 1994; pp 383-390

Thatcher RW, Krause PJ, Hrybyk M. Cortico-cortical associations and EEG coherence: a two compartmental model. Electroencephalogr Clin Neurophysiol 1986; 64:123-143

Tononi G, Edelman GM, Sporns O. Complexity and coherency: integrating information in the brain. Trends in Cognitive Sciences 1998; 2:474-484

Torres F, Faoro A, Loewenson R, Johnson E. The electroencephalogram of elderly subjects revisited. Electroencephalogr Clin Neurophysiol 1983;56:391-398

Valladares-Neto DC, Buchsbaum MS, Evans WJ, et al. EEG delta, positron emission tomography, and memory deficit in Alzheimer's disease. Neuropsychobiology 1995; 31:173-181

Van Hoesen GW. Ortical feedforward and cortical feedback neural systems in Alzheimer's disease. In: BT Hyman/C. Duyckaerts/Y. Christen (Eds.) "Connections, cognition, and Alzheimer's disease, Springer-Verlag Berlin Heidelberg 1997, pp 17-31

Visser SL, Hooijer C, Jonker C, Van Tilburg W, De Rijke W. Anterior temporal focal abnormalities in EEG in normal aged subjects; correlations with psychopathological and CT brain findings. Electroencephalogr Clin Neurophysiol 1987; 66:1-7

Visser PJ, Verhey FR, Hofman PA, Scheltens P, Jolles J. Medial temporal lobe atrophy predicts Alzheimer's disease in patients with minor cognitive impairment. J Neurol Neurosurg Psychiatry. 2002;72:491-7.

von Stein A and Sarnthein J. Different frequencies for different scales of cortical integration: from local gamma to long range alpha/theta synchronization. Int J of Psychophysiology 2000; 38: 301-313

Walker MP, Ayre GA, Cummings JL, et al. Quantifying fluctuation in dementia with Lewy bodies, Alzheimer's disease, and vascular dementia. Neurology 2000; 54:1616-1624

Whitehouse PJ, Price DL, Clark AW, Coyle JT, DeLong MR. Alzheimer disease: evidence for selective loss of cholinergic neurons in the nucleus basalis. Ann Neurol. 1981; 10:122-6.

Williamson PC, Merskey H, Morrison S, et al. Quantitative electroencephalographic correlates of cognitive decline in normal elderly subjects. Arch Neurol 1990; 47: 1185-1188

Wimo A, Winblad B, Aguero-Torres H, von Strauss E. The magnitude of dementia occurrence in the world. Alzheimer Dis Assoc Disord 2003; 17: 63-67

Wolf H, Jelic V, Gertz H-J, Nordberg A, Julin P, Wahlund L-O. A critical discussion of the role of neuroimaging in mild cognitive impairment. Acta Neurol Scand 2003; 107 [Suppl 179]:52-76

Yagyu Y, Wackermann J, Shigeta M, et al. Global dimensional complexity of multichannel EEG in mild Alzheimer's disease and age-matched controls. Dement Geriatr Cogn Disord 1997; 8:343-347

Yener GG, Leuchter AF, Jenden D, Read SL, Cummings JL, Miller BL. Quantitative EEG in frontotemporal dementia. Clin Electroencephalography 1996; 27:61-68.

In: Depression and Dementia ISBN 1-59454-114-0
Editor: Suptendra Nath Sarbadhikari, p. 305-317

Chapter 10

EVENT REALETD POTENTIALS (ERP) IN DEMENTIA AND COGNITIVE IMPAIRMENT

Fethi Idiman
Department of Neurology
Dokuz Eylül University Hospital
Izmir/Turkey

ABSTRACT

Up to now, the relationships between these potentials and neuropsychological functions such as memory, attentions, conation, expectancy, alertness etc. have been investigated. In the beginning, in normal elderly subject, the conditions under which ERPs occurred, consistent and varying features of the waves underchanging conditions of mental processing-latency, amplitude etc. were tried to be identified. Which mental processing represented by which various stimulus conditions was interpreted and changing features were evaluated through studies. Furthermore, by clinical examination and neuropsychological tests, the impaired components of mental processing were identified and which ERP changes they led to were demonstrated. At present, all these features are considered especially in early stage dementia, whether they can be helpful in reaching the diagnosis or not, and whether differential diagnosis can be made according to electrophysiological data or not. In addition, whether ERPs can be used in the evaluation of effect of drugs in therapeutical approaches or not have been investigated.

There are considerable systematic differences between normal and patient populations. In particular, the P300 component of ERPs has been widely applied in the scientific study of age-related cognitive dysfunction, because it reflects attentional and memory processes. In addition, a number of clinical studies (employing the oddball task) have indicated a probable correlation between the latencies and/or amplitudes of ERP components and changes in information processing in elderly and mental illnesses

Dementia is a common cognitive syndrome reflecting a widespread chronic progressive disease as an extension to normal aging process. In general progressive declines in memory function accompany normal aging, mild cognitive impairment (MCI) and Alzheimer's disease (AD). In Clinical practice, declines in working memory and episodic memory are observed in healthy aging relative to young subjects [12], while profound impairments in working memory and episodic memory are found in Alzheimer's disease. In addition to memory impairments, AD is also characterized by deficits in other cognitive domains including language, attention and reasoning, mild cognitive impairment (MCI) is a clinical diagnosis that characterizes elderly individuals with an isolated memory impairment more sever than in healthy aging group while other cognitive functions are normal [54].

Thus, memory impairments in the elderly can be determined in three groups as mild alterations in healthy aging, greater memory impairment in MCI, and severe memory and other cognitive deficiencies in AD. The assessment of memory impairment and accurate and early diagnosis of AD with reliable noninvasive methods is of great importance for clinical practice as much as effective and specific antidementive therapies.

Electrophysiological studies have provided some of the most direct evidence for assessing central nervous system (CNS) functions. Standardized electroencephalographic (EEG) recordings and sensory evoked potentials (EP) measures have been used clinically for many years in routine evaluations but cognitive ERPS have not yet been employed commonly in routine practice. As known, some long latency potentials which occur after rare and/or unexpected stimuli or conditional stimuli, seem to depend on cognitive processes rather than the physical characteristics of the stimulus. Therefore they are called of "Event Related Potentials" "ERPs" rather than evoked potentials. These are

1-P300 (visual auditory oddball paradigm.
2-Contingent negative variation. "CNV"
3-The other ERPs in cognitive impairments:

Readiness potential "Bereitshaftspotentials" and other movement related potentials, and Olfactory ERPs

Up to now, the relationships between these potentials and neuropsychological functions such as memory, attentions, conation, expectancy, alertness etc. have been investigated. In the beginning, in normal elderly subject, the conditions under which ERPs occurred, consistent and varying features of the waves underchanging conditions of mental processing-latency, amplitude etc. were tried to be identified. Which mental processing represented by which various stimulus conditions was interpreted and changing features were evaluated through studies. Furthermore, by clinical examination and neuropsychological tests, the impaired components of mental processing were identified and which ERP changes they led to were demonstrated. At the present, according to all these features especially in early stage dementia, whether they can be helpful in reaching the diagnosis or not, and whether differential diagnosis can be made according to electrophysiological data or not, have been considered. In addition, whether ERPs can be used in the evaluation of effect of drugs in therapeutical approaches or not have been investigated.

There are considerable systematic differences between normal and patient populations. In particular, the P300 component of ERPs has been widely applied in the scientific study of age-related cognitive dysfunction, because it reflects attentional and memory processes. In addition, a number of clinical studies (employing the oddball task) have indicated a probable correlation between the latencies and/or amplitudes of ERP components and changes in information processing in elderly and mental illnesses [1, 2, 6, 20, 26, 52].

P300 Components of ERPs in Clinical Practice

The P300 brain potential can provide information that is comparable to other clinically used biomedical assays. P300 latency is considered to be a measure of stimulus classification speed and usually non-related to response selection processes [11, 21, 22, 37, 44, 46]. Therefore, it doesn't depend on behavioral reaction time P300 latency is an index of processing time required before response generation it is a sensitive temporal measure of the neural activity underlying the processes of attention allocation and immediate memory. In addition, P300 latency is negatively correlated with mental function in normal control subject, with shorter latencies associated with superior cognitive performance [4, 6, 8, 14, 32, 33, 38, 47]. The neuropsychological tests that are best correlated with P300 laency are those that maintain attentional resources. The association is also supported by results indicating that P300 latency increases as cognitive capability decreases from demented patients [7, 10, 11, 20, 44, 51]. Thus P300 latency is directly associated with cognitive capability in both normal and patient populations.

P300 amplitude is thought to index brain activity that is required in the maintenance of working memory when the mental model of the stimulus environment is updated [5, 9, 15, 21, 33, 34, 37]. This context updating theory has its roots in Sokolov's model of the orienting response, which has been postulated to result from a change in the organism's neural representation of the stimulus [40, 43, 44, 46].

P300 amplitude is also proportional to the amount of attentional resources devoted to a given task (Wickens et al. 83, Kramer and Strayer 88) and has been associated with superior memory performance [7, 33, 50, 58, 60]. Therefore, P300 amplitude can be viewed as a measure of CNS activity that reflects the processing of in coming information when it is incorporated into memory representations of the stimulus and the context in which the stimulus occurs. Therefore variation in P300 amplitude is assumed to reflect the degree or quality of information processing.

As understood, thus, P300 amplitude and latency appear as a valuable tool for assessing cognitive function.

The P300 component might be a useful tool for investigating cognitive function in normal aging and dementia. The studies have shown that P300 peak latency is prolonged in demented patients compared to similarly aged normal subject [11, 12, 14, 15, 42, 54]. Moreover, P300 latency increases systematically as cognitive function becomes worse in dementing illness even though component size is not directly associated with the degree of mental impairment [4, 7, 37, 51]. Negative correlations between cognitive function and P300 latency have also been reported in other neurological disorders as in confusional states and posttraumatic syndromes [1, 32, 38, 45, 62]. The findings of all studies suggest that P300 may be clinically useful as an index of cognitive function although its diagnostic utility is still discussed, since Goodin et al (1978) first demonstrated the slowing of P300 event-related brain potentials with aging, a number of studies have suggested that ERPs are useful indices for assessing age-related changes in cognitive brain functions. P300 amplitude and latency can consistently discriminate disease states from control conditions. In addition, P300 component of ERPs can be useful as an effective and neuroelectric measure for evaluating therapeutic strategies involving CNS medications [23, 47, 58, 60, 61]. However, because the basic findings and methodological approaches are still being developed, additional studies that focus on increasing P300 sensitivity and discriminability are needed before clinical applications can be made on a routine basis. P300 sensitivity can be gained by taking into account biological determinants that contribute to ERP variability [3, 5, 15, 41, 45, 46] using a variety of stimuli which are processed in different ways might increase the diagnostic sensitivity of ERPs. Two distinct subtypes are recorded in all stimulus modalities for P3 component of ERPs [51, 62]. Correctly detected task relevant stimuli generate a parietal maximum P300. Whereas nontarget, deviant stimuli requiring no behavioral response generate an earlier latency fronto-central P300 (novelty P3) which is considered to be a CNS index of orienting response. Studies of scalp topography the effects of brain lesions and development suggest that different brain regions and modes of cognitive processing are utilized in response to novel and target stimuli [15, 19, 23, 40, 43, 63]. These two types of P3 are useful for investigating neural networks in specific cognitive processes.

On the other hand if we give another example for using the single peak latencies, it is generally accepted that N2 and P3 are later when the target stimulus is more difficult to discriminate and it has been reported by many researchers that the N2 and P3 latencies are generally prolonged in dementia and in AD with memory disturbances [7, 15, 36, 62]. In the other AD study, the period from the end of sensory input to stimulus discrimination has been found prolonged, this means AD patients have difficulty analyzing the meaning of stimuli. This information suggests that both the context updating process and stimulus discrimination process are delayed in AD or other dementia. On the other hand, it has been useful the differences in P300 amplitude and latency if appropriate task conditions are employed to evaluate other brain disease and psychiatric disorders such as depression, schizophrenia and alcoholism [1, 2, 4, 9, 15, 55, 61]. However some studies have shown that P300 latency can separate individuals with dementia from those with depression associated pseudodementia [5, 6, 47, 55]. In addition, P300 evaluations has provided discrimination between patients with early AD from normal healthy subjects and other controls [16] the differences in P300 amplitude and latency between AD and other control groups have been found reliable [46, 47] to differential diagnosis.

As understood, most studies on ERP in dementia or psychiatric disorders have focused on the peak latency of ERPs components on the beginning of ERPs studies, latency delays of the P300 ERP component with simple auditory oddball tasks were suggested highly sensitive and specific to dementia. But these sometimes failed to demonstrate pertinent abnormalities of the P300 component useful for the clinical diagnosis of dementia [51]. Therefore some studies have evaluated not only peak latencies of ERP components (N1 P2 N2 P3) but also interpeak latencies (IPL) (N5 P2, P2 N2 and N2 P3). Both the single peak latency and the IPL measures were useful to differentiate the pathological groups from the normal control group. In particular it can be useful for differential diagnosis of dementia although different types of dementia – *e.g.*, subcortical and cortical-may be distinguished with some features in clinical basis from each other.

Many investigators have reported that the dementia produced by different diseases may be distinguished by long latency potentials electrophysiologically [3, 4, 7, 38, 45, 46, 63]. According to their results, subcortical dementia tends to affect the earlier N1 and P2 components whereas both cortical and subcortical dementia affects the later N2 and P3 components. As known that Parkinson's disease may have cognitive impairment and a clinical dementia recognized in only 10-20% of patients above that of an age-matched population. Subtle cognitive defects are proposed to be more frequent [5, 6]. ERP is an important and susceptive method to evaluate the cognitive status of PD patients. P300 evoked by the infrequent target stimulus in oddball paradigms was well studied and its latency prolongation has been correlated with some measures of cognitive impairments in PD [7]. In recent years, in a group of nondemented PD patients and a group of normal controls, both a visual oddball paradigm and S1-S2 paradigm were employed PD patients simultaneously to evoke ERPs. Decrease of P300 amplitude in PD group was found in the S1-S2 paradigm but not in the oddball paradigm [8]. The result showed the value of this S1-S2 paradigm for detecting minor cognitive abnormalities. In general it has been suggested that P300 latency is correlated with score on cognitive tests and it may measure the cognitive changes in PD patients [4, 5, 9, 15, 27, 36, 37]. However it has also been found that the peak amplitude of P300 rather than its latency was abnormal in the patients group therefore the amplitude of P300 may decrease at first one to the cognitive decline of P300 [58] In addition it has been established that PD patients have cognitive impairment not only in late stage of the disease but also in their early stage of the disease course. As the P300 component of ERP, N270 may also be able index for revealing the minor cognitive impairment in PD patients [59].

Briefly the P300 wave is one of the cognitive components of the ERP that is used to investigate the cognitive processes and which can be used to study patient populations with a variety of psychiatric disorders. ERPs can be useful neurophysiological tool for the assessment and the clinical follow up of brain functions of subjects with memory disorders since they are sensitive to cognitive slowing which is related to aging processes and to memory impairment which are triggered by neurodegenerative pathologies [49, 53, 63]. Previous investigations with AD patients have indicated delayed P300 latencies with a standard auditory oddball compared to normal elderly controls [37, 60], whereas P300 amplitudes were found maximally decreased over frontal regions [16]. Its clinical utility has been increased by the identification of factors that contribute to the variability in its amplitude and latency. Several variables significantly influence the amplitude and latency of this wave such as age, gender, intelligence and personality. Therefore the oddball task used in many studies is relatively too easy and the study of any brain function requires the design of more complex suitable paradigms. Although its value as a diagnostic index has not been entirely established there are a number of studies on the clinical applications of P300 in the relevant literature. This wave was investigated in psychopathology, including the studies undertaken to obtain an objective diagnostic index for mental disorders and also those carried out to assess the problems concerning the interpretation of information connected with pathologies P300 associated findings on dementia, schizophrenia, depression, alcoholism, drug addiction, anxiety disorders, panic disorders and on personality disorders have been examined in detail [8,11,13,35,36,37,39,41,42]. Moreover in these studies it is concluded that P300 examinations can also assist in determining what therapeutic approach to adopt [60, 61].

"CNV" Cortical Slow Negative Shift in Cognitive Impairments

In cognitive impairments, the other long latency slow wave or ERP studied the clinical usefulness is contingent negative variation (CNV). CNV is an event related potential and a slow negative shift which occurs in a S1-S2 paradigm. According to the duration of S1-S2 interval, CNV is seen one wave as the negative shift or two waves as an orienting response "O wave" and expectancy wave "E wave". In general CNV as a negative shift was investigated in various studies and was evaluated as a neurophysiological index of cognitive dysfunctions [18, 24, 26, 34]. Mostly CNV amplitudes were measured in demented patients and nondemented controls [24, 26]. Whether the relationship between cognitive impairment and CNV amplitudes was found or not was studied [64, 65]. In many studies CNV amplitudes of demented patients were found significantly smaller than those of nondemented group [26, 33, 65]. Moreover, in some studies, a significant relationship was reported between severity of dementia and degree of amplitude reduction [18, 26]. In another study, CNV recordings were evaluated in a group of subjects affected AD at the onset of the symptoms. Recordings have been made in basal conditions and upon administration of an insignificant distracting stimulus. It has been shown that upon the administration of a distracting stimulus, marked amplitude decrease of the wave was observed in the patients compared to age-matched healthy controls [26]. About 20 years ago, The CNV recordings by Oconnor were made for different interstimulus intervals over two sessions with demented patients and normal elderly subjects. The results suggested that the amplitudes and latencies of CNV were much different for longer interstimulus interval [33]. And our study has indicated that CNV amplitudes decrease in AD patients and this finding are usually correlated with the degree of cognitive impairment [18].

Cortical topography differences suggested that the senile preparatory strategies were predominantly influenced by the extent of their initial frontal orienting response and that the senile showed less differentiation between frontal central recordings. A study of Uytdenhoef et al. has evaluated the relationship between CNV amplitude, regional cerebral blood flow (r CBF), reaction Time (RT) and MMSE (mini mental state examination) in nondemented subjects and patients with AD. The significant correlations between CNV amplitudes and rCBF, MMSE and RT have been found. Statistical analysis has shown demented from nondemented patients may distinguished with 75% accuracy [57]. Zappoli et al. have recorded and measured the CNV complex and RT to imperative (S2) signal in idiopathic cognitive impairment and AD and age-matched healthy controls. Some CNV components were obtained differently in each group. Particularly second component of CNV and postimperative negative variation (PINV) being resolution of CNV after S2 signal and RT was very prolonged. The results suggest that CNV complex and changes may constitute a valuable clue for pathophysiological brain functioning in early stage dementias [64, 65].

In addition to all studies, the usefulness of CNV was also investigated in the assessment of therapeutic efficacies. For example a study for investigating effectiveness and the usefulness of a nootropic substance cerebrolysin was made the patients with the diagnosis of moderate organic brain syndrome of different etiology and age-matched elderly controls. This was a randomized placebo-controlled double-blind study. A group patients showed significant CNV amplitude increase after ten cerebrolysin plus multivitamins infusions whereas CNV' amplitudes did not change significantly after ten infusions with multivitamins alone. Placebo group of patients presented a decrease of CNV amplitudes [25]. The results confirmed the usefulness of CNV studies by providing an index of nootropic drug effects.

According to many studies it was concluded that the CNV examinations can be useful for the assessment and following course of dementia.

THE OTHER ERPS ON COGNITIVE DISORDERS

In recent years, the N400 component of ERP has also been studied as an electrophysiological measure. In particular, its related to linguistic processes have been analyzed [35, 48]. By this way to understanding the processes underlying dementia especially AD have been tried. Nowadays electrophysiological measures of ERP-N400 seem to be a very promising tool for the study of cognitive processes that sustained the understanding and organization of language and memory. ERP-N400 are changes in voltage reflected on the scalp and which are synchronized with an observable event (e.g. speech cognition) This is a noninvasive method of monitoring brain processes and can be used to obtain electrophysiological evidence of brain functions and of psychological processes. The N400 component of ERP has been linked mainly to language processing and has been recorded in association with examples of semantic incongruence found in sentences words or visually presented figures [48]. In the scientific studies of mental processing, the value of this component of ERP was clearly illustrated.

Recently somatosensory N250 component of ERP have investigated some clinical studies Kida et al. (2003) have evaluated the components N250 and P300 of event related potentials during three kinds of somatosensory discrimination tasks one of three situation was a mental task (count condition) and another one required pressing a button to deviant stimuli as quickly as possible (motor response condition). The N250-P300 complex was only occurred by deviant stimuli in active-attended situations The N250 peak amplitude was unchanged between the count and motor response conditions whereas P300 changed. In addition the N250 latency significantly correlated with reaction time while the P300 latency did not [22]. As a result it has suggested that somatosensory N250 reflects an attentive process which is related to the temporal aspect of behavioral response.

More recently in the cognitive impairments, the other investigated ERP is N270 component. N270 is a negative potential evoked by the S1-S2 paradigm. It peaks at around 270 ms after the onset of S2 if it is presented different from S1. Because N270 is only evoked by the stimulus pairs with conflicts it is considered that N270 reflects the cognitive activity in the human brain for processing conflicts. As known cognitive impairment is a well recognized feature of idiopathic PD [59]. Although clinical dementia is recognized in only 10-20% of PD cases, subtle cognitive defects are suggested to be more frequent. ERP is an important and susceptive method to evaluate the cognitive impairment in PD patients. Wang et al employed the subtle S1-S2 paradigm to evoke potentials in nondemented PD patients and normal controls [59]. The patient group showed a delayed and a smaller N270 than the control group, and the reduction of its mean amplitude was significant. But the changes of P3 component are not consistent (un) like this. These results have indicated that PD patients as a group showed cognitive decline even in the absence of clinical dementia. N270 is a sensitive index in revealing this minor (or mild) cognitive impairment.

On the other hand, Ortiz et al. have reported that Alzheimer patients have the contralateral associated EMG responses to voluntary hand movement. They present data on the register of movement related potentials (Negative shift) and Lateralized Readiness Potential (LRP), which have shown a very fine capacity to reveal processes that occur in the motor cortex while movement execution is being prepared. The associated EMG responses have almost all the characteristics of partial errors revealed by cognitive psychology. The associated EMG responses are covert responses, so they can only be detected by EMG recordings. In addition, the appearance of this partial error changes the reaction time in the same way mainly increasing reaction time as compared with clear responses. Contrary to partial errors, the associated EMG responses do not constantly appear before the correct response. They are always after correct response. They are always after correct responses with a constant delay of 54+/-28 ms and occur with related to incorrect response preparation. All these findings have indicated that there is a specific feature in relation to inhibitory deficit in motor cortex and associated callosal pathways that avoid a correct response performance in AD patients [28].

Nowadays it has been widely accepted both visual and auditory P3 component of ERPs is sensitive to the cognitive decline occurring in old age and dementia. However new techniques such as the different modalities or different conditions in the experiment namely different paradigms have been used to increase with the aim of sensitivity. One of these is the olfactory event-related potentials (OERP). OERP have been increasingly applied in cognitive neuroscience to address basic underlying mechanisms. OERP's were evaluated to the N1/P2 and P3 components by mean amplitudes and latencies. Processing speed decreased at a constant rate over decades for the sensory (P2 latency) components. Decline in amplitude over decades was also apparent [30, 31]. However, the investigations on olfactory functional status will be needed for assessing whether they are usefulness in cognitive impairment or not.

As known that electrophysiological tests of sensory function have proved to be remarkably sensitive in the detection of subclinical disease and consequently have been of considerable assistance in the diagnosis of a variety of neurological disorders However event related potentials (ERPs) have not proved to be so sensitive terms of specific diagnosis of individual patients although they are often able to discriminate between patient groups and control groups. However such observations are of value because they provide information regarding to the nature of a disorder, even though they might not be able to identify any single patient in an experimental group as having ERPs significantly different from these observed in healthy controls. In practice the role of any clinical test is to provide complementary evidence in order to reach a diagnosis. But, few tests can be described as being "diagnostic" in their own right. Thus ERPs have many problems associated with on the clinical application. These include the broad intersubject variability of peak latencies and amplitudes in control groups, as well as the apparent nonspecifity of some ERP tests. An ERP test may usually identify abnormality in the later stages of disease in the simple conditions but the true task for the test is to identify abnormality in the later stages of disease on the simple conditions but the true task for the test is to identify abnormality in early disease when evidence of cognitive dysfunction will different and less frank than in later stages of the disorder. It is therefore, necessary to identify to cognitive deficits associated with the early stages of dementia and devise appropriate ERP tests to detect these deficits. In this context some later studies has shown that ERPs abnormalities should be investigated in particular early and late stages of dementia because ERP technique may be valuable for assessing cognitive disturbances in dementia and other mental illness, and in specific, may be useful to investigate the disturbed steps in the cognitive process of these diseases.

SUMMARY

Electrophysiological studies have provided some of the most direct evidence for assessing central nervous system (CNS) functions. Standardized electroencephalographic (EEG) recordings and sensory evoked potentials (EP) measures have been used clinically for many years in routine evaluations but cognitive ERPS have not yet been employed commonly in routine practice. As known, some long latency potentials which occur after rare and/or unexpected stimuli or conditional stimuli, seem to depend on cognitive processes rather than the physical characteristics of the stimulus. Therefore they are called of "Event Related Potentials" "ERPs" rather than evoked potentials. These are

1-P300 (visual auditory oddball paradigm.
2-Contingent negative variation. "CNV"
3-The other ERPs in cognitive impairments:

Readiness potential "Bereitshaftspotentials" and other movement related potentials, and Olfactory ERPs.

Up to now, the relationships between these potentials and neuropsychological functions such as memory, attentions, conation, expectancy, alertness etc. have been investigated. In the beginning, in normal elderly subject, the conditions under which ERPs occurred, consistent and varying features of the waves underchanging conditions of mental processing-latency, amplitude etc. were tried to be identified. Which mental processing represented by which various stimulus conditions was interpreted and changing features were evaluated through studies. Furthermore, by clinical examination and neuropsychological tests, the impaired components of mental processing were identified and which ERP changes they led to were demonstrated. At present, all these features are considered especially in early stage dementia, whether they can be helpful in reaching the diagnosis or not, and whether differential diagnosis can be made according to electrophysiological data or not. In addition, whether ERPs can be used in the evaluation of effect of drugs in therapeutical approaches or not have been investigated.

There are considerable systematic differences between normal and patient populations. In particular, the P300 component of ERPs has been widely applied in the scientific study of age-related cognitive dysfunction, because it reflects attentional and memory processes. In addition, a number of clinical studies (employing the oddball task) have indicated a probable correlation between the latencies and/or amplitudes of ERP components and changes in information processing in elderly and mental illnesses

REFERENCES

[1] Alonso-Prieto E, Lvarez-Gonzalez MA, Reyes-Verazain A, Fernande Concepcion O, Barros-Garcia E, Pando-Cabrera A. Use of event related potentials for the diagnosis and follow up of subclinical disorders of sustained attention in ischemic cerebrovascular disease. *Rev Neurol.* 2002. 1-15;34(11):1017-20.

[2] Aotsuko A, Weate SS, Drake ME, Paulson GW. Event-related potentials in parkinson's disease. *Electromyogr. Clin Neurophysiol* 1996(36) 215-220.

[3] Barrett G. Clinical application of event-related potentials in dementing illness: issues and problems. *Int J Psychophysiol.* 2000. 37(1):49-53.

[4] Benvenuto J, Jin Y, Casale M, Lynch G, Granger R. Identificaiton of diagnostic evoked response potential segment in Alzheimer's disease. *Exp Neurol.* 2002. 176(2):269-76.

[5] Beuzeron-Mangina JH, Mangina CA. Event-related brain potentials to Memory Workload and 'Analytical-Specific Perception' (Mangina-test) in patients with early Alzheimer's Disease and in normal controls. *Int J of psychophysiol* 2000(37)55-69

[6] Beuzeron-mangina JH. Intracerebral event-related potentials during memory workload. *Int. J. Psycholphysiol* 1997: 25-27.

[7] Comi G, Leocani L. Electrophysiological correlates of dementia. *Suppl Clin Neurophysiol.* 2000;53:331-6.

[8] Comi G, Leocani L. Neurophysiological imaging techniques in dementia. *Ital J Neurol Sci.* 1999;20(5 Suppl):S265-9.

[9] Fernandez-Lastra A, Morales-Rodrigues M, Penzol-Diaz J. Neurophysiological study and use of P300 evoked potentials investigation in the diagnosis and of follow-up of patients with Alzheimer's disease. *Rev Neurol.* 2001. 16-31;32(6):525-8.

[10] Ford JM, Askari N, Mathalon DM, Menon V, Gabrieli JD, Tinklenb JR, Yesavage Event-related brain potential evidence of spared knowledge in Alzheimer's disease. *Psychol Aging.* 2001. 16(1):161-76

[11] Frodl T, Hampel H, Juckel G, Burger K, Padberg F, Engel RR, Moll HJ, Hegerl U. Value of event-related P300 subcomponents in the clinical diagnosis of mild cognitive impairment and Alzheimer's Disease. *Psychophysiology.* 2002. 39(2):175-81.

[12] Golob EJ, Miranda GG, Johnson JK, Starr A. Sensory cortical interactions in aging, mild cognitive impairment, and Alzheimer's disease. *Neurobiol Aging.* 2001. 22(5):755-63.

[13] Goodin DS and Aminoff MJ. Electrophysiological differences between subtypes of dementia. *Brain* 1986(109) 1103-1113.

[14] Green J, Levey AI. Event-related potential changes in groups at increased risk f Alzheimer disease. *Arch Neurol.* 1999. 56(11):1398-1403.

[15] Hansenne M. The P300 cognitive event-related potential. II. Individual variability and clinical application in psychopathology. *Neurophysiol Clin.* 2000. 30(4):211-231.

[16] Holt LE, Raine A, Pa G, Schneider LS, Henderson W, Pollock VE. P300 topography in Alzheimer's disease. *Psychophysiology* 1995(32) 257-265

[17] Idiazabal Alecha M, Palencia Taboada AB, Sangorrin J, Espadaler-Gamissons JM. Cognitive evoked potentials in the hyperactivity attention deficit disorder. *Rev Neurol* 2002(34) 301-305.

[18] Idiman F, Contingent Negative Variation (CNV): II- Belirli Serebral Lezyonlarda.*Ege Nörolojik Bilimler Dergisi 1984* (1) 1-16.

[19] Jessen F, Kucharski C, Fries T, Papassotiropoulos A, Hoenig K, Mai W, Heun R. Sensory gating deficit expressed by a disturbed suppression the P50 event-related potential in patients in with Alzheimer's disease. *Am J Psychiatry.* 2001. 158(8):1319-21.

[20] Jimenez-Eserig A, Fernandez-Lorente J, Herrero A, Baron M, Lous de Blas G, Gobernado J. Event-related evoked potential P300 in frontotemporal dementia. *Dement Geriatr Cogn Disord.* 2002;13(1):27-32.

[21] Johnson R. Developmental evidence for modality dependent P300 generators A normative study. *Psychophysio*l 1989(26) 651-667.
[22] Kida T, Nishihira Y, Hatta A, Wasaka T. Somatosensory N250 and P300 during discrimination tasks, *Int J Psychophysiol* 2003(48) 275-283
[23] Knott V, Mohr E, Mahoney C, Engeland C, Hivitsky V. Effects of acute nicotine administration on cognitive event-related potentials in tacrine-treated and non-treated patients with Alzheimer's disease. *Neuropsychobiology*. 2002:45(3):156-60.
[24] Kochanowski J, Malara A, Broncel A, Skorupka U, Guzowska-Bart E. Clinical applications of late negative evoked potentials contingent negative variation (CNV) *Neurol Neurochir Pol.* 1999; 32 Suppl 6:187-91. (eng. abst.)
[25] Kofler B, Erhart C, Erhart P, Harrer G. The usefulness of event-related negativity in demonstrating therapeutic effects of nootropic drugs using cerebrolysin as an example. *EEG EMG verwandte*. 1990(21) 145-149 (Eng Abst)
[26] Kofler B, Harrer G, Ladurner G. Contingent negative variation (CNV) differences between cerebrovascular patients with and without dementia. *Arch Gerontol Geriatr* 1988(7) 311-318.
[27] Lijima M, Osawa M, Iwata M, Miyazaki A, Tei H. Topographic mapping of P300 and frontal cognitive function Parkinson's disease. *Behav Neurol.*2001;12(3):143-8
[28] Matsumoto R, İkeda A, Ohara S, Matsuhashi M, Baba K, Yamane F, Hori T, Mihara T, Nagamine T, Shibasaki H. Motor-related functional subdivitions of human lateral premotor cortex epicortical recording in conditional visuomotor task. *Clin neurophysiol* 2003(14) 1102-1115.
[29] Mochizuki Y, Oishi M, Takasu T. Correlations between P300 components and regional cerelbral blood flows. *J Clin Neurosci*. 2001. 8(5):407-10
[30] Morgan CD, Murphy C. Olfactory event-related potentials in Alzheimer's disease. *J Int Neuropsychol Soc.* 2002. 8(6):753-63.
[31] Murphy C, Morgan CD, Geisler MW, Wetter S, Covington JW, Madowitz MD, Nordin S, Polich JM. Olfactory event-related potentials and aging: normative data. *Int J psychophysiol* 2000(36)133-145
[32] Nakano Y, Kaseda Y, Nakamura S, Neshige R. Visual event-related potentials in progressive supranuclear plasy. *Hiroshima J Med Sci.* 2000. 49(1):37-42.
[33] Connor. Slow potential correlates of attention dysfunction in senile dementia. II.*Biol Psychol* (1980(11) 203-216.
[34] Olbrich HM, Maes H, Valerius G, Langosch JM, Gann H and Feige B. Assessing cerebral dysfunction with probe-evoked potentials in a CNV task-a study in alcoholics. *Clin Neurophysiol*. 2002(113) 815-825
[35] Olichney JM, Morris SK, Ochoa C, Salmon DP, Thal LJ, Kutas M, Iragui VJ. Abnormal verbal event related potentials in mild cognitive impairment and incipient Alzheimer's disease. *J Neurol Neurosurg Psychiatry*. 2002.73(4):377-84.
[36] Ortiz T, Fernandez A, Lopez-Ibor MI, Martinez-Castillo E, Lopez-I JJ. Inhibitory deficits in probable Alzheimer's disease. A study movement related potentials and EMG response. *Electromyogr. Clin. Neurophysiol* 1999(39) 249-255.
[37] Ortiz T, Martin Loeches M, Miguel F, Abdad EV, Puente AE. P300 latency and amplitude in diagnosis of dementia. *J Clin Psychol* 1994(50) 381-388.
[38] Osawa M. Clinically useful event-related potentials. *Rinsho Shinkeigaku*. 2001. 41(12):1168-72.

[39] Paul R, Moser D, Cohen R, Browndyke J, Zawacki T, Gordon N. Dementia severity and pattern of cognitive perpormance in vascular dementia. *Appl Neuropsychol.* 2001;8(4):211-7.

[40] Pekkonen E, Hirvonen J, Jaaskelainen IP, Kaakkola S, Huttunen J. Auditory sensory memory and the cholinergic system: implications for Alzheimer's disease. *Neuroimage* 2001(14)376-382

[41] Pekkonen E, Jousmaki V, Partanen J and Karhu J. Mismatch negativity area and age related auditory memory. *Electroencephalogr. Clin. Neurophysiol.* 1993(87) 321-325.

[42] Pekkonen E. Mismatch negativity in aging and in Alzheimer's and Parkinson's diseases. *Audiol. Neurol. Otol.* 2000(5) 216-224.

[43] Pokryszko-Dragan A, Slotwinski K, Podemski R. Modality-specific changes in P300 parameters in patients with dementia of the Alzheimer type. *Med Sci Monit.* 2003. 9(4):CR130-4.

[44] Polich J, Han A, Poceta JS, Mitler MM, Darko DF. Neuroelectric assessment of HIV: EEG, ERP, and viral load. *Int J Psychophysiol.* 2000. 38(1):97-108.

[45] Polich J, Herbst KL. P300 as a clinical assay: rationale, evaluation, and findings. *Int J Psychophysiol.* 2000. 38(1):3-19.

[46] Polich J. Pitzer A. P300 and Alzheimer's disease: oddball task difficulty and modality effects. *Electroencephalogr Clin Neurophysiol Suppl.* 1999;50:281-7.

[47] Prabhakar S, Syal P, Srivastava T. P300 in newly diagnosed non-dementing Parkinson's disease effect of dopanminergic drugs. *Neurol India.* 2000. 48(3):239-242

[48] Quiroz-G YT. N400 an electrophysiological neasure of semantic processing *Rev Neurol* 2003(36) 1176-1180.

[49] Saito H, Yamazaki H, Matsuoka H, Matsumoto K, Numachi Y, Yosh S, Ueno T, Sato M. Visual event-related potential in mild dementia of the Alzheimer's type. *Psychiatr. Clinical Neuroscience.* 2001: (55) 365-371

[50] Saito M and Ishida T. Cognitive resource model for the information processing of task-irrelevant visual stimuli. *Psychiatry and Clinical Neuroscience.* 2002(56) 145-151.

[51] Sara G, Kraiuhin C, Gordon E et al. The P300 event related potential component in the diagnosis of dementia *Aust NZ. Jmed* 1988(18) 657-660

[52] Savolainen S, Karhu J, Paakkonen A, Paljarvi L, Partanen J, Alafuzoff I, Vopalahti M. Auditory event-related potentials differentiate patients with normal pressure hydrocephalus and patients with concomitan Alzheimer's disease verified by brain biopsy. *Neuroreport.* 2001(22) 33-37

[53] Schwartz TJ, Federmeier KD, Van Petten C, Salmon DP, Kutas M. Electrophysiological analysis of context effects in Alzheimer's disease. *Neuropsychology.* 2003. 17(2):187-201.

[54] Smith, GE, Peterson RC, Parisi JE, Ivnik RJ, Kökmen E, Tangalos EG, Waring SC. Definition, course and outcome of mild cognitive impairment. *Aging, Neuropsychology and cognition* 1996(3) 141-147

[55] Sumi N, Nan'no H, Fujimoto O, Ohta Y, Takeda M. Interpeak latency of auditory event-related potentials (P300) senile depression and dementia of the Alzheimer type. *Psychiatry Clin Neurosci.* 2000. 54(6):679-84

[56] Tanaka H, Koenig T, Pascual-Marqui RD, Hirata K, Kochi K, Lehm D. Event-related potential and EEG measures in Parkinson's disease without and with dementia. *Dement Geriatr Cogn Disord.* 2000. 11(1):39-45.

[57] Uytdenhoef P, Depauw Y, Van Wettere JP, Godaux E, Bernier J, Ja J. Contingent negative variation and regional cerebral blood flow in senile dementia and cerebral aging. *Neurophysiol clin* 1988(18) 531-539.

[58] Vaney N, Chouhan S, Bhatia MS, Tandon OP. Event related evoked potentials in dementia: role of vitamin. *Indian J Physiol Pharmacol.*2002. 46(1):61-8.

[59] Wang H, Wang Y, Wang D, Lui L, Tian S, Zhang Y. Cognitive impairment in Parkinson's disease revelead by event-related potential N270. *J of Neuorol. Scienc.* 2002(194) 49-53

[60] Werber AE, Klein C, Rabey JM. Evaluation of cholinergic treatment in demented patients by P300 evoked related potentials. *Neurol Neurochir Pol.* 2001;35 Suppl 3:37-43.

[61] Werber EA, Gandelman-Marton R, Klein C, Rabey JM. The clinical use of P300 event related potentials for the evaluation of cholinesterase inhibitors treatment in demented patients. *J Neural Transm.* 2003. 110(6):659-69.

[62] Yamaguchi S, Tsuchiya H, Yamagata S, Toyoda G, Kobayashi S. Event-related brain potentials in response to novel sound in dementia. *Clin Neurophysiol.* 2000. 111(2):195-203.

[63] Yokoyama Y, Nakashima K, Shimoyama R, Urakami K, Tokashi K. Distribution of event-related potentials in patients with dementia. *Electromyogr. Clin Neurophysiol* 1995(35) 431-437.

[64] Zappoli R, Versari A, Arnetoli G, Paganini M, Muscas GC, Arneodo MG, Gangemi PF, Bartelli M, Topographic CNV activity mapping presenile mild primary cognitive decline and Alzheimer-type dementia. *Neurophysiol clin.* 1991(21) 473-483.

[65] Zappoli R, Versari A, Paganini M, Arnetoli G, Muscas GC, Gangem Arneodo MG, Poggiolini D, Zappoli F, Battagia A. Brain electrical activity (quantitative EEG and bit-mapping neurocognitive CNV components) psychometrics and clinical findings in presenite subjects with initial mild cognitive decline or probable Alzheimer type dementia. *Ital J Neurol Sci* 1995(16) 341-376

In: Depression and Dementia
Editor: Suptendra Nath Sarbadhikari, p. 319-328
ISBN 1-59454-114-0

EPILOGUE

Suptendra Nath Sarbadhikari

> The action of thinking may incidentally have other results; it may serve to amuse us … and a positive discovery … is met with ill-concealed dislike.
>
> Charles S Peirce

> … the measurement is not completed until its result enters our consciousness … the last step is, at the present state of our knowledge, shrouded in mystery.
>
> E P Wigner

> The progress of science is much slower than one anticipates. We scientists tackle only small problems.
>
> Georges Köhler, Nobel Laureate in Medicine (1984)

Depression and dementia are now rather common disorders globally. Some of the recent advances in understanding depression and dementia, and their clinical applications have been discussed by respected authors in this book. These chapters put together, also point towards the future trends of depression and dementia research and management.

The nonlinear interaction between the different subtypes of neurotransmitter receptors may form the common basis of cognitive (*e.g.*, dyslexia, dementia, schizophrenia), behavioral or affective (*e.g.* depressive) and epileptic disorders [Sarbadhikari 2004]. Vagus nerve stimulation (VNS) is an established treatment method for therapy-refractory epilepsy and also for treatment-resistant depression, as well as Alzheimer's disease [Sjogren *et al* 2002]. Stimulation of the tenth cranial nerve or Vagus causes release of a neurotransmitter Acetylcholine or ACh, which has mainly two types of receptors nicotinic and muscarinic. Nicotine (acting on Nicotinic ACh receptors or neuronal nAChRs in the Brain) is involved in the pathogenesis of Alzheimer's disease, Parkinson's disease, Depression and Schizophrenia [Mihailescu and Drucker-Collin 2000]. At the cellular level CaMK (Calmodulin Kinase, especially type II or CaMKII) and CaMKK (Calmodulin Kinase Kinase) are responsible for many of the end effects [Macpherson *et al*, 2002]. Therefore, nAChR and CaMKII seem to link a common pathway [Sarbadhikari 2004].

Similarly, a novel antiepileptic drug Levetiracetam (LEV) is now found to be quite effective in treating epilepsy. Albeit the mechanism of its action is yet to be ascertained, LEV too is believed to affect diverse pathways of epileptic, cognitive and affective disorders. In the case of LEV also, the role of calcium and its specific channel subtype (here N type) apparently point towards some final common pathway [Cramer *et al.* 2003, Bell *et al* 2002, Lukyanetz *et al* 2002].

The fields of Cognitive Psychology and Neuroscience (including Neuroinformatics and Neuroengineering) must be bridged to study our mind/brain. This may be done using computational modeling and neuroimaging. In order to bridge the fields of cognitive psychology and neuroscience, one must have a strong foundation in each of these respective fields. For over two decades cognitive psychologists have essentially rejected the notion that the brain had any relevance to the study of the mind. However, although this lack of consideration of the brain is striking, cognitive psychologists were able to explore the architecture of the mind and have established the foundation both in phenomena and methodical approaches to the study of behavior, both of which have been useful to us. On the other hand, the field of neuroscience proceeded with the idea that the mind could be understood by considering only the building blocks of the brain (*i.e.*, functioning of calcium channels in a neuron), without concern for theories of how the mind works, developed from behavioral observation. However, a strong foundation in this field has been established. Only now, after years of isolated research in cognitive psychology and neuroscience, has the bridge started to form between these two fields. The ability to use neuroimaging and neural signal processing to study the function of an intact human brain has had a huge impact on the way in which research is done in the field of cognitive neuroscience, cognitive science, and neuroscience as well. Neuroinformatics is the field that combines neuroscience and informatics research to develop and apply advanced tools and approaches essential in understanding the structure and function of the brain. Developed tools have multiple applications in the fields of machine learning, artificial intelligence and robotics, medicine and public health. The contribution of neuroinformatics (especially computational modeling) towards the better understanding of complex brain functions becomes even more important when combined with biological experiments where real data can be used to test and validate newly developed neural models. We need to comprehend the type of neural computations performed by various classes of neurons in the brain, and in particular the ones that are involved in learning and memory. Towards this target, various investigations have focused on the development and analysis of neurally inspired theoretical and machine-learning algorithms used to model memory capacity in the brain. The effects of dendritic morphology and the biophysics underlying learning induced by synaptic plasticity, on the computational (memory) capacity of pyramidal neurons and their possible role in the formation/retrieval of memories have been studied.

When dealing with a device as complex as the human brain, with nonlinear interactions between its parts, it is important to describe its functioning using equations, or by running simulations, to show that there is some empirical validity a particular idea of how the system is working. The steadfast resistance of psychologists to the use of computational modeling and mathematics has been a major drawback. Physicists have already begun to look into the issues of cognitive neuroscience using mathematics and computational modeling.

In patients suffering from cognitive disorders ranging from dyslexia to schizophrenia, neurodiagnostic testing with high-powered functional imaging techniques such as magnetic resonance imaging (MRI) and positron emission tomography (PET) can pinpoint specific areas of dysfunction in the brain. The neuropsychologists then examine the corresponding disturbances in cognition. By finding correlations between sites in the brain that are dysfunctional biologically and particular deficits of behavior, scientists are learning more about how these functions are organized in the brain in the first place. We may now view the structure and the function of the normal living human brain non-invasively. As a result, for the first time in human history we don't merely think about thinking, we can now measure it and map it. These tools for visualizing the thinking brain represent the cutting-edge of modern engineering and physics, and together with experimental questions developed by cognitive scientists and human neuroscientists, represent a stunning advance in brain research. A critical deficiency of these exciting new technologies is a paucity of appropriate image analysis tools to fully realize the vast potential of image data acquired from these revolutionary imaging systems. These new tools will enhance our ability to evaluate of the statistical significance of (possibly) active regions of interest within experimentally acquired images and signals so as to account for local spatial correlations, or to jointly model simultaneous or nearly simultaneous activations at distinct locations in the brain.

Multimodal techniques in medical imaging technology are expected in the near future to produce many new discoveries. In the field of simultaneous electroencephalography (EEG) and functional Magnetic Resonance (fMRI) recordings, the goal is of solving the extremely hard engineering problems involved in these simultaneous recordings. This combined technology also has the very appealing promise of elucidating the link between EEG, an inexpensive technology with very high temporal but low spatial resolution, and fMRI, with high spatial but low temporal resolution. [Bonmassar *et al,* 2002]

A great portion of the mammalian brain is devoted to sampling and processing sensory information generated by the animal's active exploration of its surrounding environment. These complex and vital tasks are accomplished by the cooperative action of large ensembles of neurons distributed across multiple intermediary levels of the parallel sensory pathways that connect peripheral receptors to the cortical mantle. It is necessary to understand the general computational principles underlying the dynamic interactions between populations of cortical and subcortical neurons that mediate tactile perception. To pursue this goal, new electrophysiological techniques have been advanced for carrying out long-term simultaneous recordings of the extracellular activity of hundreds of single neurons distributed across multiple levels of somatosensory and motor pathways in behaving animals. Such experimental paradigms are used in combination with multivariate statistical techniques, computer graphics, and neural network models to analyze the spatiotemporal structure of neuronal ensemble activity and its correlation with different aspects of exploratory tactile behaviors.

Computational modeling and experimental verification should go hand in hand. May be in another few years both the approaches would meet exactly midway to give us a firm bridge over the vast river of ignorance regarding the brain dynamics. Bremner *et al* [2003] propose a neural circuitry for depression in this manner.

For example, techniques that are helpful in representing spatiotemporal processes at one scale (e.g., multiple units) may be useful at other scales (*e.g.*, fMRI). By bringing together experts who use different approaches and technologies across a range of experimental model systems, the target should be to enhance understanding on how different scales of observation and organization are linked.

Finally, for assessing Brain Dynamics in various conditions of mental health and disease, a hybrid or fusion approach will to be more fruitful by combining one or more of these approaches [Sarbadhikari and Pal, 2002; Sarbadhikari and Chakrabarty 2001].

- Two or more modalities like EEG (electrophysiological) and fMRI (neurochemical and anatomical).
- Linear (FFT) and nonlinear (D2; L1) approaches.
- Cognitive Psychological (Top down, behavioral) with Neurophysiological (Bottom up) approaches.
- Global with Local (and Hemispheric) approaches.
- Proper (*e.g.*, MANOVA) statistical analyses with computer simulations.

Now, let us briefly discuss what the authors have tried to convey through their respective chapters.

Pradhan *et al* (Chapter 1) believe that the living systems are inherently nonlinear and complex in nature. However, surprisingly many biologists and medical professionals are unaware of the power, magic and beauty of nonlinear science that underlies living processes. The recent developments in the physics of complex systems encompassing nonlinear dynamics and the theory of chaos have considerably altered our perception and analysis of many complex systems, including that of the human brain. This new scientific revolution has silently pervaded all disciplines and emerged as the frontier of research today. It is also heralded as the third most important discovery of man after relativity and quantum mechanics. The importance of emerging trends of nonlinear dynamics and chaos to neurobiology is presented and discussed in the context of various states of consciousness, behavior and psychopathology. They review the physical and dynamical aspect of brain's electrical activity from this new perspective and indicate possible future directions like replacing the phenomenological approach of EEG interpretation by a model-driven approach for better understanding of EEG waveforms and rhythms. The developments in nonlinear dynamics and its application to EEG may be helpful for realistic modeling of various neuro-oscillatory phenomena. It may help in the construction of physiologically realistic mathematical models that simulate brain activities and allow prediction as to how they may be affected by experimental manipulations. Nonlinear dynamics may produce tools for feature extraction, EEG data compression and analysis. Its methodology is also of importance in analyzing other oscillatory and transitional states of brain activity seen in epilepsy, task loaded attentional states, cognitive task performance and in various states of consciousness and behaviors which have been most difficult to be discerned in background EEG activities. This newly gained insight of chaotic dynamics of brain is a significant departure from the earlier stochastic visualization.

Tan (Chapter 2) has outlined the grounds of a new theory, to explain the mind-brain-body triad in health and disease. This is the *psychomotor theory*. First, he has briefly analyzed the historical development of the relationship between mind and brain, which is being discussed since more than a few thousand years. The tight junctions between psychological and motor systems were subjected to a detailed analysis using examples in health and disease. The feedback circuits between mind, brain, and body were shown to occur within the mind-brain-body triad, in normal states, and psycho-neural diseases. It was stated that psychiatric signs and symptoms are coupled with motor disturbances; neurological diseases are coupled with psychological disturbances; changes in cortical and spinal motor-system activity may influence mind-brain-body triad, and *vice versa.* Accordingly, a psychomotor theory was created to explain the psychomotor coupling in health and disease, stating that, not the mind-brain duality or unity, but the mind-brain-body triad as a functional unit is essential in health and disease, since mind does not end in the brain, but further controls movements, in a reciprocal manner; mental and motor events share the same neural substrate, cortical and spinal motor neurons; mental events emerging from the motoneuronal system is strongly coupled with the unity of the mind-brain-body triad. So, the psychomotor theory rejects the mind-brain duality, instead, advances the unity of the psychomotor system, which will have important consequences in understanding and improving the human mind, brain, and body in health and disease.

Lateralization describes the way the two cerebral hemispheres differ structurally and functionally to give rise to sidedness in individuals. Electrophysiological, behavioral, hormonal, anatomical, and neurochemical changes in depression and dementia are well documented. The overall idea that evolves from lateralization studies is that there seems to be some final common pathway. Albeit it may not be evident apparently, recent studies appear to point towards such missing link(s), which I have humbly tried to assimilate in Chapter 3.

In Chapter 4, Chakrabarti discusses the roles of neurotransmitters in depression since this group of diseases is associated with significant morbidity in younger age group. Prevalence of these important mental diseases in the community is assessed by ICD-10 and DSM-IV based diagnostic criteria. However, these diagnostic criteria are not adequate for estimation of susceptibility and vulnerability of a subset of population to these disorders, so that preventive interventions could be initiated at an early age. A more accurate prediction of susceptibility to these diseases can be carried out by correlation of life events with biomarker epidemiology, which estimates presence of certain biochemical and genetic changes in the susceptible population detectable before the onset of the disease. For example, child abuse is associated with markedly elevated rates of major depression (MDD) in child, adolescent and adult cohorts. Studies have demonstrated that stress early in life can alter the development of multiple neurotransmitter systems and promote structural and functional alterations in brain regions similar to those seen in adults with depression. Clinical studies, also, suggest that long-term neurobiological changes associated with early stress can be modified by familial / genetic factors, the quality of the subsequent care giving environment, and pharmacological interventions. There is considerable evidence that the serotonergic system, involved in depression, is partly under genetic control and yet unknown genetic factors mediate the risk for suicidal behavior independently of the genetic factors responsible for the heritability of MDD associated with suicide. Similarly, increasing evidence supports an important role for metals like copper in neurodegenerative diseases like Alzheimer's disease (AD) and Creutzfeldt-Jakob disease (CJD). Moreover, Familial Alzheimer's disease (FAD) is now linked to at least three genes encoding the amyloid precursor protein (APP) on chromosome 21 and presenilin 1 and 2 on chromosome 14 and 1, respectively. Also, common polymorphisms of the apolipoprotein E gene influence the risk and age of onset of Alzheimer's disease. He examines the currently available neurochemical and genetic evidences and their correlation with life events from population based studies, which could be useful in screening susceptibility to depression. He also attempts further to set up criteria for susceptibility, which would help designing early interventions in prevention of depression.

Sharma (Chapter 5) says that stress, depending on its magnitude and severity, alters neurochemical transmission in the central nervous system (CNS) and induces breakdown of the blood-brain barrier (BBB) leading to Alzheimer's diseases and related neurodegenerative disorders. Expression of heat shock proteins (HSPs) in the CNS is another common finding in stressful situations. Thus, a possible inter-relationship between breakdown of the BBB, HSP expression and neuronal damage appears quite likely. Evidence presented in this chapter clearly suggests that the BBB disruption during stress is instrumental in causing selective neural injury leading to long-term consequences on the brain function. Alterations in fluid microenvironment of the brain together with edema formation lead to several cellular and molecular changes in the brain resulting in HSP induction, cell injury and/or cell death. Restoration of normal BBB function in hyperthermia or other CNS diseases by drugs could be a promising approach to minimize neurodegenerative changes. Taken together, it appears that BBB seems to be the gateway for brain dysfunction and development of neurological disorders leading to neurodegeneration.

In Chapter 6, Subodh and Mandal feel that the concept of distinct functional specialization of the two sides of the human brain is helpful in understanding the brain-behavior relationship in general, and specifically in psychiatric illness. Left hemisphere superiority in cognitive functions and right hemisphere advantage, although less clear-cut, for affect processing have generally been accepted. Empirical support for right hemisphere superiority in emotional processing has been drawn from studies conducted on both normal and clinical subjects. Clinical studies in this regard were mostly conducted on brain-damaged patients, and a few on psychiatric patients, mainly schizophrenics. Very few studies were conducted on patients with affective disorders. Although the research techniques that utilize the differential specialization of the cerebral hemispheres in processing emotional cues have to be methodologically improved for providing more conclusive results, some observations may be helpful in resolving some of the neuropsychiatric issues. In their chapter, they examined studies that have reflected hemispheric asymmetry in patients with depressive illness. The chapter is divided into three sections. The first section accounts the lateralization of affect. The second section deals with the lateralization studies in depression (behavioral, electrophysiological, functional imaging and brain lesions). Finally, they present general comments and recommendations for future research.

Their chapter is different from mine in the sense that they have restricted the chapter to depression only, but have stressed more on functional imaging and brain lesion (along with behavioral) studies. This chapter, along with mine, underscores the need for a fusion of approaches for studying diseases of the brain.

Kumar (Chapter 7) believes that at a time when we have either conquered or controlled most of other illnesses depression is emerging as a significant health problem. There is considerable evidence that depression is growing and it is predicted that it will continue to do so in the near future causing significant mortality and morbidity. Significant advances have been made in the biology of depression both regarding the etiology and treatment. Antidepressants, ECT (electroconvulsive therapy) and Light therapy are the main biological methods of treatment while vagal nerve stimulation (VNS) and repetitive transcranial magnetic stimulation (rTMS) are being evaluated. Selective serotonergic reuptake inhibitors offered a significant advance in our understanding of how modern antidepressant medication can be found. Selective noradrenergic reuptake inhibitors have been added as another powerful weapon in the collection of modern psycho-pharmacologist. These drugs are thought to be better not only because they may have an earlier onset of action compared to older drugs but also because they may help with social functioning. Treatment of depression may be particularly challenging in cases where refractory depression develops, atypical features of depression are present or in patients with chronic depression. Special consideration needs to be made for treating depression in women at different phases in their reproductive life, in the elderly and in children. It is possible that treating depression aggressively may improve the future course and prognosis.

Jeong (Chapter 8) feels that Nonlinear dynamical analysis (NDA) has been extensively applied to a variety of physiological data for the last two decades. One of its major contributions is to the EEG in patients with dementias, particularly Alzheimer's disease (AD). The hallmark of nonlinear EEG abnormalities in demented patients is the globally decreased complexity of EEG patterns and a prominent decrease in information transmission among cortical areas quantified by information-theoretic measures like mutual information. These findings might be associated with functional disconnections among cortical areas resulting from death of cortical neurons, axonal pathology, cholinergic deficits and thus decreased nonlinear processes underlying cortical dynamics in dementias. While the average diagnostic accuracy of EEG for dementias using conventional analyses is currently about 80%, it has been shown that NDA of EEG recordings might contribute to the improvement of the accuracy of differential diagnosis of dementias and early detection in the preclinical stage. This chapter introduces the concepts and algorithms of NDA and focuses on primary findings of EEG abnormalities in dementia patients obtained from NDA. He suggests that NDA provides not only potentially valuable diagnostic information but also a deeper understanding of neuropathological mechanisms underlying dementias in ways that are not possible by conventional spectral analyses.

In Chapter 9, Jelic cautions that in order to look into the future and evaluate progress, one has to be aware of what has been done in the past. This chapter aims to show that the methodology of diagnostic, clinical research does not follow the same pace of development for new diagnostic techniques. Recent evidence-based review by The Diagnosis of Dementia Committee addressed major issues in the diagnosis of dementia and in the resulting practice parameter on dementia did not consider qEEG (quantitative or quantified EEG) among the laboratory tests that could improve diagnostic accuracy of dementing illness or be used in the presymptomatic detection of the disease [Knopman *et al.*, 2001]. One of the problems that qEEG brings as a potential useful investigation in clinical reality, is the multitude of parameters it produces and there is still no agreement across the studies which could be the best candidate for potential discrimination of patients. Various authors do not use exactly same inclusion criteria (spectrum of tested patients not specified in detail), analyzing technique (reference electrode choice, arbitrary montage selections) or EEG parameters. Therefore, so far it has been impossible to make a metaanalysis for validation purposes. More prospective, preferably multicentric, studies on unselected and larger samples are needed for the validation of respective techniques. Implications of this evidence-based aspect are twofold: optimal clinical practice based on the best available evidence and selection of the most promising areas of the future research. So far, none of the qEEG parameters has been proven to be sufficiently reliable to be used for diagnosing individual patients. Multivariate approach should be used to evaluate the added value of qEEG in combination with another diagnostic technique. So far, the attitude was mainly win-lose approach trying to establish the diagnostic supremacy of one technique. However, the characteristics of a disease process are a tension between the pathophysiological cascade of events on one side and neuronal repair and compensation mechanisms on the other side. In other words, natural history of the disease is determined not only by what has been lost, but also by what has been left during the disease process. Therefore, besides the development of the tests which show accurately how much the brain has been affected structurally and functionally, attempts should be made towards the procedures that reflect how much of brain function has been left and towards understanding the cognitive brain reserve which delays clinical manifestation of the dementia. Could varying figures on sensitivities derived from EEG studies in dementia be discussed and explained in this way? Obviously, a larger number of prospective studies is needed not only aiming to confirm the dementia diagnosis from a longitudinal perspective, but also to reveal a heterogeneous nature of disease progression. It seems that we are facing a new era where neurodegenerative diseases, including dementia, will not be defined as clinicopathological entities but as a processes with overlapping pathogenic mechanisms. Could we, therefore, in differential diagnosis expect optimal specificity with respect to patients groups classified clinically into different dementia syndromes? A clinically important question with respect to new emerging methods of qEEG analysis is that whether these new methods have any significant diagnostic value at all. So far, diagnostic accuracies of non-linear parameters do not show any additional advantage over the conventional parameters. It should be further explored what is their functional significance and if they could add any complementary information to the diagnostic process. Finally, if any of qEEG variables is going to be validated and established as a biomarker of a disease with sufficiently high sensitivity and specificity, it could be incorporated in the algorithmic approach used in presymptomatic/preclinical detection of the disease (dementia or depression). This approach is a major avenue of future research.

The apparent disagreement on the emphasis between these two chapters by Jeong and Jelic is resulting from a perspective of a clinician (latter) who expects to get an accurate and reliable assessment tool for each individual patient on one side (an evidence-based approach necessary for any consensus statement in the future) and on the other side a researcher (former) developing new analyzing techniques and fascinating research results which are optimized for highly selected and, in general, small clinical samples. Although there is a lot of converging evidence from the studies performed so far, one has to address their methodological limitations with a constructive criticism in order to give guidelines for future research. Jelic has suggested that to some extent in her chapter. under the headline "Methodological criteria for a diagnostic test" and in the starting sentence from her concluding paragraph: "In contrast to other chapters that are introducing new ways of qEEG analysis, this chapter aimed to show that the methodology of diagnostic, clinical research does not follow the same pace of development for new diagnostic techniques."

In Chapter 10, Idiman says that Electrophysiological studies have provided some of the most direct evidence for assessing central nervous system (CNS) functions. Standardized EEG recordings and sensory evoked potentials (EP) measures have been used clinically for many years in routine evaluations but cognitive ERPs have not yet been employed commonly in routine practice. As known, some long latency potentials which occur after rare and/or unexpected stimuli or conditional stimuli seem to depend on cognitive processes rather than the physical characteristics of the stimulus. Therefore they are called of "Event Related Potentials" (ERP)s rather than evoked potentials. These are: (A) P300 (visual auditory oddball paradigm); (B) Contingent negative variation. "CNV"; (C) The other ERPs in cognitive impairments, like, Readiness potential "Bereitshaftspotentials" and other movement related potentials, and Olfactory ERPs. Till now, the relationships between these potentials and neuropsychological functions such as memory, attentions, conation, expectancy, alertness have been investigated. In the beginning, in normal elderly subject, the conditions under which ERPs occurred, consistent and varying features of the waves underchanging conditions of mental processing-latency, and amplitude were tried to be identified. The mental processing represented by specific stimulus conditions was interpreted and changing features were evaluated through studies. Furthermore, by clinical examination and neuropsychological tests, the impaired components of mental processing were identified and which ERP changes they led to were demonstrated. At present, all these features are considered especially in early stage dementia, whether they can be helpful in reaching the diagnosis or not, and whether differential diagnosis can be made according to electrophysiological data or not. In addition, whether ERPs can be used in the evaluation of effect of drugs in therapeutical approaches or not have been investigated. There are considerable systematic differences between normal and patient populations. In particular, the P300 component of ERPs has been widely applied in the scientific study of age-related cognitive dysfunction, because it reflects attentional and memory processes. In addition, a number of clinical studies (employing the oddball task) have indicated a probable correlation between the latencies and/or amplitudes of ERP components and changes in information processing in elderly and mental illnesses.

The essence of this book can thus be summarized as follows.

Most of the mechanisms of brain action, in health, as well as diseases like depression and dementia, are nonlinear. The psychomotor theory can shed some light on the brain-mind-body interaction in health and disease. Specific neurotransmitters through their different receptor subtypes ultimately act along some final common pathway, in a lateralized fashion to produce depression and dementia. The currently available neurochemical and genetic evidences and their correlation with life events from population based studies, may be useful in screening susceptibility to dementia and depression. Further, criteria may be set up for susceptibility to these diseases and they might help designing early interventions in prevention of depression and dementia. The breakdown of the BBB (Blood brain barrier) through Heat Shock Protein (HSP) is also responsible for many neurodegenerative diseases. Aggressive and individualized management of patients suffering from depression and dementia may be the most promising gift of medical science and technology to humanity. Nonlinear dynamic analysis (NDA) of EEG (electroencephalography) may aid in the differential diagnosis of dementias. However, the methodologies have to be standardized further to make it clinically acceptable universally. ERPs (event related potentials in EEG) can be of great help in diagnosis and also assessing prognosis of dementias. Finally, fusion or hybrid techniques, especially those incorporating fMRI or functional magnetic resonance imaging (along with qEEG or quantitative EEG) can be of immense help in diagnosing, managing and predicting the prognosis of depression and dementia.

The most noteworthy point (elaborately discussed by Jelic, as well as Subodh and Mandal) is that methodological standardization is an absolute prerequisite for reaching any firm conclusion, especially diagnostic ones. This is truer in the cases of heterogeneous groups of disorders like depression and dementia.

It should be investigated whether all the results obtained from studies (described in this book) can be correlated with clinical and behavioral changes in affective disorders (*e.g.*, depression); and behavioral or cognitive (*e.g.*, dyslexia, schizophrenia, dementia) disorders. Moreover, nonlinear modeling on the basis of cellular neurotransmitter (receptor subtype) and HSP (heat shock protein) changes may be able to predict our behavior more correctly, especially in the cases mentioned. Population based screening for depression and dementia, based on neurochemical and genetic markers could also hold promise in future.

References

I have not mentioned the chapters in this book in the list of references here.

Bell C, Vanderlinden H, Hiersemenzel R, Otoul C, Nutt D, Wilson S; The effects of levetiracetam on objective and subjective sleep parameters in healthy volunteers and patients with partial epilepsy; *J Sleep Res.* 2002; **11:**255–263.

Bonmassar G, *et al*, Motion and Ballistocardiogram artifact removal for interleaved EEG and fMRI recordings; *Neuroimage*, 2002, **16:** 1127–1141

Bremner JD, *et al*, Regional brain metabolic correlates of alpha-methylparatyrosine-induced depressive symptoms: implications for the neural circuitry of depression, *JAMA*, 2003, **289:** 3125-34.

Cramer JA, De Rue K, Devinsky O, Edrich P, Trimble MR; A systematic review of the behavioral effects of levetiracetam in adults with epilepsy, cognitive disorders, or an anxiety disorder during clinical trials; *Epilepsy Behav.,* 2003; **4:** 124–132.

Knopman DS, DeKosky ST, Cummings JL, *et al.*, Practice parameter: Diagnosis of dementia (an evidence-based review). Report of the quality standards subcommittee of the American Academy of Neurology, *Neurology,* 2001; **56**:1143-1153

Lukyanetz EA, Shkryl VM, Kostyuk PG; Selective blockade of N-type calcium channels by levetiracetam; *Epilepsia;* 2002; **43:** 9–18.

Macpherson P, *et al*, Protein Kinase C and Calcium/Calmodulin-activated Protein Kinase II (CaMK II) Suppress Nicotinic Acetylcholine Receptor Gene Expression in Mammalian Muscle: A specific role for camk ii in activity-dependent gene expression, *J. Biol. Chem.*, 2002, **277:** 15638-46

Mihailescu S and Drucker-Colin R; Nicotine, Brain Nicotinic Receptors and Neuropsychiatric Disorders; *Arch. Med. Res.*, 2000, **31:** 131–144.

Sarbadhikari S.N. and Chakrabarty K, Chaos in the brain: a short review alluding to epilepsy, depression, exercise and lateralization, *Med. Eng. Phys*, 2001, **23:** 445–455.

Sarbadhikari S.N. and Pal S.K.; Automated Techniques for identifying depression from EEG, In, Leondes C T, Ed, Handbook of Computational Methods in Biomaterials, Biotechnology and Biomedical systems, Kluwer Academic Publishers, 2002, Vol. 4, Chapter 3: 51–81.

Sarbadhikari SN, Balancing the Brain Activity: Putative links between Epileptic, Cognitive and Affective Disorders, In Benjamin SM, Ed, Focus on Epilepsy Research, Nova Science Publishers, Hauppauge, USA, 2004: 309 – 367.

Sjogren M J C, *et al*; Cognition-Enhancing Effect of Vagus Nerve Stimulation in Patients With Alzheimer's Disease: A Pilot Study; *J Clin Psychiatry* 2002; 63: 972–980.

INDEX

A

B

C

D

E

F

G

H

I

J

K

L

M

N

O

P

Q

R

S

V

W

Z